An Essential Guide to Food and Nutrition

An Essential Guide to Food and Nutrition

Editor: Margo Field

Callisto Reference

www.callistoreference.com

Callisto Reference,
118-35 Queens Blvd., Suite 400,
Forest Hills, NY 11375, USA

Visit us on the World Wide Web at:
www.callistoreference.com

ISBN: 978-1-63239-998-4 (Hardback)

The publisher's policy is to use permanent paper from mills that operate a sustainable forestry policy. Furthermore, the publisher ensures that the text paper and cover boards used have met acceptable environmental accreditation standards.

Printed in China.

Cataloging-in-Publication Data

An essential guide to food and nutrition / edited by Margo Field.
p. cm.
Includes bibliographical references and index.
ISBN 978-1-63239-998-4
1. Food. 2. Nutrition. I. Field, Margo.
RA601 .E77 2018
363.192--dc23

Table of Contents

Preface IX

Chapter 1 **An Okinawan-based Nordic diet improves anthropometry, metabolic control, and health-related quality of life in Scandinavian patients with type 2 diabetes** 1
Gassan Darwiche, Peter Höglund, Bodil Roth, Ewa Larsson, Trygve Sjöberg, Björn Wohlfart, Stig Steen and Bodil Ohlsson

Chapter 2 ***In vivo* protein quality of selected cereal-based staple foods enriched with soybean proteins** 16
Laura Acevedo-Pacheco and Sergio O. Serna-Saldvíar

Chapter 3 **Dietary tryptophan depletion in humans using a simplified two amino acid formula** 25
Maike Linden, Katrin Helmbold, Janina Kempf, Shabnam Sippas, Christian Filss, Karl-Josef Langen, Albrecht Eisert and Florian Daniel Zepf

Chapter 4 **Enhanced nutrition improves growth and increases blood adiponectin concentrations in very low birth weight infants** 40
Elin W. Blakstad, Sissel J. Moltu, Britt Nakstad, Marit B. Veierød, Kenneth Strømmen, Pétur B. Júlíusson, Astrid N. Almaas, Arild E. Rønnestad, Kristin Brække, Christian A. Drevon and Per O. Iversen

Chapter 5 **Fish consumption pattern among adults of different ethnics in Peninsular Malaysia** 51
Nurul Izzah Ahmad, Wan Rozita Wan Mahiyuddin, Tengku Rozaina Tengku Mohamad, Cheong Yoon Ling, Siti Fatimah Daud, Nasriyah Che Hussein, Nor Aini Abdullah, Rafiza Shaharudin and Lokman Hakim Sulaiman

Chapter 6 **Correlates of fruit, vegetable, soft drink, and snack intake among adolescents: the ESSENS study** 66
Mekdes K. Gebremariam, Sigrun Henjum, Laura Terragni and Liv Elin Torheim

Chapter 7 **Meals based on vegetable protein sources (beans and peas) are more satiating than meals based on animal protein sources (veal and pork) - a randomized cross-over meal test study** 75
Marlene D. Kristensen, Nathalie T. Bendsen, Sheena M. Christensen, Arne Astrup and Anne Raben

Chapter 8 **Enhanced polyunsaturated fatty acids production in *Mortierella alpina* by SSF and the enrichment in chicken breasts** 84
Shengli Yang and Hui Zhang

Chapter 9 **Metabolic effects of quail eggs in diabetes-induced rats: comparison with chicken eggs** ... 92
Eric Lontchi-Yimagou, Agatha Tanya, Carine Tchankou, Judith Ngondi and Julius Oben

Chapter 10 **Effects of royal jelly supplementation on regulatory T cells in children with SLE** ... 99
Asmaa M. Zahran, Khalid I. Elsayh, Khaled Saad, Esraa M. A. Eloseily, Naglaa S. Osman, Mohamd A. Alblihed, Gamal Badr and Mohamed H. Mahmoud

Chapter 11 **Chronic leucine supplementation improves lipid metabolism in C57BL/6J mice fed with a high-fat/cholesterol diet** ... 109
Jun Jiao, Shu-Fen Han, Wei Zhang, Jia-Ying Xu, Xing Tong, Xue-Bin Yin, Lin-Xi Yuan and Li-Qiang Qin

Chapter 12 **Plasma phospholipid pentadecanoic acid, EPA, and DHA, and the frequency of dairy and fish product intake in young children** ... 119
Nicolai A. Lund-Blix, Kjersti S. Rønningen, Håkon Bøås, German Tapia and Lene F. Andersen

Chapter 13 **Effects of stachyose on absorption and transportation of tea catechins in mice: possible role of Phase II metabolic enzymes and efflux transporters inhibition by stachyose** ... 127
Wenfeng Li, Yalong Lu, Di Huang, Xiao Han and Xingbin Yang

Chapter 14 **Development of a Mediterranean diet score adapted to Japan and its relation to obesity risk** ... 137
Masao Kanauchi and Kimiko Kanauchi

Chapter 15 **Food sources of energy and nutrients in Finnish girls and boys 6-8 years of age - the PANIC study** ... 144
Aino-Maija Eloranta, Taisa Venäläinen, Sonja Soininen, Henna Jalkanen, Sanna Kiiskinen, Ursula Schwab, Timo A. Lakka and Virpi Lindi

Chapter 16 **Dietary apigenin potentiates the inhibitory effect of interferon-α on cancer cell viability through inhibition of 26S proteasome-mediated interferon receptor degradation** ... 156
Sheng Li, Li-juan Yang, Ping Wang, Yu-jiao He, Jun-mei Huang, Han-wei Liu, Xiao-fei Shen and Fei Wang

Chapter 17 **School meal provision, health, and cognitive function in a Nordic setting - the ProMeal-study: description of methodology and the Nordic context** ... 168
Maria Waling, Anna S. Olafsdottir, Hanna Lagström, Hege Wergedahl, Bert Jonsson, Cecilia Olsson, Eldbjørg Fossgard, Asle Holthe, Sanna Talvia, Ingibjorg Gunnarsdottir and Agneta Hörnell

Chapter 18 **Zolfino landrace (*Phaseolus vulgaris* L.) from Pratomagno: general and specific features of a functional food** ... 179
Francesco Balestri, Rossella Rotondo, Roberta Moschini, Mario Pellegrino, Mario Cappiello, Vito Barracco, Livia Misuri, Carlo Sorce, Andrea Andreucci, Antonella Del-Corso and Umberto Mura

Chapter 19 **Twelve-week-conjugated linoleic acid supplementation has no effects on the selected markers of atherosclerosis in obese and overweight women** 190
Monika Dus-Zuchowska, Edyta Madry, Patrycja Krzyzanowska, Paweł Bogdanski and Jaroslaw Walkowiak

Permissions

List of Contributors

Index

Preface

This book has been a concerted effort by a group of academicians, researchers and scientists, who have contributed their research works for the realization of the book. This book has materialized in the wake of emerging advancements and innovations in this field. Therefore, the need of the hour was to compile all the required researches and disseminate the knowledge to a broad spectrum of people comprising of students, researchers and specialists of the field.

Food and nutrition include the study of food processing, deterioration causes, etc. by applying the elements of biology, engineering and science. Nutrition science also includes the study of the topics like catabolism, absorption, assimilation, biosynthesis, etc. This book aims to equip students and experts with the advanced topics and upcoming concepts in the area of food and nutrition science. It brings forth some of the most innovative concepts and elucidates the unexplored aspects of this subject. The book presents researches and studies performed by experts across the globe. It is a vital tool for all researching or studying food and nutrition science as it gives incredible insights into emerging trends and concepts of this field.

At the end of the preface, I would like to thank the authors for their brilliant chapters and the publisher for guiding us all-through the making of the book till its final stage. Also, I would like to thank my family for providing the support and encouragement throughout my academic career and research projects.

Editor

An Okinawan-based Nordic diet improves anthropometry, metabolic control, and health-related quality of life in Scandinavian patients with type 2 diabetes: a pilot trial

Gassan Darwiche[1,2*], Peter Höglund[3,4], Bodil Roth[1,2], Ewa Larsson[4,5], Trygve Sjöberg[4,5], Björn Wohlfart[4,5], Stig Steen[4,5] and Bodil Ohlsson[1,2]

[1]Department of Clinical Sciences, Division of Internal Medicine, Lund University, Lund, Sweden; [2]Skåne University Hospital, Malmö, Sweden; [3]Department of Laboratory Medicine, Division of Clinical Chemistry & Pharmacology, Lund University, Lund, Sweden; [4]Skåne University Hospital, Lund, Sweden; [5]Department of Cardiothoracic Surgery, Clinical Sciences Lund, Lund University, Lund, Sweden

Abstract

Background: Our hypothesis was that a modified diet would improve blood glucose control with beneficial impact on weight management and overall health in established diabetes.

Objective: This prospective interventional study investigated the clinical effect of an Okinawan-based Nordic diet on anthropometry, metabolic control, and health-related quality of life (HRQoL) in Scandinavian type 2 diabetes patients.

Design: Food was prepared and delivered to 30 type 2 diabetes patients. Clinical information along with data on HRQoL, blood samples, and urine samples were collected during 12 weeks of diet interventions, with follow-up 16 weeks after diet completion.

Results: After 12 weeks of dietary intervention, a reduction in body weight (7%) ($p < 0.001$), body mass index ($p < 0.001$), and waist circumference (7.0 cm) ($p < 0.001$) was seen. Improved levels of proinsulin ($p = 0.005$), insulin ($p = 0.011$), and fasting plasma glucose ($p < 0.001$) were found already after 2 weeks; these improved levels remained after 12 weeks when lowered levels of C-peptide ($p = 0.015$), triglycerides ($p = 0.009$), total cholesterol ($p = 0.001$), and low-density lipoprotein-cholesterol ($p = 0.041$) were also observed. Insulin resistance homeostasis model assessment for insulin resistance was lowered throughout the study, with a 20% reduction in hemoglobin A1c levels ($p < 0.001$) at week 12, despite reduced anti-diabetes treatment. Lowered systolic blood pressure (9.6 mmHg) ($p < 0.001$), diastolic blood pressure (2.7 mmHg) ($p < 0.001$), and heart and respiratory rates ($p < 0.001$) were accompanied by decreased cortisol levels ($p = 0.015$) and improvement in HRQoL. At follow-up, increased levels of high-density lipoprotein-cholesterol were found ($p = 0.003$).

Conclusion: This interventional study demonstrates a considerable improvement of anthropometric and metabolic parameters and HRQoL in Scandinavian type 2 diabetes patients when introducing a modified Okinawan-based Nordic diet, independently of exercise or other interventions. Through these dietary changes, anti-diabetes treatment could be decreased or cancelled.

Keywords: *anthropometry; metabolic control; interventional study; type 2 diabetes; Okinawan diet; Nordic diet; quality of life*

The pandemic of type 2 diabetes mellitus and obesity, driven by an increasing worldwide adoption of energy-dense diets and sedentary lifestyles, is associated with significant comorbidities and health-care costs and represents two of the biggest global health challenges of the modern world (1). Obesity plays a central role in occurrence of various diseases such as hyperinsulinemia, hyperglycemia, and dyslipidemia, and it has been strongly associated with insulin resistance in both normoglycemic subjects and individuals with type 2 diabetes mellitus (2). Insulin resistance exacerbates chronic hyperinsulinemia favoring anabolic metabolism that renders increased body weight, fosters carbohydrate cravings, and promotes insulin resistance, further promoting anabolic metabolism (3). Dietary intervention capable of lowering the insulin demand, improving insulin sensitivity, or both, is likely to reduce the incidence of disorders related to insulin resistance, as indicated by interventional studies (4, 5). These studies suggest weight reduction based on diet and exercise modifications to be important factors to reduce the risk of diabetes development. Whether dietary changes alone can play a crucial role in the prevention of diabetes is less clear, because it is difficult to determine the individual effectiveness of diet, independently of physical activity and weight loss.

The important features of healthy dietary patterns include a high intake of whole-grain and non-processed, plant-derived foods and a lower intake of red meat, meat products, sweets, salt, high-fat dairy, and refined grains and are shared by Mediterranean and Okinawan diets (6). These diets have been shown to improve metabolism, inflammation, and cardiovascular health in the population (7). Residents of Okinawa, the southernmost prefecture of Japan, are known for their long average life expectancy and high number of centenarians, with an accompanying low risk of age-associated diseases. Much of the longevity advantage in Okinawa is thought to be related to a healthy lifestyle. Part of this healthy lifestyle includes the traditional diet (8) that is low in calories yet nutritionally dense, particularly with regard to vitamins, minerals, and phytonutrients in the form of antioxidants and flavonoids (9).

Recently, our research group showed that an Okinawan-based single meal could promote a more favorable postprandial metabolic response and more pronounced satiety than a traditional meal in healthy subjects (10). Interventional studies investigating the effect of an Okinawan-based diet on Scandinavian type 2 diabetes patients has to our knowledge never been done previously. The aim of this study was to investigate the clinical effect of a modified Okinawan-based Nordic diet on anthropometry, metabolic control, and health-related quality of life (HRQoL) in Scandinavian type 2 diabetes subjects.

Materials and methods

The subjects were treated according to the Helsinki declaration and the study was approved by the Regional Ethics Review Board at Lund University (2014/460). All subjects gave their written, informed consent before entering the study, and the study was monitored by an external monitor and registered at ClinicalTrials.gov data base (NCT02405806).

Study population

Thirty clinically diagnosed type 2 diabetes patients aged between 18 and 70 years were recruited at a primary health care centre in southern Sweden. Patients were to have both parents inborn in Scandinavia, to avoid possible influence of ethnicity on the study results. They were included in the study independently of body mass index (BMI) or anti-diabetes treatment regimen. Overall exclusion criteria were severe food allergy; type 1 diabetes; a prior major gastrointestinal surgery; and severe heart, pulmonary, cardiovascular, malignant, or psychiatric diseases. Patients with severe liver insufficiency, defined as spontaneous international normalized ratio (INR) > 1.1, or severe renal insufficiency, defined as estimated glomerular filtration rate (eGFR) < 30 mL/min/1.73 m^2, were excluded (Fig. 1). The study started on February 2, 2015 and ended on September 18, 2015.

Study design

The trial was designed as a clinical prospective study and was conducted during 12 weeks after introduction of an Okinawan-based Nordic diet, followed by another

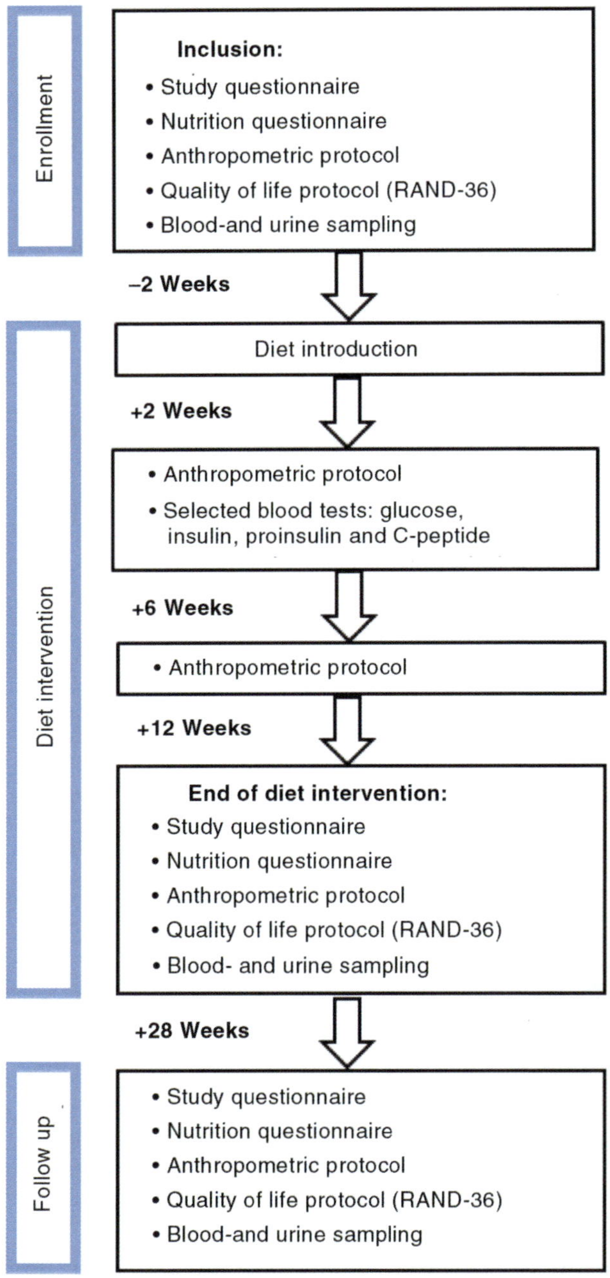

Fig. 1. Flowchart of the design and phases of the Okinawan-based Nordic diet intervention study. Diet introduction followed a 2 week run-in period (2 weeks). The participants were followed up 16 weeks after the end of dietary intervention.

16 weeks when participants were allowed to choose their own diet. Before entering the study, the patients were invited to an information meeting about the food composition and meal order. The subjects underwent a 2-week run-in period and were then followed by regular visits at 2, 6, 12, and 28 weeks after diet introduction, meeting the team of physicians and one nutritionist (Fig. 1).

A self-administered study questionnaire; nutrition questionnaire; and a HRQoL questionnaire, Research and Development 36-Item Health Survey (RAND-36) (11), along with information sheet and consent form, were sent home to the subjects and later collected and checked during their first visit. At the initial visit, the subjects underwent a clinical examination, and anthropometric data were collected along with blood and urine samples. All participants were instructed by a nutritionist (EL) on how to prepare their breakfast, based on the data from the nutrition questionnaire. Ready-made food for lunch, dinner, and snacks was delivered in a cooler bag to the subjects at home, three times a week and free of charge, along with written information and recipes for the final meal preparation. The participants were encouraged to maintain their regular physical activity habits throughout the intervention. No new dietary supplements such as fish oil, probiotics, or multivitamin drugs were allowed to be introduced during the study period. At most, one visit to a restaurant or change to another diet per week was allowed. Journeys or a stay for a long period at another place had to be discussed with the principal investigator (PI). Smoking habits were not changed during the study. Maximal intake of alcoholic beverages was set to 30 g ethanol/week. The nutritionist had a close contact with the subjects to support them and enhance compliance as much as possible.

At 2 weeks, anthropometric and clinical measurements were checked along with selected blood tests including fasting plasma glucose, C-peptide, insulin, and proinsulin, and a dietary follow-up was carried out with the ability to adjust the diet for energy content and composition when required. Anthropometric and clinical data were re-collected at half-time after 6 weeks. At completion of the dietary intervention at week 12 and at follow-up at week 28, a slightly shorter follow-up version of the study questionnaire, the nutrition questionnaire, the HRQoL questionnaire RAND-36 were administered, and anthropometric and clinical data and blood and urine samples were collected.

Assessment of anthropometry and clinical variables

The investigation took place at Skåne University Hospital in Malmö. Assessments of standard physical and clinical variables were done under identical conditions by two clinically experienced physicians (BO and GD). Physical examination included cardiopulmonary, abdominal, and neurological examination as well as measurement of blood pressure, pulse, respiratory rate, weight, height, waist circumference, and assessment of BMI (kg/m^2). Blood pressure was measured in the supine position after a 5-min rest with the arm at the level of the heart. Height was measured to the nearest centimeter, and weight to the nearest kilogram in subjects wearing light clothes, but not shoes, and BMI was calculated. Normal weight was defined as BMI <25 kg/m^2, overweight as BMI ≥ 25 kg/m^2 but <30 kg/m^2, and obesity as BMI ≥ 30 kg/m^2 (12). Waist circumference was measured to the nearest centimeter in a standing position after a gentle expiration, midway between the lower border of the rib cage and the superior border of the iliac crest (13). In addition, questions about intake of dietary supplements, vitamins, and probiotics; changes in medication; physical activity or routines; and any extraordinary events of daily life were completed.

Diets

The meals and snacks were planned together with the kitchen of Igelösa Life Science AB and delivered to the subjects regularly free of charge, along with recipes and instructions on how to prepare the food. The breakfast was exempt; the subjects had to buy breakfast themselves. Three alternatives were suggested, depending on their ordinary breakfast ingested, described in the nutrition questionnaire. The diet was based on the traditional Okinawan diet (6, 14), but it was modified and developed in the kitchen to suit the Nordic diet with tastes and food components suitable for the Nordic population. The meal composition was close to a moderately low carbohydrate-rich diet, one of four recommended diets from the Swedish National Food Agency for patients with diabetes (15). These recommendations are also in line with international recommendations (16, 17). The diet consists of ordinary raws, but with minimal industrial processing. The food is based on traditional Nordic raws, for example, whole grains, vegetables, leguminous, root crops, fat fish, birds, fruits, berries, and nuts (Table 1). Simultaneously, the amount of sugar, white flour, read meat, processed meat, and dairy products is limited. Actually, to promote a low glycemic response, the content of high glycemic index (GI) foods was reduced radically (e.g. white flour and sugar) in favor of nutrients with low impact on the blood sugar (Table 1). The diet has a good nutritional supply including a mean calorie intake of about 1,900 kcal/day. The participants were allowed to eat three meals a day including breakfast, lunch, and dinner, and two snacks between meals consisting of a variety of fruits, berries, and seeds (Table 1). Organic food items were preferred whenever possible. At occurrence of cravings, the subjects were instructed to eat a third snack (e.g. carrots, boiled eggs, mackerel in tomato sauce, or cottage cheese with berries) to avoid eating fast carbohydrates. Gently chopped raw vegetables and green salad were to be ingested with the main meals; 100 g at breakfast, 150 g at lunch, and

Table 1. Description of food items included in each food group in the Okinawan-based Nordic diet

Food group	
Root vegetables	Hot or cold. Red or yellow carrots as snacks or incorporated in the dish. Parsnips, parsley root, rutabaga, celery root, beetroot, artichoke, or sweet potatoes as part of the dishes.
Potatoes	Shredded in potatoes burger, fried raw.
Vegetables	Onion, leek, garlic, cabbage, cauliflower, broccoli, squash, eggplant, fennel, spinach, various types of salad, tomato, pepper, cucumber, mushroom, and asparagus.
Legumes	Fresh: green peas, sweet peas, and soybean (edamame). Dried: white and black beans, kidney beans, and lentils.
Nuts	Walnuts, almonds, and cashews.
Seeds	Sunflower seeds, pumpkin seeds, linseed, and sesame seed, as part of snacks served with fruits and berries.
Fruits and berries	Apple, orange, pear, strawberry, blueberry, lingonberry, dried apricots, and prunes. Coconut milk was used for cooking.
Meat products and poultry	Chicken, rooster, turkey, game meat (hart and deer), and ground beef.
Fish and seafood	Salmon, codfish, plaice, mackerel, herring, and prawns.
Egg	Eggs were used for cooking and as snacks.
Dairy products	Low-fat drinking milk (maximum 1.5% fat), filmjölk (a Swedish fermented product similar to yogurt) and low-fat yogurt (1.5% fat), hard cheese (17% fat), parmesan cheese, cottage cheese, and quark. Whipped cream (36% fat) and soy cream used for cooking, and Turkish yogurt (10% fat).
Fat and oil	Vegetable oil including rapeseed oil, sesame oil, and olive oil for cooking and dressing. Vegetable fat spread (60% fat) for bread.
Rice	Whole-grain rice and black Thai rice. A maximum of half a deciliter of uncooked rice per serving.
Cereals	Rolled oats, rye flakes, whole-grain whole-kernel rye, oat, barley, and wheat. Bread rich in whole grain, a maximum of two slices per day. Whole-grain pasta, bean paste, millet, oat bran, quinoa, and rye flour.
Beverages/liquids (non-alcoholic)	Recommended free amount of tap water or mineral water with the meals. Light products to be avoided. Tea, filtered coffee, or instant coffee.
Spices	Own preference with restrictions on salt.
Sweets and desserts	Homemade dark chocolate ($>70\%$), bean truffles, coconut flakes, ginger, and prune cake. No refined sugar or sweetener was used, but instead natural sweet foods such as prunes, pears, and occasionally honey.
Alcoholic beverages	Maximal intake of alcoholic beverages was set to 30 g ethanol/week.

150 g at dinner. The participants were instructed always to start with the vegetables and to eat slowly. Nutrition information is given in Table 2. Most participants had irregular meal intake, and many did not eat any breakfast, before entry in the study.

Study questionnaire

A validated study questionnaire, originally designed for the Malmö Preventive Project (18) and later slightly modified for the great population cohort of Malmö Diet and Cancer Study (19), was used for data collection. It contains questions about ordinary lifestyle factors and socioeconomic factors including information on origin, marital status, education, occupation, diet, and physical activity. In addition, a history of tobacco smoking, snuff habits, and alcohol consumption is included. The questions also cover a medical history of previous illness, disorders, or surgical operations; allergies; current medications; intake of dietary supplements and probiotics; menstrual and reproductive history; use of exogenous hormones for contraception and postmenopausal replacement therapy; and data on heredity factors.

Nutrition questionnaire

A nutrition questionnaire was used at recruitment to collect information on ordinary food habits and energy intake. This basic information was used by the nutritionist to individually design the breakfast, together with the participants (Table 3). The questionnaire was repeated at the end of the intervention and at follow-up.

Health-related quality of life questionnaire (RAND-36)

The validated self-report questionnaire: RAND 36-Item Health Survey was applied to evaluate quality of life (11). This instrument has been used to measure HRQoL in many various diseases, and normal references values are available (20). It comprises 36 items that assess eight health concepts: physical functioning, role limitations caused by general health perceptions, physical health problems, role limitations caused by emotional problems, social functioning, emotional well-being, energy/fatigue, and pain. The percentage scores range from 0% (lowest or worst possible level of functioning) to 100% (highest or best possible level of functioning). The few minor differences between 36-Item Short-Form Health Survey (SF-36) and RAND-36 have been described by Hays et al. (21).

Table 2. Nutrition composition and daily mean intake of energy, nutrients, and food components of the modified Okinawan-based Nordic diet, compared with NNR 2012

Nutritional value	Unit	Calculated value	E%	Recommended NNR 2012
Total energy	kcal	1,866	–	–
Energy (excluding beverages)	kcal	1,629	–	–
Protein	g	95.0	23	10–20 E%
Fat	g	63.9	35	25–40 E%
Saturated fatty acids	g	18.7	10	<10 E%
Polyunsaturated fatty acids	g	14.9	8	5–10 E%
Mono-unsaturated fatty acids	g	17.8	10	10–20 E%
Carbohydrates	g	168.4	42	45–60 E%
Sucrose	g	23.5	6	<10 E%
Dietary fiber	g	35.9	4	25–35 g
α-Tocopherol	mg	1.9	–	–
β-Carotene	μg	9902.1	–	–
Retinol	μg	259.7	–	–
Vitamin A	μg	139.9	–	700
Vitamin D	μg	8.8	–	10
Vitamin E	mg	11.4	–	8
Thiamine	mg	1.1	–	1.1
Riboflavin	mg	1.2	–	1.2
Niacin equivalent	mg	34.5	–	14
Niacin	mg	19.7	–	14
Vitamin B6	mg	2.1	–	1.2
Folate	μg	386.1	–	300
Vitamin B12	μg	10.4	–	2
Vitamin C	mg	303.0	–	75
Sodium	mg	2401.1	–	2,300
Potassium	mg	3385.6	–	3,100
Phosphorus	mg	1446.7	–	600
Calcium	mg	840.4	–	800
Iron	mg	10.7	–	15
Magnesium	mg	317.4		280
Zinc	mg	9.7		7
Iodine	μg	34.9		150
Selenium	μg	61.0		50

NNR = Nordic nutrition recommendations.
The daily average calorie content of the meals is given in kilocalories, and the energy percentage (E%) is presented for protein, fat, saturated fatty acids, polyunsaturated fatty acids, mono-unsaturated fatty acids, carbohydrates, and sucrose. The results are calculated on the intake of a normal week. Recommendations for a traditional diet according to the NNR are shown for comparison (15). Recommendations for total daily energy intake are not given because they are individual and differ between subjects. Vitamins A and D and iodine may be underestimated due to lack of data.

Blood samples

Venous blood samples were taken in the morning between 07:45 and 09:00 h after a 10-h fast. All samples consisted of whole blood drained into 6-mL serum separation tubes, plasma separation tubes, and BD Microtainer tubes with EDTA (BD Biosciences, Franklin Lakes, NJ). Blood chemistries were analyzed continually during the study. Remaining samples were stored at −80°C after immediate cooling and centrifugation of the blood at 3,000 rpm for 5 min, for later analyses.

Blood chemistries at baseline and at weeks 12 and 28 included blood count (hemoglobin, leukocytes, and thrombocytes), iron status (iron, total iron-binding capacity, and transferrin), C-reactive protein [CRP], kidney function tests (calcium (Ca), magnesium (Mg), potassium (K), sodium (Na), creatinine, and eGFR), liver function tests (alanine transaminase, aspartate aminotransferase, alkaline phosphatase, gamma glutamyl transpeptidase [GGT], bilirubin, albumin, and INR), cobalamin, and folate. Metabolic analyses measured were C-peptide, insulin, glucose, glycosylated hemoglobin A1c (HbA1c), and lipid profile (cholesterol, high-density lipoprotein [HDL], low-density lipoprotein [LDL], and triglyceride), and apolipoproteins A1 and B. Apolipoproteins A1 and B were used to calculate the apolipoprotein B/apolipoprotein A1 ratio as a risk predictor for cardiovascular events. Homeostasis model assessment for insulin resistance (HOMA2-IR) was calculated using the HOMA2 calculator version 2.2.3 (22, 23). As recommended by the HOMA2 calculator software, observations with extreme values of fasting plasma glucose (<3 or >25 mmol/L), serum C-peptide (<0.2 or >3.5 nmol/L), or both, were excluded. Serum insulin and C-peptide levels were determined using the one-step immune-complex sandwich assay with electrochemiluminescence immunoassay detection technique based on ruthenium derivatives (Elecsys® insulin and C-peptide, Roche Diagnostics Ltd., Switzerland). Circulating stress markers were assessed by cortisol and thyroid-stimulating hormone (TSH). All samples were analyzed by standard methods at the Department of Clinical Chemistry, Skåne University Hospital, Malmö, Sweden.

At baseline and at week 2, fasting glucose, C-peptide, insulin, and proinsulin were measured. Proinsulin in serum was measured at the Department of Clinical Chemistry, Karolinska University Hospital, Stockholm, Sweden by an enzyme-linked immunosorbent assay (Proinsulin ELISA, Mercodia AB, Uppsala, Sweden) that uses a solid phase two-site enzyme immunoassay for photometric quantification of human proinsulin. There is no cross-reactivity with insulin or C-peptide.

Urinary analysis for microalbuminuria

Urinary albumin and creatinine were measured using the Cobas Integra system (Roche Diagnostics Ltd., Rotkreuz, Switzerland). Urinary albumin was measured by the immunoturbidimetric method and urinary creatinine by the kinetic Jaffe reaction. The albumin/creatinine ratio was used to estimate microalbuminuria levels obtained from spot urine samples in the morning. Albuminuria was defined as the ratio of urine albumin to creatinine of ≥3.0 g/mol.

Table 3. Mean energy composition of the individual breakfast meals over the course of the study ($n = 30$)

	Breakfast at baseline					Breakfast at week 12				
Subject no.	Energy (kcal)	Protein (g/E%)	Fat (g/E%)	Carbs (g/E%)	Fiber (g/E%)	Energy (kcal)	Protein (g/E%)	Fat (g/E%)	Carbs (g/E%)	Fiber (g/E%)
1	488	22/18	33/59	25/20	6/2	331	17/21	17/46	24/30	7/4
2	184	7/15	3/15	29/64	6/7	258	13/20	10/33	27/42	7/5
3	301	12/16	22/63	14/19	3/2	267	16/24	15/50	15/23	4/3
4	191	10/20	12/55	11/24	0.7/0.7	420	28/28	16/34	37/36	5/2
5	209	8/16	5/21	31/60	5/5	248	10/17	8/28	30/49	8/6
6	241	8/14	5/17	38/64	8/6	81	3/15	2/26	10/52	3/8
7	515	20/16	21/36	55/43	12/5	362	24/27	13/33	33/37	5/3
8	230	10/18	11/40	22/39	3/2	537	33/25	19/32	53/40	8/3
9	526	26/20	24/40	49/38	5/2	309	23/30	10/29	31/41	5/3
10	260	9/14	12/41	28/43	3/2	248	14/23	9/30	26/42	5/5
11	119	7/24	6/41	9/30	3/5	131	8/25	7/44	8/26	3/5
12	298	10/13	9/26	43/58	5/3	–	–	–	–	–
13	328	16/19	3/9	56/70	5/3	310	13/17	10/29	39/51	5/3
14	443	18/16	20/41	45/41	5/2	141	8/22	6/40	12/35	3/3
15	332	11/14	8/22	51/62	4/2	221	16/30	5/21	25/46	4/4
16	213	7/13	3/13	36/69	5/5	253	15/24	9/32	24/39	6/5
17	291	10/14	14/43	28/40	8/5	537	15/12	33/55	40/31	9/3
18	497	21/17	27/48	41/34	4/1	188	11/24	4/19	14/30	4/4
19	300	12/16	13/38	31/43	10/6	385	18/19	15/35	42/44	8/4
20	343	13/16	16/40	33/40	8/4	175	9/21	9/44	14/32	4/4
21	383	15/16	11/26	51/54	8/4	299	10/13	6/17	49/67	8/5
22	590	25/17	29/44	55/38	4/1	–	–	–	–	–
23	390	17/17	11/26	51/53	8.5/4	364	14/16	15/37	38/42	9/5
24	555	19/14	26/42	56/41	11/4	488	25/21	15/27	58/48	9/3
25	502	25/20	18/32	57/46	5/2	341	19/23	17/43	27/32	5/3
26	212	10/19	4/17	31/59	6/5	265	15/23	3/11	39/60	9/6
27	465	20/18	18/32	53/46	4/2	355	24/27	14/35	31/36	5/3
28	290	15/21	17/53	18/25	2/1	–	–	–	–	–
29	153	6/17	3/19	24/65	4/4	305	15/20	9/27	38/51	8/5
30	454	21/19	16/31	52/47	7/3	374	20/21	11/26	45/50	7/3

Two subjects (12 and 22) did not complete the study, and one subject (28) did not submit the logbook at the end of the study.

Statistical analyses

A power analysis was performed based on previous studies of occasional subjects, and we found that at most nine subjects were needed to demonstrate clinically important differences in HbA1c, total cholesterol, systolic blood pressure, and weight and 18 subjects to demonstrate clinically important differences in diastolic blood pressure with 80% power at 5% significance level. We included 30 patients to take into account drop-outs. We tested hypotheses with linear mixed effect models to analyze continuous variables, with random intercept and unstructured covariance's for repeated measures within a patient, with visits as nominal fixed effect, using baseline as reference. We assumed that missing observations were unrelated to the observed value; that is, they were missing at random. In these analyses, predicted mean values and their 95% confidence limits are presented, together with estimates of changes from baseline and 95% confidence limits and p values for the changes. Descriptive statistics are presented as means and standard deviations for continuous variables and as counts or frequencies for categorical variables. Statistical calculations were done with MATLAB R2015a (The MathWorks Inc., Natick, MA). A p value <0.05 is considered statistically significant.

Results

Adherence to the diet and study protocol

The trial was initiated with 30 subjects. One of the subjects missed the 2-week follow-up, but otherwise completed the study. Two participants withdrew from the study at the half-time follow-up after 6 weeks: one because of inability to adapt to the new diet and the other because of work-related time constraints. Final samples were taken at withdrawal. Data obtained from non-completers and subjects with transitory infection ($n = 4$), surgery ($n = 2$), or depression ($n = 2$) during the study period were not excluded. Baseline data collected at the time of the first clinical visit are given in Table 4.

The meals were well received by the majority of subjects. However, after 2 weeks, five subjects had to increase the caloric content of the food by an average of 146 kcal/day (distributed as 6 g of protein; 7 g of fat, of which 2 g was saturated fat; and 14 g of carbohydrates, including 2.5 g of dietary fiber) due to rapid weight loss. Higher energy requirements were identified related to physical activity at work and leisure time. All of these subjects went back at their own request to the initial calorie content of the meals after another 4 weeks at the half-time follow-up, as they felt sufficiently satiated. Four other subjects, all with irritable bowel syndrome, had to reduce the fiber content, whole-grain and root fruit content, or both, of the food because of troublesome bloating, abdominal pain, acid reflux, constipation, and in one case even diarrhea. In these cases, the protein content of the food was increased to maintain ordinary amount of calories, and at the half-time follow-up, the exaggerated symptoms were normalized. A reduction by half of the amount of whole grains entailed an increase in the protein proportion of 60 kcal/day.

Although encouraged to maintain their regular physical activity habits throughout the study period (Table 4), nine subjects had increased, and another four subjects had reduced, their regular physical activity by one level (e.g. from moderate exercise during leisure to moderate regular exercise during leisure or the opposite) at the end of the study.

Anthropometric and clinical analyses

A progressive significant body weight reduction was seen at 2, 6, and 12 weeks after introduction of the new diet. The mean reduction of body weight and waist circumference at 12 weeks was 6.2 kg ($p < 0.001$) and 7.0 cm ($p < 0.001$), respectively. This weight loss was equivalent to 7% of total body weight at baseline. Mean BMI was reduced from 29.9 kg/m^2 at baseline to 28.4 kg/m^2 after 12 weeks ($p < 0.001$), and 53% of the obese subjects ($n = 15$) went from obesity to overweight, and 25% of the overweight subjects ($n = 12$) went from overweight to normal weight. Despite some increase, the mean weight, BMI, and waist circumference remained significantly lower compared with baseline at 16 weeks after completion of dietary intervention (Table 5).

Table 4. Patient characteristics at inclusion

Sex (female/male)	17/13	Antihypertensive medication (%)	63
Age (years)	57.5 ± 8.2	Lipid-lowering medication (%)	47
BMI (kg/m^2)	29.9 ± 4.1	IBS (%)	13
Education (%)		Diabetes duration (years)	10.4 ± 7.6
Primary school	16	HbA1c (mmol/mol)	61.6 ± 17.6
High school	57	Diabetes management (%)	
College	27	Diet alone	7
Occupation (%)		Metformin	40
Employed	67	Sulfonylurea	3
Retired	17	Sulfonylurea and metformin	7
Sick leave	13	DPP-4 inhibitor and metformin	3
Unemployed	3	Metformin and insulin	27
Smokers (%)	23	Insulin	13
Snuff users (%)	23	Diabetes complication (%)	
Frequency of alcohol intake (%)		Retinopathy	27
None	10	Nephropathy	17
Once a month or less	50	Neuropathy	30
2–4 times a month	27	Gastroparesis	3
2–3 times a week	13	Macroangiopathy	17
Physical activity (%)			
Sedentary leisure time	7		
Moderate exercise during leisure	53		
Moderate regular exercise during leisure	27		
Regular exercise and training	13		

$n = 30$. BMI = body mass index, IBS = irritable bowel syndrome, HbA1c = glycosylated hemoglobin, DPP-4 = dipeptidyl peptidase-4. Age, BMI, total energy intake, diabetes duration, and HbA1c values are presented as means ± standard deviation, and other values are presented as percentages.

Table 5. Anthropometric analyses

Variable	Mean	Lower	Upper	Mean change	Lower	Upper	p
Weight (kg)							
Baseline	89.8	84.5	95.1	–	–	–	–
Week 2	86.7	81.4	92.1	−3.03	−3.61	−2.45	<0.001
Week 6	85.1	79.8	90.5	−4.66	−5.61	−3.72	<0.001
Week 12	83.6	78.1	89.0	−6.20	−7.61	−4.78	<0.001
Week 28	85.4	79.7	91.1	−4.40	−6.57	−2.24	<0.001
BMI (kg/m^2)							
Baseline	29.9	28.4	31.3	–	–	–	–
Week 2	28.9	27.4	30.4	−1.00	−1.18	−0.81	<0.001
Week 6	28.3	26.8	29.8	−1.53	−1.83	−1.23	<0.001
Week 12	27.8	26.3	29.4	−2.05	−0.52	−1.57	<0.001
Week 28	28.4	26.8	30.0	−1.47	−2.13	−0.82	<0.001
Waist circumference (cm)							
Baseline	107.3	103.4	111.2	–	–	–	–
Week 2	104.1	99.6	108.6	−3.19	−5.53	−0.85	0.008
Week 6	102.6	98.6	106.6	−4.67	5.88	−3.47	<0.001
Week 12	100.3	96.1	104.4	−7.02	−8.62	−5.42	<0.001
Week 28	101.7	97.6	105.9	−5.54	−7.11	−3.96	<0.001
Heart rate (beats/min)							
Baseline	80.50	77.13	83.87	–	–	–	–
Week 2	72.48	68.33	76.63	−8.02	−11.41	−4.63	<0.001
Week 6	68.73	64.30	73.16	−11.77	−15.50	−8.05	<0.001
Week 12	67.27	62.77	71.77	−13.23	−17.04	−9.42	<0.001
Week 28	67.88	63.32	72.44	−12.62	−16.50	−8.74	<0.001
Systolic blood pressure (mmHg)							
Baseline	140.17	134.72	145.61				
Week 2	136.63	130.20	143.06	−3.54	−7.65	0.58	0.091
Week 6	132.96	126.58	139.34	−7.21	−11.25	−3.17	<0.001
Week 12	130.55	124.39	136.71	−9.62	−13.30	−5.93	<0.001
Week 28	139.74	133.84	145.65	−0.42	−3.65	2.81	0.796
Diastolic blood pressure (mmHg)							
Baseline	82.33	78.73	85.93	–	–	–	–
Week 2	77.78	73.79	81.77	−1.58	−1.54	−0.62	0.001
Week 6	76.29	72.49	80.08	−1.55	−2.43	−0.68	<0.001
Week 12	74.88	71.03	78.73	−2.70	−3.57	−1.84	<0.001
Week 28	78.74	74.76	82.72	−1.75	−2.78	−0.72	0.001
Respiratory rate (breaths/min)							
Baseline	17.30	16.34	18.26	–	–	–	–
Week 2	15.72	14.64	16.80	−1.58	−2.54	−0.62	0.001
Week 6	15.75	14.74	16.75	−1.55	−2.43	−0.68	<0.001
Week 12	14.60	13.60	15.59	−2.70	−3.57	−1.84	<0.001
Week 28	15.55	14.40	16.69	−1.75	−2.78	−0.72	0.001

BMI = body mass index.

$n = 30$. The mean values, mean changes, and 95% confidence interval with upper and lower limits are presented for anthropometric parameters at inclusion (baseline); at 2, 6, and 12 weeks after introduction of diet intervention; and at 16 weeks after the end of diet intervention (week 28). Comparisons were made between each time point and baseline by using linear mixed effect models. A value of $p < 0.05$ was considered statistically significant.

There were no changes in lipid-lowering or antihypertensive medication, except titration of enalapril from 10 to 15 mg in one case at the start of the study. A significant reduction in the systolic and diastolic blood pressure could be seen after 2, 6, and 12 weeks. The diastolic blood pressure remained lower compared with baseline after

28 weeks of follow-up (Table 5). A significant progressive mean reduction in the heart and respiratory rates could be seen already 2 weeks after the diet introduction, persisting during the following weeks of intervention and 16 weeks after completion of dietary intervention (Table 5).

Metabolic biomarkers

During dietary intervention, there was a significant reduction in the mean fasting plasma glucose values already after 2 weeks ($p < 0.001$), and these levels were maintained until the end of the intervention, when the mean level of HbA1c was reduced by 20% ($p < 0.001$). At week 28, the mean level of HbA1c remained lower than at baseline (Table 6). There was a 43% reduction of proinsulin levels ($p = 0.005$) and insulin levels ($p = 0.011$) after 2 weeks and a significant reduction in C-peptide levels after 12 weeks ($p = 0.015$). These reductions were followed by reduced insulin resistance after 2 weeks, which remained after 28 weeks (Table 6). None of the participants increased their anti-diabetes treatment during the study. However, in 15 cases, the anti-diabetes medication had to be reduced gradually during the study period, and in two cases, including one on insulin treatment, the medication was cancelled. These reductions persisted 16 weeks later. Out of the remaining 12 diabetes patients on insulin, three got their insulin therapy cancelled and another eight had their insulin doses reduced by $27.6 \pm 16.4\%$ on average. During the dietary intervention period, there was also a significant reduction in cortisol levels ($p = 0.015$), but this reduction did not remain at the 28-week follow-up (Table 6).

Twelve weeks after the dietary introduction, a significant improvement was seen in the lipid profile for triglycerides ($p = 0.009$), total cholesterol ($p = 0.001$), and LDL-cholesterol ($p = 0.041$) (Table 6). This improvement did not remain at the follow-up, 16 weeks afterward. In contrast, a significant increase was observed for HDL-cholesterol at this time ($p = 0.003$) (Table 6). The mean reduction in GGT was 0.23 μkat/L ($p = 0.016$) at the end of the intervention period. No significant changes in the albumin/creatinine ratio or the apolipoprotein B/apolipoprotein A1 ratio was seen during or after diet intervention. Blood count, iron status tests, CRP, kidney function tests, liver function tests (except for GGT), TSH, cobalamin, and folate were not affected during the study period (data not shown).

Health-related quality of life

Compared with baseline, the mean scores for the RAND-36 scale improved and were significantly higher for physical functioning ($p < 0.001$), general health ($p < 0.001$), vitality ($p = 0.011$), social functioning ($p = 0.001$), and mental health ($p = 0.003$) after 12 weeks. The largest increase was in the social functioning and physical functioning scales. The increase in the mean scores for the vitality scale peaked at 16 weeks after the end of diet intervention ($p < 0.001$). Even though the other scale scores had declined at this point, the mean increase in physical functioning, general health, and social functioning were still significantly improved relative to baseline (Table 7).

Discussion

This is the first study to investigate the effects of a modified Okinawan-based Nordic diet in Scandinavian type 2 diabetes subjects. In this 12-week intervention, the dietary intervention led to significant reductions in weight and waist circumference. Beneficial effects in metabolic parameters were achieved, including improvement in glucose-insulin homeostasis, insulin resistance, and lipid homeostasis during reduction of anti-diabetes treatment. The blood pressure was lowered and progressive reductions in the heart and respiratory rates were seen, along with reduction in cortisol levels and improvement of HRQoL.

Most data about food and nutrition are based on epidemiological studies or experimental studies using test solutions or substitution of one or two substances. Few studies are performed as interventional studies on complete meals. Consequently, there is a good understanding of individual food groups' positive impacts on metabolic and cardiovascular risk factors, but there is no uniform general dietary strategy to prevent diabetes (24). Dietary interventions recommended by the European Society of Cardiology; the European Association for the Study of Diabetes, Diabetes and Nutrition Study Group (17); and the American Diabetes Association (16) emphasize an appropriate intake of total energy and a diet in which fruits, vegetables, whole-grain cereals, legumes, and low-fat protein sources predominate. Specific dietary recommendations include limiting saturated and trans fats and alcohol intake, monitoring carbohydrate consumption, and increasing dietary fiber and foods containing whole grains. The traditional dietary pattern in Okinawa encompasses high consumption of vegetables and legumes (mostly soy in origin); moderate consumption of fish products; low consumption of meat, meat products, and dairy products; and moderate alcohol consumption. The caloric intake is low, but the diet is rich in omega-3 fats, has a high monounsaturated-to-saturated fat ratio, and emphasis on low GI carbohydrates (14).

Low GI diets are associated with lower risk of type 2 diabetes and heart disease (25) and can be useful in the management of glucose levels in patients with diabetes (26). Whole-grain cereals and legumes have been reported to be generally associated with health-beneficial effects (27) including postprandial blood glucose control and reduction in the levels of circulating inflammatory biomarkers (28). Furthermore, epidemiological and clinical studies demonstrate that intake of dietary fiber and whole grains is inversely related to obesity (29), type 2 diabetes

Table 6. Metabolic control and biomarkers for disease risk

Variable	Mean	Lower	Upper	Mean change	Lower	Upper	p
Fasting glucose (mmol/L)							
Baseline	9.71	8.54	10.87	–	–	–	–
Week 2	7.90	6.62	9.18	−1.81	−2.51	−1.11	<0.001
Week 12	7.91	6.55	9.27	−1.80	−2.63	−0.96	<0.001
Week 28	9.28	7.71	10.85	−0.42	−1.58	0.73	0.466
HbA1c (mmol/mol)							
Baseline	61.57	56.42	66.72	–	–	–	–
Week 12	49.20	44.02	54.38	−12.37	−16.40	−8.33	<0.001
Week 28	54.36	48.83	59.90	−7.20	−11.68	−2.72	0.002
Proinsulin (pmol/L)							
Baseline	23.84	16.70	30.98	–	–	–	–
Week 2	13.69	6.46	20.92	−10.15	−17.15	−3.15	0.005
Insulin (mIU/L)							
Baseline	15.53	12.72	18.35	–	–	–	–
Week 2	12.73	9.89	15.57	−2.81	−4.96	−0.66	0.011
Week 12	11.67	8.85	14.48	−3.87	−5.99	−1.75	<0.001
Week 28	12.78	9.32	16.24	−2.75	−5.67	0.16	0.064
C-peptide (nmol/L)							
Baseline	0.99	0.81	1.17	–	–	–	–
Week 2	0.92	0.73	1.12	−0.07	−0.17	0.04	0.208
Week 12	0.88	0.69	1.07	−0.11	−0.21	−0.02	0.015
Week 28	0.88	0.66	1.09	−0.11	−0.25	0.02	0.108
HOMA2-IR (U)							
Baseline	3.00	2.50	3.51	–	–	–	–
Week 2	2.53	1.96	3.09	−0.48	−0.85	−0.11	0.012
Week 12	2.37	1.82	2.91	−0.64	−0.98	−0.30	<0.001
Week 28	2.61	2.05	3.16	−0.40	−0.75	−0.05	0.025
Cortisol (nmol/L)							
Baseline	367	337	397	–	–	–	–
Week 12	325	290	360	−41.20	−74.07	−8.34	0.015
Week 28	348	315	382	−18.34	−49.73	13.06	0.249
Triglycerides (mmol/L)							
Baseline	1.79	1.41	2.16	–	–	–	–
Week 12	1.49	1.09	1.89	−0.30	−0.52	−0.08	0.009
Week 28	1.96	1.46	2.46	0.17	−0.20	0.54	0.367
Cholesterol (mmol/L)							
Baseline	4.65	4.36	4.95	–	–	–	–
Week 12	4.22	3.87	4.57	−0.44	−0.69	−0.18	0.001
Week 28	4.71	4.37	5.05	0.06	−0.18	0.30	0.636
HDL (mmol/L)							
Baseline	1.22	1.10	1.35	–	–	–	–
Week 12	1.19	1.05	1.32	−0.04	−0.10	0.03	0.267
Week 28	1.34	1.20	1.47	0.11	0.04	0.18	0.003
LDL (mmol/L)							
Baseline	2.92	2.62	3.22	–	–	–	–
Week 12	2.68	2.33	3.03	−0.24	−0.48	−0.01	0.041
Week 28	2.82	2.49	3.16	−0.10	−0.30	0.11	0.356

Table 6. (Continued)

Variable	Mean	Lower	Upper	Mean change	Lower	Upper	p
GGT (μkat/L)							
Baseline	0.80	0.53	1.07	–	–	–	–
Week 12	0.58	0.30	0.85	−0.23	−0.41	−0.04	0.016
Week 28	0.53	0.17	0.89	−0.27	−0.57	0.03	0.073

HbA1c = hemoglobin A1c, HOMA2-IR = homeostasis model assessment for insulin resistance, HDL = high-density lipoprotein; LDL = low-density lipoprotein, GGT = gamma glutamyl transpeptidase.
$n = 30$ subjects. The mean values, mean changes, and 95% confidence interval with upper and lower limits are given for fasting blood values of glucose and HbA1c; fasting serum levels of proinsulin, insulin, and C-peptide; insulin resistance as measured by HOMA2-IR (one missing value); and fasting plasma values of cortisol, triglycerides, cholesterol, HDL, LDL and GGT. Values are shown at inclusion (baseline); 2, 6 and 12 weeks after diet intervention; and 16 weeks after the end of diet intervention (week 28). Comparisons were made between each time point and baseline by using linear mixed effect models. A value of $p < 0.05$ is considered statistically significant.

(30), cancer (31), and cardiovascular disease (32). Dietary fiber's beneficial influence on obesity has been attributed to a decreased caloric density of the foods, reducing the energy intake over time (29); decreased nutrient absorption (33); increased satiety (28); and a slower rate of food ingestion (34). The composition of indigestible carbohydrates has also been shown to diminish episodes of hyperglycemia and related metabolic risk variables through a mechanism involving colonic fermentation (28). Consequently, it has been suggested that low-GI foods, which in addition are rich in whole-grain constituents, could be particularly advantageous to diminish risk factors associated with insulin resistance (28).

Despite a mean calorie intake of 1,900 kcal/day in the Okinawan-based diet, the average weight reduction was 6.2 kg after 12 weeks, representing 7% of total body weight. Research shows that modest weight loss of 5–10% is associated with improved health outcomes, including lower blood glucose levels, lower blood pressure, and improved lipid levels (35). Observational studies have reported that weight loss more than 5 kg over a 10-year period reduced the risk of diabetes by 50% or more (36). One reason to the present described weight reduction may be an increased satiety found already after a single meal of the diet compared with a traditional meal (10). The Okinawan-based diet composition with more fiber and greater food volume demands more chewing, thereby constituting a slower eating pattern with increased mastication and slower gastric emptying (37), factors that all induce less feeling of hunger and desire to eat (38). Because of the lower carbohydrate content, energy composition is optimized by a higher proportion of protein. Protein is the most satiating nutrient, and high-protein intake directly activates the arcuate nucleus and nucleus tracts solitaries in the brain, resulting in a suppressed food intake and delayed gastric emptying (39). The concomitant reduction in waist circumference and GGT in this study indicate that weight loss was related to a decrease in abdominal obesity (40). This may be of importance, because a strong relationship between central obesity and cardiovascular disease has been found (41).

During the dietary intervention, the mean fasting plasma glucose values were significantly reduced along with reduced insulin resistance, and decreased HbA1c levels at the end of the intervention period, despite a considerable gradual reduction in anti-diabetes medication. Preproinsulin is processed to proinsulin, before conversion to insulin and C-peptide and stored in secretary granules, awaiting release on demand. If the demand for insulin triggered by insulin resistance reaches a certain threshold, an insufficiency of the cleavage capacity of β cells leads to an increased secretion of intact proinsulin in addition to the desired insulin molecule (42). A large cross-sectional study has confirmed that intact proinsulin is a highly specific marker for insulin resistance (43). Proinsulin and C-peptide have been demonstrated to be cardiovascular risk factors by stimulating plasminogen activator inhibitor-1 secretion to block fibrinolysis (44) and by pro-inflammatory and pro-atherogenic effects (42, 45). The markedly reduced levels of C-peptide, insulin, and proinsulin already 2 weeks after the dietary introduction suggest a rapid reduction of insulin resistance, as indicated by the results for HOMA2-IR. These immediate responses may rather depend on dietary changes than by weight changes, because only a single meal of the Okinawan diet attenuated postprandial levels of glucose, glucose-dependent insulinotropic polypeptide (GIP), C-peptide, and insulin in comparison with a traditional meal (10). Significant improvement was seen in the lipid profile for triglyceride, total cholesterol, and LDL-cholesterol in the present study, although the fat content was higher than recommended in traditional diabetes diet (16). This may depend on the improved glucose-insulin homeostasis and lower levels of GIP, because GIP together with hyperinsulinemia

Table 7. Evaluation of quality of life using RAND 36-Item Health Survey

Variable	Mean	Lower	Upper	Mean change	Lower	Upper	*p*
Physical functioning							
Baseline	75.7	69.3	82.1	–	–	–	–
Week 12	86.5	80.1	92.9	10.8	4.9	16.7	<0.001
Week 28	85.3	78.4	92.2	9.6	3.2	16.1	0.004
Physical role functioning							
Baseline	74.2	60.7	87.6	–	–	–	–
Week 12	78.3	64.9	91.8	4.2	−9.8	18.1	0.555
Week 28	73.3	57.7	88.8	−0.9	−16.9	15.1	0.911
Bodily pain							
Baseline	72.8	62.9	82.8	–	–	–	–
Week 12	79.7	69.1	90.3	6.9	−1.6	15.3	0.109
Week 28	80.3	69.1	91.5	7.5	−1.8	16.7	0.112
General health							
Baseline	58.7	51.2	66.1	–	–	–	–
Week 12	68.7	60.4	76.9	10.0	4.2	15.8	<0.001
Week 28	67.7	58.9	76.5	9.0	2.5	15.5	0.007
Vitality							
Baseline	56.2	48.1	64.3	–	–	–	–
Week 12	66.7	56.2	77.1	10.5	2.5	18.5	0.011
Week 28	68.4	59.3	77.5	12.2	6.1	18.4	<0.001
Social functioning							
Baseline	78.4	70.6	86.3	–	–	–	–
Week 12	89.3	79.8	98.8	10.9	4.3	17.4	0.001
Week 28	87.4	77.4	97.3	8.9	1.8	16.1	0.015
Emotional role functioning							
Baseline	81.1	71.3	90.9	–	–	–	–
Week 12	84.5	71.6	97.3	3.4	−9.1	15.8	0.592
Week 28	83.8	69.7	97.8	2.7	−11.0	16.3	0.699
Mental health							
Baseline	73.2	67.0	79.4	–	–	–	–
Week 12	82.0	75.3	88.7	8.8	3.2	14.4	0.003
Week 28	78.6	71.8	85.3	5.4	−0.4	11.1	0.067

$n = 30$. The percentage scores range from 0% (lowest or worst possible level of functioning) to 100% (highest or best possible level of functioning). The mean values, mean changes, and 95% confidence interval with upper and lower limits are given for eight health concepts at inclusion (baseline); 12 weeks after diet intervention; and 16 weeks after the end of diet intervention (week 28). Comparisons were made between each time point and baseline by using linear mixed effect models. A value of $p < 0.05$ is considered statistically significant.

and hyperglycemia is strongly involved in lipid regulation in humans (46).

A significant reduction in cortisol levels could be observed, along with a progressive reduction in the heart and respiratory rates and lowering in systolic and diastolic blood pressure. Activation of the sympatho-adrenal medullary (SAM) system and the hypothalamo-pituitary-adrenal (HPA) axis increases cortisol levels, blood pressure and heart rate (47). Excessive activation of these pathways in response to physiological challenges, including food intake, has been linked to the development of numerous chronic diseases including cardiovascular disease, type 2 diabetes, anxiety, and depression (48). There are several potential mechanisms behind the observed phenomena of lowered stress levels in the present study. Animal studies suggest that obesity can be associated with increased HPA axis and SAM system in responses to stress (49), and human studies have shown that adiposity in men is associated with hyperactivity of the HPA axis after ingestion of a standardized meal consisting of 22% protein, 53% carbohydrates, and 25% fat (50). One study has shown that intake of meals with high carbohydrate content results in a significantly higher HPA axis response in women with predominant visceral body fat distribution, compared with women with peripheral body fat distribution and normal-weighted healthy controls (51). Both the weight reduction and the lower carbohydrate load in the Okinawan-based Nordic diet may have contributed to the reduced stress level. Furthermore, data indicate a strong relationship between obesity and HRQoL, and even a small weight reduction leads to significant improvements in HRQoL (52).

Although caloric restriction is an effective method of losing body weight and body fat, it becomes more challenging if compliance to the diet cannot be maintained. The impact of home delivery and the pre-portioned meals may have contributed to adherence to dietary restrictions during intervention. However, on the 16-week follow-up after diet intervention, the weight, BMI, waist circumference, insulin resistance, and HbA1c remained significantly lower than at baseline, even with sustained reduction in anti-diabetes treatment. Also, diastolic blood pressure and heart and respiratory rates remained lower than at baseline, and a significant increase in HDL-cholesterol was observed at this time. This delayed effect in the improvement of HDL-cholesterol is difficult to explain, but it could be attributed to a continued generally healthier dietary pattern, increased physical activity after the completion of the dietary intervention, or both. Actually, we assume these residual beneficial effects in part to be related to subject's adoption to changed eating habits (e.g. changing breakfast habits, diminished meal size, continuing eating fruit and vegetables, and regular meals). Participants were instructed always to start with the vegetables, to eat slowly and to drink water with the meals, to induce satiety and less intake of energy-rich food. Evidence to this advice comes from studies in which increasing the vegetable portion on the plate by substituting it for meat and grain significantly increased vegetable intake and reduced the energy intake (53, 54).

It remains to determine to what extent the beneficial role depends on dietary composition or weight reduction. Even though some of our findings support an influence of dietary changes, including an immediate metabolic response after diet introduction the first weeks in line with a single meal evaluation of Okinawan-based diet and traditional diet (10), we presume additional beneficial effects as a result of weight changes. A limitation of the present study was that no control group was included. It is a challenge to construct an appropriate control group in open, non-blinded studies. Instead, the participants were characterized at baseline and followed during and after diet intervention, thus being their own controls. A control group provides some evidence that changes occurring over time were not the result of natural temporal trends or of unmeasured events that occurred contemporaneously with the exposure under study. A similar diet interventional study, using a control group advised to follow their habitual diet and physical activity, did however not show any effects on these controls (55). Furthermore, these patients were already scheduled for regular, clinical follow-ups at their primary care center. Thus, the psychological benefit of being enrolled in a clinical study should be less than if patients without an established clinical contact had been included.

In conclusion, a modified Okinawan-based Nordic diet seems to be well accepted by the participants and the beneficial health effects is considerable in type 2 diabetes. The dietary intervention led to significant reductions in anthropometric and metabolic parameters with an improvement of HRQoL. Further studies have to be conducted to examine its potential to be applied for practical use in a larger Scandinavian population to reduce the risk for metabolic syndrome and associated diseases.

Authors' contribution

The study was conducted by two separate teams, in conjunction with each other. The dietary concept was developed by SS, EL, TS, and BW.

The study design was set up by GD, PH, and BO. GD and BO ran the study. BO was PI and financed the clinical parts of the study. BR and EL performed data collection and monitored the study. PH performed the statistical analyses. GD wrote the manuscript. All authors contributed to the writing of the manuscript by constructive criticism and the final version was approved by all authors.

Acknowledgements

This study was supported by grants from Hans-Gabriel and Alice Trolle Wachtmeister's Foundation for Medical Research, King Gustaf V:s and Queen Victoria Free Maison's Foundation, Dir Albert Påhlsson's Foundation, Development Foundation of Region Skåne, and Foundation of Skåne University Hospital. We acknowledge the staff at Igelösa Life Science AB, Lund, for supplying and preparing the meals and the staff at the Internal Medicine Research Group, Skåne University Hospital, Malmö, for assistance to perform this study.

Conflict of interest and funding

SS is the founder of Igelösa Life Science AB. The other authors have no conflicts of interest.

References

1. International Diabetes Federation (2015). IDF diabetes Atlas. 7 ed. Brussels, Belgium: International Diabetes Federation.
2. Rexrode KM, Manson JE, Hennekens CH. Obesity and cardiovascular disease. Curr Opin Cardiol 1996; 11: 490–5.
3. Heller RF. Hyperinsulinemic obesity and carbohydrate addiction: the missing link is the carbohydrate frequency factor. Med Hypotheses 1994; 42: 307–12.
4. Knowler WC, Barrett-Connor E, Fowler SE, Hamman RF, Lachin JM, Walker EA, et al. Diabetes Prevention Program Research Group. Reduction in the incidence of type 2 diabetes with lifestyle intervention or metformin. N Engl J Med 2002; 346: 393–403.
5. Ramachandran A, Snehalatha C, Mary S, Mukesh B, Bhaskar AD, Vijay V. Indian Diabetes Prevention Programme (IDPP). The Indian diabetes prevention programme shows that lifestyle modification and metformin prevent type 2 diabetes in Asian

Indian subjects with impaired glucose tolerance (IDPP-1). Diabetologia 2006; 49: 289–97.
6. Willcox DC, Scapagnini G, Willcox BJ. Healthy aging diets other than the Mediterranean: a focus on the Okinawan diet. Mech Ageing Dev 2014; 136: 148–62.
7. O'Keefe JH, Gheewala NM, O'Keefe JO. Dietary strategies for improving post-prandial glucose, lipids, inflammation, and cardiovascular health. J Am Coll Cardiol 2008; 51: 249–55.
8. Suzuki M, Willcox BJ, Willcox DC. Implications from and for food cultures for cardiovascular disease: longevity. Asia Pac J Clin Nutr 2001; 10: 165–71.
9. Willcox BJ, Willcox DC, Todoriki H, Fujiyoshi A, Yano K, He Q, et al. Caloric restriction, the traditional Okinawan diet and healthy aging: the diet of the world's longest-lived people and its potential impact on morbidity and lifespan. Ann N Y Acad Sci 2007; 1114: 434–55.
10. Ohlsson B, Höglund P, Roth B, Darwiche G. Modification of a traditional breakfast leads to increased satiety along with attenuated plasma increments of glucose, C-peptide, insulin, and GIP in humans. Nutr Res 2016; 36: 359–68.
11. Garratt A, Schmidt L, Mackintosh A, Fitzpatrick R. Quality of life measurement: bibliographic study of patient assessed health outcome measures. BMJ 2002; 324: 1417.
12. World Health Organization (WHO). BMI classification. Global database on body mass index 2015. Available from: http://apps.who.int/bmi/index.jsp?introPage=intro_3.html [cited 4 February 2016].
13. Clinical guidelines on the identification, evaluation, and treatment of overweight and obesity in adults – the evidence report. National Institutes of Health. Obes Res 1998; 6: 51S–209S.
14. Willcox DC, Willcox BJ, Todoriki H, Suzuki M. The Okinawan diet: health implications of a low-calorie, nutrient-dense, antioxidant-rich dietary pattern low in glycemic load. J Am Coll Nutr 2009; 28: 500S–16S.
15. Nordic Council of Ministers (2014). Nordic nutrition recommendations 2012: integrating nutrition and physical activity. Copenhagen K: Nord, Nordic Council of Ministers. doi: http://dx.doi.org/10.6027/nord2014-002
16. American Diabetes Association, Bantle JP, Wylie-Rosett J, Albright AL, Apovian CM, Clark NG, et al. Nutrition recommendations and interventions for diabetes: a position statement of the American Diabetes Association. Diabetes Care 2008; 31: S61–78.
17. Task Force on diabetes, pre-diabetes, and cardiovascular diseases of the European Society of Cardiology (ESC); European Association for the Study of Diabetes (EASD), Rydén L, Grant PJ, Anker SD, Berne C, et al. ESC guidelines on diabetes, pre-diabetes, and cardiovascular diseases developed in collaboration with the EASD – summary. Diab Vasc Dis Res 2014; 11: 133–73.
18. Berglund G, Eriksson KF, Israelsson B, Kjellström T, Lindgärde F, Mattiasson I, et al. Cardiovacsular risk groups and mortality in an urban Swedish male population: the Malmö preventive project. J Intern Med 1996; 239: 489–97.
19. Manjer J, Carlsson S, Elmståhl S, Gullberg B, Janzon L, Lindström M, et al. The Malmö diet and cancer study: representativity, cancer incidence and mortality in participants and non-participants. Eur J Cancer Prev 2001; 10: 489–99.
20. Aalto AM, Aro AR, Teperi J. RAND-36 as a measure of health-related quality of life. Reliability, construct validity and reference values in the Finnish general population. Helsinki: National Research and Development Centre for Welfare and Health; 1999.
21. Hays RD, Sherbourne CD, Mazel RM. The RAND 36-item health survey 1.0. Health Econ 1993; 2: 217–27.
22. Diabetes Trials Unit TOCfD. Endocrinology and metabolism 2016 HOMA2 calculator. Oxford, UK: The University of Oxford. Available from: http://www.dtu.ox.ac.uk/homacalculator/ [cited 12 January 2016].
23. Levy JC, Matthews DR, Hermans MP. Correct homeostasis model assessment (HOMA) evaluation uses the computer program. Diabetes Care 1998; 21: 2191–2.
24. Ley SH, Hamdy O, Mohan V, Hu FB. Prevention and management of type 2 diabetes: dietary components and nutritional strategies. Lancet 2014; 383: 1999–2007.
25. Barclay AW, Petocz P, McMillan-Price J, Flood VM, Prvan T, Mitchell P, et al. Glycemic index, glycemic load and chronic disease risk – a meta-analysis of observational studies. Am J Clin Nutr 2008; 87: 627–37.
26. Brand-Miller J, Hayne S, Petocz P, Colagiuri S. Low-glycemic index diets in the management of diabetes – a meta-analysis of randomized controlled trials. Diabetes Care 2003; 26: 2261–7.
27. Venn BJ, Perry T, Green TJ, Skeaff CM, Aitken W, Moore NJ, et al. The effect of increasing consumption of pulses and whole grains in obese people: a randomized controlled trial. J Am Coll Nutr 2010; 29: 365–72.
28. Nilsson AC, Östman EM, Holst JJ, Björck IM. Including indigestible carbohydrates in the evening meal of healthy subjects improves glucose tolerance, lowers inflammatory markers, and increases satiety after a subsequent standardized breakfast. J Nutr 2008; 138: 732–9.
29. Tucker LA, Thomas KS. Increasing total fiber intake reduces risk of weight and fat gains in women. J Nutr 2009; 139: 576–81.
30. Meyer KA, Kushi LH, Jacobs DR, Jr., Slavin J, Sellers TA, Folsom AR. Carbohydrates, dietary fiber, and incident type 2 diabetes in older women. Am J Clin Nutr 2000; 71: 921–30.
31. Park Y, Brinton LA, Subar AF, Hollenbeck A, Schatzkin A. Dietary fiber intake and risk of breast cancer in postmenopausal women: the National Institutes of Health-AARP diet and health study. Am J Clin Nutr 2009; 90: 664–71.
32. Streppel MT, Ocke MC, Boshuizen HC, Kok FJ, Kromhout D. Dietary fiber intake in relation to coronary heart disease and all-cause mortality over 40 y: the Zutphen study. Am J Clin Nutr. 2008; 88: 1119–25.
33. Lattimer JM, Haub MD. Effects of dietary fiber and its components on metabolic health. Nutrients 2010; 2: 1266–89.
34. Kimm SY. The role of dietary fiber in the development and treatment of childhood obesity. Pediatrics 1995; 96: 1010–14.
35. Wing RR, Lang W, Wadden TA, Safford M, Knowler WC, Bertoni AG, et al. Benefits of modest weight loss in improving cardiovascular risk factors in overweight and obese individuals with type 2 diabetes. Diabetes Care 2011; 34: 1481–6.
36. Colditz GA, Willett WC, Rotnitzky A, Manson JE. Weight gain as a risk factor for clinical diabetes mellitus in women. Ann Intern Med 1995; 122: 481–6.
37. Benini L, Castellani G, Brighenti F, Heaton KW, Brentegani MT, Casiraghi MC, et al. Gastric emptying of a solid meal is accelerated by the removal of dietary fibre naturally present in food. Gut 1995; 36: 825–30.
38. Zhu Y, Hsu WH, Hollis JH. Increasing the number of masticatory cycles is associated with reduced appetite and altered postprandial plasma concentrations of gut hormones, insulin and glucose. Br J Nutr 2013; 110: 384–90.
39. Cecil JE, Francis J, Read NW. Comparison of the effects of a high-fat and high-carbohydrate soup delivered orally and intragastrically on gastric emptying, appetite, and eating behaviour. Physiol Behav 1999; 67: 299–306.
40. D'Onise K, McDermott RA, Campbell SK. Benefits of modest weight or waist circumference loss in a remote North Queensland indigenous population. Aust N Z J Public Health 2013; 37: 345–9.

41. Yusuf S, Hawken S, Ounpuu S, Dans T, Avezum A, Lanas F, et al. Effect of potentially modifiable risk factors associated with myocardial infarction in 52 countries (the INTERHEART study): case-control study. Lancet 2004; 364: 937–52.
42. Marx N, Walcher D, Raichle C, Aleksic M, Bach H, Grüb M, et al. C-peptide colocalizes with macrophages in early atherosclerotic lesions of diabetic subjects and induces monocytes chemotaxis *in vitro*. Arterioscler Thromb Vasc Biol 2004; 24: 540–5.
43. Forst T, Standl E, Hohberg C, Konrad T, Schulze J, Strotmann HJ, et al. IRIS II study: the IRIS II score – assessment of a new clinical algorithm for the classification of insulin resistance in patients with Type 2 diabetes. Diabet Med 2004; 21: 1149–53.
44. Eliasson M, Røder ME, Dinesen B, Evrin PE, Lindahl B. Proinsulin, intact insulin, and fibrinolytic variables and fibrinogen in healthy subjects. A population study. Diabetes Care 1997; 20: 1252–5.
45. Vasic D, Marx N, Sukhova G, Bach H, Durst R, Grüb M, et al. C-peptide promotes lesion development in a mouse model of arteriosclerosis. J Cell Mol Med 2012; 16: 927–35.
46. Asmar M, Simonsen L, Madsbad S, Stallknecht B, Holst JJ, Bülow J. Glucose-dependent insulinotropic polypeptide may enhance fatty acid re-esterification in subcutaneous abdominal adipose tissue in lean humans. Diabetes 2010; 59: 2160–3.
47. Elenkov IJ, Chrousos GP. Stress hormones, proinflammatory and antiinflammatory cytokines, and autoimmunity. Ann N Y Acad Sci 2002; 966: 290–303.
48. Chrousos GP. Stress and disorders of the stress system. Nat Rev Endocrinol 2009; 5: 374–81.
49. Tilbrook AJ, Rivalland EAT, Turner AI, Lambert GW, Clarke IJ. Responses of the hypothalamopituitary adrenal axis and the sympathoadrenal system to isolation/restraint stress in sheep of different adiposity. Neuroendocrinology 2008; 87: 193–205.
50. Jayasinghe SU, Torres SJ, Nowson CA, Tilbrook AJ, Turner AI. Cortisol, alpha amylase, blood pressure and heart rate responses to food intake in men aged 50–70 years: importance of adiposity. BMC Obes 2014; 1: 14.
51. Vicennati V, Ceroni L, Gagliardi L, Gambineri A, Pasquali R. Response of the hypothalamic-pituitary-adrenocortical axis to high-protein/fat and high-carbohydrate meals in women with different obesity phenotypes. J Clin Endocrinol Metab 2002; 87: 3984–8.
52. Fontaine KR, Barofsky I. Obesity and health-related quality of life. Obes Rev 2001; 2: 173–82.
53. Rolls BJ, Roe LS, Meengs JS. Portion size can be used strategically to increase vegetable consumption in adults. Am J Clin Nutr 2010; 91: 913–22.
54. Rolls BJ, Roe LS, Meengs JS. Salad and satiety: energy density and portion size of a first course salad affect energy intake at lunch. J Am Diet Assoc 2004; 104: 1570–6.
55. Adamsson V, Reumark A, Fredriksson IB, Hammarström E, Vessby B, Johansson G, et al. Effects of a healthy Nordic diet on cardiovascular risk factors in hypercholesterolaemic subjects: a randomized controlled trial (NORDIET). J Intern Med 2011; 269: 150–9.

*Gassan Darwiche
Department of Clinical Sciences
Skåne University Hospital
SE-205 02 Malmö
Sweden
Email: ghassan.darwiche@med.lu.se

2

In vivo protein quality of selected cereal-based staple foods enriched with soybean proteins

Laura Acevedo-Pacheco and Sergio O. Serna-Saldívar*

Centro de Biotecnología-FEMSA, Escuela de Ingeniería y Ciencias, Tecnológico de Monterrey, Monterrey, México

Abstract

Background: One way to diminish protein malnutrition in children is by enriching cereal-based flours for the manufacturing of maize tortillas, wheat flour tortillas, and yeast-leavened breads, which are widely consumed among low socio-economic groups.

Objective: The aim was to determine and compare the essential amino acid (EAA) scores, protein digestibility corrected amino acid scores (PDCAAS), and *in vivo* protein quality (protein digestibility, protein efficiency ratio (PER), biological values (BV), and net protein utilization (NPU) values) of regular versus soybean-fortified maize tortillas, yeast-leavened bread, and wheat flour tortillas.

Design: To comparatively assess differences in protein quality among maize tortillas, wheat flour tortillas, and yeast-leavened breads, EAA compositions and *in vivo* studies with weanling rats were performed. The experimental diets based on regular or soybean-fortified food products were compared with a casein-based diet. Food intake, weight gains, PER, dry matter and protein digestibility, BV, NPU, and PDCAAS were assessed. The soybean-fortified tortillas contained 6% of defatted soybean flour, whereas the yeast-leavened bread flour contained 4.5% of soybean concentrate.

Results: The soybean-fortified tortillas and bread contained higher amounts of lysine and tryptophan, which improved their EAA scores and PDCAAS. Rats fed diets based on soybean-fortified maize or wheat tortillas gained considerably more weight and had better BV and NPU values compared with counterparts fed with respective regular products. As a result, fortified maize tortillas and wheat flour tortillas improved PER from 0.73 to 1.64 and 0.69 to 1.77, respectively. The PER improvement was not as evident in rats fed the enriched yeast-leavened bread because the formulation contained sugar that decreased lysine availability possibly to Maillard reactions.

Conclusions: The proposed enrichment of cereal-based foods with soybean proteins greatly improved PDCAAS, animal growth, nitrogen retention, and PER primarily in both maize and wheat flour tortillas. Therefore, these foods can help to diminish protein malnutrition among children who greatly depend on cereals as the main protein dietary source.

Keywords: *soybean proteins*; *maize tortillas*; *wheat flour tortillas*; *bread*; *PDCAAS*; *protein efficiency ratio*; *nitrogen retention*

Responsible Editor: Per Ole Iversen, University of Oslo, Norway.

Malnutrition could be solved globally by enrichment and fortification of food products with high-quality proteins and micronutrients (1, 2). According to Food and Agriculture Organization (FAO), 11.3% of the global population (805 million) were chronically malnourished in 2012–2014 (3). The easiest way to assist low socio-economic groups is to enrich flours at mill level with low-cost protein supplements that complement their essential amino acid (EAA) scores. The World Health Organization (WHO) estimated that in 2013, 98.9 million children younger than age 5 were underweight, from which 97.9 million inhabited developing countries (4).

It has been proposed that a solution to this problem is to increase the amount of protein in cereal staple foods (wheat, rice, and maize). These cereals provide most of the calories (more than 60%) and protein (about 50%) consumed in the average diet. Therefore, these staples are ideally suited for nutritional enrichment (5–7). In 2013, world production of all cereals was approximately 2,781 million tons. The FAO states that wheat, rice, and maize constitute more than 80% of the global cereal production (8). In Mexico, maize tortillas, wheat flour tortillas, and table bread are the basic cereal foods of the diet especially among low socio-economic groups.

Unfortunately, maize-based tortillas and wheat-based bakery items lack the EAA lysine as well as optimum levels of relevant micronutrients such as iron, zinc, and vitamins A, D, E, and B12 (6, 7, 9).

Soybean (*Glycine max*) is the main legume produced worldwide. In 2013, more than 276 million tons were globally produced (8). Soybeans are a rich source of high-quality protein similar in terms of protein digestibility corrected amino acid scores (PDCAAS) to meat and dairy proteins. In addition, soybean products contain micronutrients and bioactive compounds such as isoflavones, flavonoids, saponins, both soluble and insoluble dietary fiber, and folic acid (10, 11). The industrial manufacturing of soybeans yields important products such as full-fat meals, oil, defatted meals, texturized proteins, concentrates, isolates, and soybean milk. The different array of soybean protein products contain from 40 to 90% protein with a good EAA score (12, 13). More importantly, soybean proteins provide high amounts of EAA that are found in lower concentrations in most cereals, making these proteins ideal sources to fortify these foods (14). From the processing point of view, different soybean proteins possess a range of functional properties such as gelling, emulsifying, foaming, water, and oil holding capacities (15).

Previous studies have shown that wheat bread, maize tortillas, and wheat flour tortillas can be successfully fortified with different soybean proteins without affecting sensory acceptance. These products contained 23–30% more protein compared to regular counterparts as well as an improved EAA score (9, 16, 17). To the best of our knowledge, there are no studies evaluating *in vivo* protein quality of soybean-fortified maize and wheat flour tortillas and bread at the same time. Thus, the aim of this research was to determine and compare the *in vivo* protein quality (animal growth and nitrogen retention) and the EAA scores of regular maize tortillas, yeast-leavened bread, and wheat flour tortillas compared with counterparts fortified with soybean proteins. Weanling rats were used because they have similar EAA requirements to infants and they are considered as a good model for protein quality studies (18).

Materials and methods

Chemical analyses of food products and diets

Compositions of animal-formulated diets are shown in Table 1. Foods were chemically characterized for moisture, protein, ether extract, crude fiber, and ash with the American Association of Cereal Chemists International (AACC) approved methods, respectively (44-15.02, 46-13.01, 30-20.01, 32-10.01, 08-01.01) (19). The nitrogen-free extract (NFE) was calculated by difference, whereas the energy values of regular and soybean-fortified foods were determined according to the Atwater coefficient by multiplying the NFE and protein content by 4 kcal/g and ether extract by 9.

Amino acid score and PDCAAS of food products

The complete EAA scores of regular and fortified tortillas and yeast-leavened breads were obtained following the Association of Official Analytical Chemists (AOAC) Official Method 982.30 E(a) (20). Briefly, the amino acid composition of all foods was determined by HPLC system (1525 binary pump, waters, Milford MA, USA) equipped with a 3.9×150 mm AccQ-Taq C18 column bonded with endcapped octadecylsilane, a fluorescence detector (Waters 2475 multi fluorescence), and an autosampler (Waters 717 plus). The concentration of particular amino acids was calculated by comparing with standards. The PDCAAS were calculated from the limiting EAA related to the requirement for children multiplied by the *in vivo* protein digestibility data estimated with weanling rats (21). The PDCAAS is recognized by the FAO/WHO and the US Food and Drug Administration as the preferred quick method for the estimation of protein quality.

Preparation of diets

Maize flour tortillas and wheat flour tortillas were manufactured with composite flours containing approximately 6.0% of defatted soybean meal with a protein dispersibility index (PDI) of 23.2 ± 0.11, whereas the yeast-leavened table bread with a bread flour containing 4.5% soybean protein concentrate with a PDI of 52 ± 0.5. The preparation and characteristics of these regular and soybean-fortified cereal-based foods are detailed by Chuck-Hernández et al., Perez-Carrillo et al., and Lazo-Velez et al. (9, 16, 17). The regular and soybean-fortified products were dehydrated in a convention oven set at 50°C for 8 h and then ground in a Wiley mill equipped with a 2 mm sieve. The ground products were chemically characterized before diet formulation. Diets were formulated to contain 10% protein (1.6% nitrogen) according to the official PER AOAC 960.48 method (20). Diets were blended for 10 min in a Hobart mixer equipped with a paddle with the starch, vegetable oil, mineral premix (AIN 76), vitamin premix (AIN 76), and cellulose in order to contain equal amounts of corn oil, calories, and fiber. The control diet had similar composition to the experimental diets and contained casein (AIN high nitrogen) as the only source of protein. Diets were packed in sealed plastic bags and stored in a freezer (−20°C) until the beginning of the animal study and then transferred to a refrigerator (5°C).

Animal study design and protein efficiency ratio bioassay

Assessment of the protein efficiency ratio (PER) was performed according to the official procedures recommended by the AOAC Official Method 960.48 (20). The protocol for this study (2013-Re-009) was approved by the Tecnológico de Monterrey Animal Care Committee and is based on international standards. Fifty-six weanling male Wistar rats (Bioinvert-Mexico) of approximately 21 days of age were housed in individual metabolic cages at a temperature of 22°C and a 12:12 light–dark cycle. They were acclimated to the new environment for 2 days. Rats were distributed to eight blocks according to their initial body weight. Each block had seven animals assigned to the seven different treatments. A total of 56 animals were used (8 blocks and 7 treatments) and fed *ad libitum* for 28 days. The control diet (CSD) contained casein as the source of protein, whereas the six experimental diets included regular or soybean-fortified tortillas or yeast-leavened bread. The experimental diets were named as maize tortilla diet (MTD), wheat flour tortillas diet (WTD), yeast-leavened bread diet (BRD), soybean-fortified maize tortillas diet (SMTD), soybean-fortified wheat flour tortillas diet (SWTD), and soybean-fortified yeast-leavened bread diet (SBRD) (Table 1). Food intake and body weights were measured every 2 weeks for the duration of the study. Experimental and adjusted PER values were calculated using the following equations: Experimental PER = weight gain/protein intake and adjusted PER = (2.5/Experimental PER value of the control casein) × (Experimental PER values of the respective treatment).

Animal study for determination of nitrogen retention
Feces and urine were collected daily from day 14 until day 28 and immediately placed in a freezer at a temperature of −20°C. Food intake was carefully monitored for this period of time. In order to prevent urine nitrogen losses due to microbial contamination, urine containers were supplemented daily with 1 ml HCl (1:1). After 14 consecutive days of feces and urine collection, nitrogen was analyzed in feed, dried feces and urine following the AACC Official Kjeldahl Method 46–13:01 (19). Apparent protein digestibility, biological value (BV) and net protein utilization (NPU) were calculated using the following equations: % Protein digestibility = [[(Food intake) (% Nitrogen in Food)] − [(Feces) (% Nitrogen in Feces)]/[(Food intake) (% Nitrogen in Food)]] × 100, % BV = [[(Food intake) (% Nitrogen in Food)] − [(Feces) (% Nitrogen in Feces) − [(Urine) × (% Nitrogen in Urine)]]/[[(Food intake) (% Nitrogen in Food)] − [(Feces) (%Nitrogen in Feces)]] × 100 and % NPU Value = [(% Protein Digestibility) × (% BV)]/100.

Statistical analyses
Body weight, food intake, protein intake, PER, dry matter digestibility, protein digestibility, BV, and NPU values were analyzed using analysis of variance (ANOVA) for randomized block design followed by a Duncan's Multiple Range post-hoc test. Level of significance was declared at $p < 0.05$. Pearson correlation coefficients were calculated with the aim to identify significant relationships ($p < 0.05$) between nitrogen retention data, animal growth (PER), and PDCAAS. All statistical analyses were performed using the computer software Minitab16.

Results

Chemical composition of regular and soybean-fortified products
Formulation and chemical composition of the regular and soybean-fortified tortillas and yeast-leavened bread

Table 1. Formulation of regular and soybean-fortified cereal-based diets offered to weanling rats during the animal studies[1]

	Casein	Maize tortillas		Yeast-leavened bread		Wheat flour tortillas	
Ingredient (g/100 g)	CSD	MTD	SMTD	BRD	SBRD	WTD	SWTD
Corn oil	8.00	7.62	7.06	5.47	6.13	0	3.84
Water	0	0.29	1.55	0.62	0	2.97	2.19
Minerals AIN-76	3.50	3.50	3.50	3.50	3.50	3.50	3.50
Vitamins AIN-76	1.00	1.00	1.00	1.00	1.00	1.00	1.00
Cellulose	1.00	0	0	0.07	0.12	0.50	0.55
Casein	11.60	–	–	–	–	–	–
Starch	64.90	–	8.84	14.86	30.00	3.12	27.88
Sucrose	10.00	–	–	–	–	–	–
Maize tortillas	–	87.59	–	–	–	–	–
Soybean-fortified maize tortillas	–	–	78.05	–	–	–	–
Yeast-leavened bread	–	–	–	74.48	–	–	–
Soybean-fortified bread	–	–	–	–	59.25	–	–
Wheat flour tortillas	–	–	–	–	–	88.91	–
Soybean-fortified wheat flour tortillas	–	–	–	–	–	–	61.04

[1]CSD, casein control diet; MTD, maize tortillas diet; SMTD, soybean-fortified maize tortillas diet; BRD, yeast-leavened bread; SBRD, soybean-fortified bread; WTD, wheat flour tortillas; SWTD, soybean-fortified wheat tortillas. Diets were formulated according to the PER protocol to contain 10% crude protein, 8% crude fat, and 1% crude fiber. In addition, they were supplemented with 1% vitamins and 3.5% mineral premix.

are summarized in Tables 1 and 2, respectively. The enriched cereal products containing 4.5 or 6.0% soybean concentrate or defatted soybean flour provided approximately 20% more protein, but similar amounts of energy compared to regular counterparts. The wheat flour tortillas contained higher calorie content (448.30 and 443.80 kcal/100 g) compared with maize tortillas (397.50 and 395.80 kcal/100 g). The addition of soybean protein to fortified foods increased the protein:calorie ratio compared to the respective regular counterparts (Table 2). It is worth mentioning that all experimental diets were formulated to contain equal amounts of protein, crude fat, crude fiber, and non-fibrous carbohydrates so the only sources of variation were the amino acid score and other not measured compounds present in soybeans like, for example, isoflavones (which were, however, not in the focus of this study).

The amino acid compositions of the six foods are shown in Table 2. All fortified products were characterized by improved EAA composition especially in terms of lysine, tryptophan, and threonine. For instance, the most limiting amino acid lysine improved its concentration from 2.5 g/100 g protein (mean of lysine of MT, BR and WT) to around 3.4 g/100 g protein (mean of soybean-fortified counterparts). The regular and soybean-fortified maize tortillas contained 0.72 and 0.93 g of tryptophan (the second most limiting amino acid) per 100 g protein, respectively (Table 2). In this particular product, The amino acid score of lysine improved from 49 to 64 after soybean enrichment. Likewise, the EAA scores of soybean-fortified wheat flour tortillas and yeast-leavened bread improved in about 15 units (Table 3).

Animal growth performance (PER bioassay)

The results related to total diet intake and PER are summarized in Table 4. The daily food intake ranged from 6.23 to 11.52 g/d in groups of rats fed the experimental diets and averaged 13.41 g/d in the group fed the control casein diet (Table 4). Animals fed the soybean-fortified diets consumed significantly higher quantities of food (approximately 28% more) compared to their counterparts fed regular diets. Rats fed with soybean-fortified maize or wheat tortillas-based diets gained 1.86 and 2.28 g/day, respectively, while animals fed respective regular diets gained 0.47 and 0.59 g/day. Likewise, animals fed the soybean-fortified bread diet gained 0.74 g/day while their counterparts fed regular bread gained only

Table 2. Chemical composition, caloric value, and amino acid composition of regular maize tortillas, wheat flour tortillas, and yeast-leavened bread foods fortified with soybean proteins[1,2]

	Maize tortillas		Yeast-leavened bread		Wheat flour tortillas	
	MT	SMT	BR	SBR	WT	SWT
Proximate composition, %						
Crude protein (N*6.25)	9.17±0.45	11.52±0.01	9.30±0.82	11.55±0.31	7.95±0.17	9.84±1.81
Crude fat	1.0±0.01	0.9±0.10	2.21±0.32	2.14±0.12	10.5±1.15	9.72±0.06
Crude fiber	1.7±0.14	2.0±0.07	0.4±0.28	0.5±1.84	0.2±1.41	0.3±0.49
Ash	0.8±0.02	0.9±0.02	1.4±0.10	1.4±0.11	1.2±0.05	1.3±0.07
Nitrogen-free extract[2]	87.33	84.68	86.69	84.41	80.15	78.84
Energy Value[3] (kcal/100 g)	397.50	395.80	405.65	405.00	448.30	443.80
Protein:calorie ratio (g protein/100 Kcal)	2.30	2.91	2.29	2.85	1.77	2.21
Amino acids (g/100 g protein)						
Threonine	3.62	3.70	2.75	2.97	2.75	3.01
Valine	4.83	4.85	4.12	4.27	4.12	4.28
Isoleucine	3.62	3.89	3.61	3.84	3.61	3.83
Leucine	13.03	11.83	6.95	7.19	6.95	7.17
Lysine	2.90	3.73	2.32	3.23	2.32	3.19
Histidine	2.90	2.83	2.06	2.19	2.06	2.18
Tryptophan	0.72	0.93	1.37	1.38	1.37	1.42
Methionine + Cysteine	3.98	3.72	3.78	3.50	3.78	3.60
Phenylalanine + Tyrosine	7.60	7.88	7.12	7.52	7.12	7.46

[1]MT, maize tortillas; SMT, soybean-fortified maize tortillas; BR, yeast-leavened bread; SBR, soybean-fortified bread; WT, wheat flour tortillas; SWT, soybean-fortified wheat tortillas. Values are means ± SD and are expressed on dry matter basis, $n = 3$. The average moisture content of foods were: 51.79 ± 1.25 for MT, 47.70 ± 0.67 for SMT, 36.2 ± 1.18 for BR, 37.30 ± 1.43 for SBR, 29.04 ± 0.82 for WT and 30.62 ± 0.96 for SWT.
[2]NFE = nitrogen-free extract that gives an indication of non-fibrous carbohydrates (starch plus sugars).
[3]Calculated using the Atwater coefficient.

Table 3. Effect of soybean enrichment on amino acid scores of maize tortillas, yeast-leavened bread, and wheat flour tortillas foods[1]

Amino acids	Food agriculture Organization/World Health Organization Requirement 2–5 years infant	Maize tortilla		Yeast-leavened bread		Wheat flour tortilla	
		MT	SMT	BR	SBR	WT	SWT
Threonine	3.4	106	109	80	87	80	88
Valine	3.5	137	138	117	122	117	122
Isoleucine	2.8	129	138	128	137	128	136
Leucine	6.6	197	179	105	108	105	108
Lysine	5.8	**49**	**64**	**40**	**55**	**40**	**55**
Histidine	1.9	152	149	108	115	108	114
Tryptophan	1.1	65	84	124	125	124	129
Methionine + Cysteine	2.5	159	148	151	140	151	144
Phenylalanine + Tyrosine	6.3	120	125	113	119	113	118

[1]MT, maize tortillas; SMT, soybean-fortified maize tortillas; BR, yeast-leavened bread; SBR, soybean-fortified bread; WT, wheat flour tortillas; SWT, soybean-fortified wheat tortillas. Amino acid scores calculated based on the Food and Agriculture Organization/World Health Organization requirement for 2–5 years infant. Values highlighted on bold letters depict the limiting amino acid.

0.16 g/day. These differences in average daily gains were highly significant. Food intake, final body weight, daily weight gain, protein intake, and PER values were significantly higher ($p < 0.05$) in casein and all soybean-fortified diets compared to the regular diets. The adjusted PER of the regular maize and wheat flour tortillas were 70 and 72 lower, respectively, compared to casein. On the other hand, the PER of these soybean-fortified products were 34 and 29 lower compared to casein.

The average adjusted PER of the regular diets ranged from 0.2 to 0.7, whereas for soybean-fortified diets from 0.9 to 1.8. Therefore, the PERs of weanling rats fed with fortified diets were at least twice as high compared with animals fed their respective regular diets.

As shown in Table 4, animals fed the control casein diet had the highest adjusted PER. The adjusted PER values of the soybean-fortified maize and WTDs were 1.64 and 1.77, respectively (71 and 66% of the adjusted PER of the casein diet, respectively). The lowest PER values corresponded to rats fed the bread diets (regular and fortified).

Nitrogen retention study

Dry matter and apparent protein digestibility, nitrogen retention values (BV and NPU), and PDCAAS are depicted in Table 5. As expected, animals fed with the casein-based diet had the highest dry matter and protein digestibility values and PDCAAS (97, 91, and 91% respectively).

Table 4. Effect of soybean protein enrichment of maize tortillas, yeast-leavened bread, and wheat flour tortillas on the growth and protein efficiency ratios (PER) of weanling rats fed formulated diets[1,2]

	Diets						
	Control casein	Maize tortillas		Yeast-leavened bread		Wheat flour tortillas	
	CSD	MTD	SMTD	BRD	SBRD	WTD	SWTD
Initial weight (g)	47.5 ± 5.0 a	47.7 ± 5.2 a	45.6 ± 5.4 a	45.6 ± 5.5 a	46.4 ± 5.3 a	45.6 ± 5.1 a	45.7 ± 5.7 a
Final weight (g)	157.2 ± 11.4 a	60.9 ± 11.5 e	97.8 ± 12.6 c	50.2 ± 8.6 f	67.1 ± 11.0 d	62.2 ± 7.2 e	109.5 ± 17.8 b
Average daily gain (g)	3.9 ± 0.4 a	0.47 ± 0.3 e	1.9 ± 0.4 c	0.2 ± 0.2 f	0.7 ± 0.3 d	0.6 ± 0.1 e	2.3 ± 0.4 b
Food intake (g/day)	13.4 ± 1.4 a	6.8 ± 1.3 e	10.1 ± 1.5 c	6.2 ± 1.3 f	7.1 ± 1.7 d	7.6 ± 0.9 d	11.5 ± 2.2 b
Protein intake (g/day)	1.2 ± 0.1 a	0.5 ± 0.1 f	0.9 ± 0.1 c	0.6 ± 0.1 e	0.6 ± 0.2 d	0.7 ± 0.1 d	1.0 ± 0.2 b
Experimental PER	3.2 ± 0.2 a	0.9 ± 0.4 e	2.1 ± 0.3 c	0.3 ± 0.2 f	1.2 ± 0.3 d	0.9 ± 0.1 e	2.3 ± 0.1 b
Adjusted PER	2.50 a	0.73 e	1.64 c	0.22 f	0.89 d	0.69 e	1.77 b
FER	0.29 ± 0.11	0.07 ± 0.08	0.19 ± 0.02	0.03 ± 0.03	0.10 ± 0.03	0.08 ± 0.01	0.20 ± 0.01

[1]MTD, maize tortillas; SMTD, soybean-fortified maize tortillas; BRD, yeast-leavened bread; SBRD, soybean-fortified bread; WTD, wheat flour tortillas; SWTD, soybean-fortified wheat tortillas; FER, Food Efficiency Ratio. Values are averages ± SD of eight observations except for the control and regular maize tortillas treatments that experienced the death of one animal.

[2]Means denoting different letter(s) within rows are statistically different ($p < 0.05$).

Table 5. Effect of soybean protein enrichment of maize tortillas, yeast-leavened bread, and wheat flour tortillas on dry matter and protein digestibilities, nitrogen retention, and protein digestibility corrected amino acid scores (PDCAAS) estimated with weanling rats fed formulated diets[1,2]

	Diets						
	Control casein	Maize tortillas		Yeast-leavened bread		Wheat flour tortillas	
	CSD	MTD	SMTD	BRD	SBRD	WTD	SWTD
Dry matter digestibility (%)	96.5±0.4 a	89.3±2.4 d	90.8±0.8 d	94.6±0.9 b	94.6±1.9 b	90.6±0.1 d	92.3±0.5 c
Protein digestibility (%)	91.3±1.0 a	72.5±4.7 e	78.8±2.2 d	83.2±2.1 bc	84.8±2.2 b	81.4±2.8 c	83.0±1.6 bc
Biological value (%)	71.0±5.5 a	56.0±9.5 bc	72.4±13.1 a	44.5±17.1 d	52.2±11.2 c	57.9±8.6 bc	61.8±9.9 b
Net protein utilization value (%)	64.0±4.5 a	40.5±6.8 de	57.1±10.8 b	37.3±15.1 e	44.3±10.0 d	47.1±7.2 cd	51.4±8.3 bc
PDCAAS[3]	91.26	35.53	50.44	33.26	46.61	32.57	45.64

[1]MTD, maize tortillas; SMTD, soybean-fortified maize tortillas; BRD, yeast-leavened bread; SBRD, soybean-fortified bread; WTD, wheat flour tortillas; SWTD, soybean-fortified wheat tortillas. Values are averages ± SD of eight observations except for the control and regular maize tortillas treatments that experienced the death of one animal.

[2]Means denoting different letter(s) within rows are statistically different ($p < 0.05$).

[3]Protein digestibility corrected amino acid score. Calculated by multiplying protein digestibility by amino acid score (refer to Table 3).

The NPU and PER values were positively correlated with PDCAAS ($r = 0.85$ and $r = 0.87$, respectively, $p < 0.05$). Therefore, all soybean-fortified products had higher nitrogen retention and PDCAAS values compared to their respective regular counterparts. The data clearly showed that the proposed soybean enrichment favored nitrogen retention estimated as BV and NPU; and animal growth estimated with the PER assay. Interestingly, the casein-based or the SMTDs showed similar BV (71 and 72%, respectively). The NPU value and PDCAAS scores of the fortified maize tortillas diet were 1.4 times higher compared to its regular counterpart. Among treatments, the BRD was with the lowest BV and NPU scores.

Discussion

Results of this study clearly indicate that the proposed soybean enrichment intervention greatly improved EAA, PDCAAS, animal growth, and nitrogen retention values in a weanling rat model. According to the FAO, wheat and maize provided worldwide 526 and 146 kcal/day and 15.9 and 3.5 g/day protein in 2011, respectively (8). In Latin America, maize plays a more important role. For instance, maize, mainly in the form of tortillas and related products, provides 928 kcal/day and 26 g protein/day for the average Mexican.

The wheat flour tortillas contained the highest amount of energy due to the addition of shortening in the formulation. The ratio of protein to calories clearly favored the soybean-fortified products because of the protein enrichment (Table 2).

All fortified products were characterized by improved EAA composition especially in terms of lysine, tryptophan, and threonine because soybean is a rich source of these EAA. Soybean is especially rich in lysine and tryptophan. Defatted soybean flour containing around 50% protein provides approximately 10 times more lysine and tryptophan compared with regular maize tortilla flour. Therefore, the addition of only 6% soybean flour greatly improved the contents of these two limiting EAA. The same trend was observed with the lysine content of the wheat-based enriched products (Tables 2 and 3). The second limiting EAA in wheat flour tortillas and table bread was threonine. The enrichment with soybean proteins also slightly improved the amounts of this particular amino acid. The significant improvements in the EAA scores with similar levels of the soybean enrichment in maize tortillas, wheat flour tortillas, and table bread were previously documented by many authors (6, 7, 22–28).

Animals fed the casein- and soybean-fortified products consumed higher amounts of food compared with animals fed regular products due to the better EAA scores. Previous studies clearly indicated lower food intakes in animals consuming low-protein quality diets (6, 22, 24, 27, 28). The higher food intake plus the better EAA score of the soybean-fortified products improved caloric intake and greatly upgraded weight gains and PER (Table 4). An enhanced protein and energy intake would promote a faster recovery of children affected by protein calorie malnutrition, marasmus, or kwashiorkor. According to the WHO, a stronger formula that achieve energy and protein intake for catch-up growth in severe malnutrition patients should provide 100 kcal and 2.9 protein per 100 ml (29). All the soybean-fortified foods contained protein:calorie ratios varying from 2.2 to 2.9 g protein/100 kcal (Table 2), which are higher compared to the values ranging from 1.8 to 2.3, observed in regular counterparts. The improved protein calorie ratios of soybean-fortified foods were slightly lower or equal to the recommended values to combat protein-energy malnutrition (29). As expected, animals fed the casein control diet had the best protein digestibly, BV, NPU, PDCAAS, and PER values. Animals fed the soybean-fortified maize or wheat flour tortillas had about 30% less PER compared to counterparts fed the casein-based diet. This difference is attributed to a higher rate of protein digestibility (Table 5), and better EAA score and PDCAAS of casein-fortified compared with soybean-fortified products. However, from the practical point of view, casein costs about five times more than commercial defatted soybean flours used for the production of both types of tortillas and about twice as more compared to a soybean protein concentrate which was used for the production of enriched bread. Therefore, the intervention with soybean products is more recommended in terms of cost benefit.

Weanling rats fed with the soybean-fortified maize and soybean-fortified wheat tortilla diets gained 52.2 and 63.8 g during the 28-day growth trial compared with counterparts fed with regular products which gained 13.2 and 16.6 g, respectively. A similar trend in weight gain was evident in a study in which rats fed with fortified tortillas with 8% of defatted soybean meal and 4% of defatted sesame meal had weight gains 2.5 times higher compared with counterparts fed the control maize tortillas (28). Also Gonzalez Agramon and Serna Saldivar reported weight gains in weanling rats three times higher when they were fed with soybean-fortified wheat flour tortillas in comparison with animals fed regular wheat flour tortillas (23). These authors attributed the improved performance to the higher retention of nitrogen, which was mainly anabolized into body weight (23).

The higher PER values of the soybean-fortified maize and wheat tortillas were closer to the observed PER of animals fed the control diet. Previously, Chavez and Chavez reported that the PER of tortillas containing 6% of defatted soybean flour was 80% higher in comparison to the casein-based diet. In this study, the PER value of SMTD equaled 66% of PER value of casein (24). Moreover, weanling rats fed with soybean-fortified wheat flour tortillas had twice as high PER values when compared with rats fed with the unfortified tortillas (23). As shown in Table 4, rats fed the fortified wheat flour tortillas had average daily gains of 2.28 g while rats fed the regular WTD had an average daily gain of 0.59 g.

As shown in murine models, the proposed soybean enrichment of maize tortillas not only improves nitrogen retention and growth performance but also brain development of animals (6, 7, 25, 26).

Interestingly, animals fed the BRD diet were the ones that ended with the lowest gains and PERs. This occurred despite the fact that bread was fermented with dried yeast (2% based on flour weight), which is known to have adequate levels of all EAAs especially lysine (8 g/100 g of protein) (30). It is important to mention that among the cereal-based products tested herein, the bread formulation was the only food item containing supplemented sugar (5.5% based on flour weight) that is known to lower lysine bioavailability after thermal treatments such as the one applied during baking (17). Thus, the yeast-leavened bread-based diet was the treatment with the lowest BV and NPU scores. It is well known that sugars can interact with proteins and form Maillard compounds, interfering with lysine availability (31, 32). Apparently the level of heat treatment during baking probably affected amino acid bioavailability and protein digestibility (32, 33). There are some strategies to avoid the observed negative impact of sugar on protein quality. Prolonged fermentation time can lead to conversion of higher amounts of sugar into non-browning reaction metabolites. The other possible strategy is to employ leaner formulations in terms of supplemented sugars. French baguettes, pita, or Arabic flat breads and Chinese steamed breads, commonly produced with sugar-free formulations, should benefit more after soybean protein supplementation.

According to Mahmoodi et al., sugar negatively affected protein quality of soybean-fortified bread by decreasing the food efficiency ratio (FER) values estimated with rats (27). The 7% defatted soybean-fortified bread had a FER value of 0.18 ± 0.01 whereas the same bread with 3% sugar had a significantly lower FER value (0.12 ± 0.02). Concomitantly, in our study we found that bread supplemented with 4.5% soybean concentrate showed a FER value of 0.10 ± 0.03 (Table 4) similar to Mahmoodi et al. (27).

The casein-based diet had the highest dry matter digestibility, apparent protein digestibility, and PDCAAS values, because casein possesses high digestibility and a complete EAA score, which increases nitrogen retention and, therefore, animal growth (23, 34).

It is important to mention that soybean products contain significant amounts of isoflavones that are known to prevent oxidative stress, chronic diseases, cancer and that possess weak estrogenic activity (35, 36). The defatted soybean flour and concentrate contain about 150 and 95 mg isoflavones/100 g, respectively (37). The isoflavone concentration in tortillas and bread is approximately 15 times lower because the wheat or nixtamalized flours were supplemented with 6% of defatted soybean flour or 4.5% of concentrate. Giampietro et al. concluded that soybean isoflavones did not significantly affect hormonal balance of children in a human intervention study (38).

Conclusions

The addition of approximately 6% of defatted soybean flour to maize tortillas or wheat flour tortillas greatly improved the protein:calorie ratio, lysine and tryptophan contents, PER, nitrogen retention values, and PDCAAS. This protein quality improvement effect was not as evident in the yeast-leavened bread probably because its formulation contained sugar that upon baking reduced lysine bioavailability. Hence, intake of cereal-based soybean-fortified products, particularly those produced with sugar-free formulations, can benefit millions of people, especially children living in developing countries around the globe, who experience growth stunt due to the lack of good quality protein in their diets.

Acknowledgment

The authors acknowledge the United States Soybean Export Council (USSEC) for providing the array of soybean samples and sponsoring this research.

Conflict of interest and funding

None of the authors had any personal or financial conflict of interest.

References

1. Van den Briel T, Webb P. Fighting world hunger through micronutrient fortification programs. Food Technol 2003; 57: 44–7.
2. Okezie B. World food security: the role of postharvest technology. Food Technol 1998; 52: 64–9.
3. Food and Agriculture Organization (2014). International Fund for Agricultural Development and World Food Programme. The state of food insecurity in the world. Strengthening the enabling environment for food security and nutrition. Rome, Italy. Available from: http://www.fao.org/publications/sofi/2014/es/ [cited 4 February 2015].
4. World Health Organization (2015). Available from: http://apps.who.int/gho/data/?theme=main [cited 18 February 2015].
5. Serna-Saldivar SO, Lopez-Ahumada G, Ortega-Ramirez R, Abril-Dominguez R. Effect of sodium stearoyl-2-lactylate on the rheological and baking properties of bread fortified with defatted soybean and sesame meal. J Food Sci 1988; 53: 211–14.
6. Amaya-Guerra CA, Alanis-Guzman MG, Serna-Saldívar SO. Effects of soybean fortification on protein quality of tortilla based diet from regular and quality protein maize. Plant Foods Hum Nutr 2004; 59: 45–50.
7. Amaya-Guerra C, Serna-Saldívar SO, Alanis-Guzman MG. Soybean fortification and enrichment of regular and quality protein maize tortillas affects brain development and maze performance of rats. Br J Nutr 2006; 96: 161–8.
8. Food and Agriculture Organization (2016). Available from: http://faostat.fao.org [cited 10 February 2016].
9. Chuck-Hernández C, Perez-Carrillo E, Soria-Hernández C, Serna-Saldívar SO. Functionality and organoleptic properties of maize tortillas enriched with five different soybean proteins. Cereal Chem 2015; 92: 341–9.
10. Pereira Lobato LP, Iakmiu Camargo Pereira AE, Lazaretti MM, Barbosa DS, Carreira CM, Mandarino JM, et al. Snack bars with high soy protein and isoflavone content for use in diets to control dyslipidaemia. Int J Food Sci Nutr 2012; 61: 49–58.
11. Erdman JW. Soy protein and cardiovascular disease: a statement for healthcare professionals from the nutrition committee of the AHA. Circulation 2000; 102: 2555–9.
12. Ribotta PD, Arnulphi SA, León AE, Añón MC. Effect of soybean addition on the rheological properties and breadmaking quality of wheat flour. J Sci Food Agric 2005; 85: 1889–96.
13. Karr-Lilienthal LK, Bauer LL, Utterback PL, Zinn KE, Frazier RL, Parsons CM, et al. Chemical composition and nutritional quality of soy bean meals prepared by extruder/expeller processing for use in poultry diets. J Agric Food Chem 2006; 54: 8108–14.
14. Serna-Saldivar SO. Los cereales en la nutrición humana. Química, almacenamiento e industrialización de los cereales. 2nd ed. México: AGT Editor SA; 2013.
15. Nishinari K, Fang Y, Guo S, Phillips GO. Soy proteins: a review on composition, aggregation and emulsification. Food Hydrocoll 2014; 39: 301–18.
16. Perez-Carrillo E, Chew-Guevara AA, Heredia Olea E, Chuck-Hernandez C, Serna-Saldívar SO. Evaluation of the functionality of five different soybean proteins in hot-press wheat flour tortillas. Cereal Chem 2015; 92: 98–104.
17. Lazo-Vélez MA, Chuck-Hernandez C, Serna-Saldívar SO. Evaluation of the functionality of five different soybean proteins in yeast-leavened pan breads. J Cereal Sci 2015; 64: 63–9.
18. Kurpad AV. Protein. Quality and sources. In: Caballero B, ed. Encyclopedia of human nutrition. Vol. 4, 3rd ed. Oxford: Academic Press; 2013, pp. 123–30.
19. AACC (1999). American Association of Cereal Chemists International. Approved methods of analysis. Methods: 44–15.02 moisture air-oven methods, 46–13.01 crude protein micro-Kjeldahl method, 30–20.01 crude fat in grain and stock feeds, 32–10.01 crude fiber in flours, feeds and feedstuffs, 08–01.01ash basic method. 11th ed. Saint Paul, MN: The Saint Pauls Association.
20. AOAC (2012). Official methods of analysis of AOAC international. Method 982.30 E(a), acid hydrolysis. Method 960.48, protein efficiency ratio. 19th ed. Gaithersburg, MD: Association of Official Analytical Chemists.
21. Schaafsma G. The protein digestibility-corrected amino acid score. J Nutr 2000; 130: 18655–75.
22. Serna-Saldívar SO, Canett R, Vargas J, González M, Bedolla S, Medina C. Effect of soybean and sesame addition on the nutritional value of maize and decorticated sorghum tortillas produced by extrusion cooking. Cereal Chem 1988; 65: 44–8.
23. Gonzalez-Agramon M, Serna-Saldivar SO. Effect of defatted soybean and soybean isolate fortification on the nutritional, physical, chemical and sensory properties of wheat flour tortillas. J Food Sci 1988; 53: 793–7.
24. Chavez A, de Chavez M. La Tortilla de Alto Valor Nutritivo, 1st ed. Mexico: McGraw Hill; 2004.
25. Stylianopoulos C, Serna-Saldívar SO, Arteaga-MacKinney G. Effects of fortification and enrichment of maize tortillas on growth and brain development of rats throughout two generations. Cereal Chem 2002; 79: 85–91.
26. Figueroa-Cárdenas JD, Acero-Godínez MG, Vasco-Méndez NL, Lozano-Guzmán A, Flores-Acosta LM. Nutritional quality of nixtamal tortillas fortified with vitamins and soy proteins. Int J Food Sci Nutr 2003; 54: 189–200.
27. Mahmoodi MR, Mashayekh M, Entezari MH. Fortification of wheat bread with 3–7% defatted soy flour improves formulation, organoleptic characteristics, and rat growth rate. Int J Prev Med 2014; 5: 37–45.
28. Serna-Saldivar SO, Abril-Dominguez JR, Lopez-Ahumada G, Ortega-Ramirez R. Nutritional evaluation of table bread fortified with defatted soybean and sesame meals. Arch Latinoam Nutr 1999; 49: 260–4.

29. World Health Organization (2000). Severe malnutrition. In: Management of the child with a serious infection or severe malnutrition. Geneva, Switzerland: WHO, pp. 80–91.
30. Yamada EA, Sgarbieri VC. Yeast (*Saccharomyces cerevisiae*) protein concentrate: preparation, chemical composition, and nutritional and functional properties. J Agric Food Chem 2005; 53: 3931–6.
31. Serrem CA, de Kock HL, Taylor JRN. Nutritional quality, sensory quality and consumer acceptability of sorghum and bread wheat biscuits fortified with defatted soy flour. Int J Food Sci Technol 2011; 46: 74–83.
32. Pasini G, Simonato B, Giannattasio M, Peruffo ADB, Curioni A. Modifications of wheat flour proteins during *in vitro* digestion of bread dough, crumb, and crust: an electrophoretic and immunological study. J Agric Food Chem 2001; 49: 2254–61.
33. Pope LL, Karr-Lilienthal LK, Utterback PL, Bruce KJ, Merchen NR, Parsons CM, et al. Altering the bed depth in the desolventizer/toaster (DT) used in soybean meal preparation affects protein quality and amino acid digestibility by cecectomized rosters. Anim Feed Sci Technol 2007; 133: 275–85.
34. Wouters AG, Rombouts I, Lagrain B, Delcour JA. Impact of casein and egg white proteins on the structure of wheat gluten based protein rich food. J Sci Food Agric 2016; 96(3): 757–63.
35. Messina MJ. Legumes and soybeans: overview of their nutritional profiles and health effects. Am J Clin Nutr 1999; 70: 439–50.
36. Tham DM, Gardner CD, Haskell WL. Potential health benefits of dietary phytoestrogens: a review of the clinical, epidemiological, and mechanistic evidence. J Clin Endocrinol Metab 1998; 88: 2223–35.
37. Bhagwat S, Haytowitz DB, Holden JM. 2008 USDA Database for the Isoflavone Content of Selected Foods. U.S. Department of Agriculture Agricultural Research Service. Beltsville Human Nutrition Research Center Nutrient Data Laboratory. Available from: http://www.ars.usda.gov/nutrientdata [cited 4 May 2016].
38. Giampietro PG, Bruno G, Furocolo G, Casati A, Brunetti E, Spadoni GL, et al. Soy protein formulas in children: no hormonal effects in long-term feeding. J Pediatr Endocrinol Metab 2004; 17: 191–6.

*Sergio O. Serna Saldívar
School of Engineering and Sciences
Tecnológico de Monterrey
Av. Eugenio Garza Sada 2501 Sur Monterrey, N.L. CP 64849
México
Email: sserna@itesm.mx

3

Dietary tryptophan depletion in humans using a simplified two amino acid formula

Maike Linden[1,2], Katrin Helmbold[1,2], Janina Kempf[1,2,3], Shabnam Sippas[1,2,3], Christian Filss[4], Karl-Josef Langen[4,5,6], Albrecht Eisert[7] and Florian Daniel Zepf[1,2,8,9]*

[1]Clinic for Child and Adolescent Psychiatry, Psychosomatics and Psychotherapy, RWTH Aachen University, Aachen, Germany; [2]JARA Translational Brain Medicine, Jülich Aachen Research Alliance, Jülich, Germany; [3]Faculty of Arts and Social Sciences, Maastricht University, Maastricht, The Netherlands; [4]Section JARA-Brain, Jülich-Aachen Research Alliance (JARA), Jülich, Germany; [5]Institute of Neuroscience and Medicine (INM-3, -4, -5), Research Centre Jülich, Jülich, Germany; [6]Department of Nuclear Medicine, RWTH Aachen University Hospital, Aachen, Germany; [7]Department of Pharmacy, RWTH Aachen University, Aachen, Germany; [8]Centre and Discipline of Child and Adolescent Psychiatry, Psychosomatics and Psychotherapy, School of Psychiatry and Clinical Neurosciences & School of Paediatrics and Child Health, Faculty of Medicine, Dentistry and Health Sciences, The University of Western Australia, Perth, Australia; [9]Specialised Child and Adolescent Mental Health Services (CAMHS), Department of Health in Western Australia, Perth, Australia

Abstract

Background: Acute tryptophan depletion (ATD) is a well-established dietary method in translational brain research used to briefly lower central nervous serotonin (5-hydroxytryptamine (5-HT)) synthesis. A simplified two amino acid ATD formula ($ATD_{PHE/LEU}$) was developed while reducing the overall amount of amino acids (AAs), with the objective of administration especially in children and adolescents in future studies.
Objective: This study investigated tryptophan (TRP) influx rates across the blood-brain barrier (BBB) after dietary $ATD_{PHE/LEU}$ administration relative to the ATD Moja-De protocol that has been established for use in children and adolescents.
Design: Seventy-two healthy adults (50% females) were randomized into four groups and administered ATD Moja-De, its TRP-balanced control condition (BAL), $ATD_{PHE/LEU}$, or its respective control mixture ($BAL_{PHE/LEU}$) in a counterbalanced, double-blind, between-subjects design. Blood samples were collected at baseline and at hourly intervals for 6 h after AA intake. Questionnaires about mood, taste, and challenge tolerance were completed at fixed time points.
Results: Both challenge mixtures significantly reduced central nervous TRP influx as calculated by Michaelis–Menten kinetics relative to baseline and the respective control conditions with only mild and comparable side effects. A greater decline in TRP influx over the BBB after $ATD_{PHE/LEU}$ administration when compared with ATD Moja-De was detected without group effects for taste, challenge tolerance, and mood. There was unintended initial short increase in plasma TRP concentrations observed after $ATD_{PHE/LEU}$ intake, and a possible redistribution between free and protein-bound TRP triggered by protein synthesis stimulated by the ingested AAs may account for this finding. Moreover, a decline in TRP influx after $BAL_{PHE/LEU}$ administration over a 6-h period was observed, and the large amount of PHE in the $BAL_{PHE/LEU}$ mixture may be a possible explanation for this particular phenomenon, which could have led to an unexpected increase in displacement of TRP at the BBB in this control condition.
Conclusions: This pilot study provides preliminary evidence for the possibility of lowering TRP influx as calculated by Michaelis–Menten kinetics into the brain by using a simplified ATD protocol in humans. The simplified composition of only two AAs, the lower overall AA amount, and the appropriate tolerance are characteristics of the newly developed $ATD_{PHE/LEU}$ protocol. Future studies focusing on the effects of the $ATD_{PHE/LEU}$ protocol and its respective control condition on CSF 5-HIAA concentrations, as well as neurochemical studies in rodents, are needed to further validate this newly developed AA mixture before definite conclusions about its usability in ATD-related research in humans, its specificity, and additional effects can be made.

Keywords: *serotonin*; *amino acids*; *dietary tryptophan depletion*; *influx rate*; *Michaelis–Menten kinetics*; *humans*

Acute tryptophan depletion (ATD) is an established dietary challenge procedure used to investigate the central nervous effects of the neurotransmitter serotonin (5-hydroxytryptamine (5-HT)) in humans and rodents by a short term and reversible reduction in the brain 5-HT synthesis rate. This method has been commonly used in translational brain research for more than 25 years and is of both clinical and scientific relevance, particularly because 5-HT modulates an extensive range of physiological and behavioral functions (1). Moreover, it is known to be involved in the pathogenesis and pathophysiology of a variety of different behaviors and neuropsychiatric disorders, including affective, eating, and attention deficit hyperactivity disorders (2–13).

ATD is accomplished through the administration of a mixture of large neutral amino acids (LNAAs) lacking tryptophan (TRP). Because 5-HT is not able to pass the blood-brain barrier (BBB), it is synthesized from its physiological precursor, the amino acid (AA) TRP, in the brain. A small proportion of TRP reaches the central nervous system through passive diffusion. The majority of free TRP uses the active transport system L-1, a carrier in the capillary cell plasma membrane specialized for the transportation of all LNAAs, to cross the BBB (14). An affinity to the aforementioned AA, increased by 100–1,000 times, characterizes the BBB-specific type of the L-1 system (15). Moreover, L-systems differing in these and other properties can be found in all cell types in the human body (e.g. gastrointestinal tractus and hepatic and renal tissues). The uptake of TRP into the brain using L-1, which is saturated under physiological conditions, marks a facilitated diffusion that follows Michaelis–Menten kinetics with competitive substrate inhibition of the LNAAs at the common transporter (15–17). When orally administering a beverage of LNAAs lacking TRP, it was shown that TRP plasma concentrations decline because of increased protein synthesis in the liver, which is induced by the administered AA load. Based on preliminary findings in rats (18), this is thought to be an underlying principle of the ATD challenge procedure introduced by Young et al. because of reduced substrate availability for brain 5-HT synthesis with regard to reduced plasma TRP levels. Moreover, ATD makes use of the outlined competitive substrate inhibition, resulting in a diminished uptake of endogenous TRP into the central nervous system at L-1 (19–23). Specifically, the administered AAs compete with endogenous TRP at L-1 for uptake into the central nervous system. The synthesis of 5-HT in the brain comprises two steps: first, the hydroxylation of TRP by the tryptophan hydroxylase 2 (TPH2) into 5-hydroxytryptophan, followed by a 5-hydroxytryptophan decarboxylase catalysis in the second step, which leads to 5-HT (24, 25). TPH2 is involved in the rate-limiting step of the central nervous 5-HT synthesis pathway, with TPH2 showing a saturation of approximately 50% under physiological conditions (26). As a consequence, reduced substrate availability of TRP due to competing mechanisms at the L-1 when other AAs are administered leads to a lowered central nervous 5-HT synthesis rate. As outlined above, AA administration is thought to induce restricted 5-HT synthesis by stimulating protein synthesis in the liver with the consumption of additional TRP from plasma stores (26, 27).

The history of ATD development is characterized by a variety of modifications of the respective AA mixtures. In 1977, Concu et al. (28) applied the ATD technique to humans using 18.2 g of a TRP-free mixture (containing L-glycine, L-lysine (LYS), L-methionine (MET), L-phenylalanine (PHE), L-leucine (LEU), L-isoleucine (ILE), L-threonine (THR), and L-valine (VAL)). They detected a decline in serum TRP by 42% in healthy men (29). Moja et al. (30) also tested a similar formulation, lacking glycine, in healthy male subjects. In their study, plasma TRP decreased to ~35% of the initial level following the administration of an AA dose of 36.6 g. Most of the published ATD studies refer to a protocol introduced by Young et al. (31). Young and colleagues used a 100 g mixture of 15 amino acids (nine LNAA and six non-essential AAs) and found a 76% decrease in plasma TRP. This formulation can cause a large range of side effects (such as nausea, vomiting, headache, and dizziness), which were also reported in other ATD studies (2, 20, 32–35). Dougherty et al. (21) found that reducing the amino acid dose to only 50 g helped diminish observed side effects while implying a slightly less robust depletion when compared with the 100 g formulation.

ATD Moja-De, a modification of the formulation by Moja et al. (30), was developed in 2002 (36, 37) with the aim of establishing a body weight-adapted dosing regimen that can be used in minors. This concept does not only help to reduce side effects to a tolerable level but also allows the application of ATD Moja-De to children and adolescents as well as adults, opening further developmental research perspectives for future studies. Moreover, ATD Moja-De is the only available ATD formulation to date that has been shown to decrease brain 5-HT in mice (38).

Based on the above mentioned developments, we decided to establish a new formulation, called $ATD_{PHE/LEU}$, for optimizing TRP depletion procedures in healthy adult humans. Once data in adult humans are obtained as proposed in this study, this formulation could potentially be used for future studies in children and adolescents. Our motivation was to introduce a new protocol for a possible later use in children and adolescents allowing a reduction of the overall AA amount and a less complex composition, leading to a solid depletion magnitude while reducing or maintaining the very low side effects established in ATD Moja-De. Hence, a new protocol was developed based on mathematical considerations and existing data that showed differing affinities of competing AAs to L-1 (16), thus impacting TRP influx over the BBB to the greatest extent. $ATD_{PHE/LEU}$ was intended to consist of two AAs, PHE and LEU, as these show the highest affinities to the L-1 transporting enzyme of all competing LNAAs (16, 36). Therefore, based on a recent study confirming the effectiveness of a similar simplified protocol in a mouse model (12), we expected adequate stimulation of protein synthesis in the liver (thus leading to a decline in plasma TRP) and a more effective displacement of TRP by PHE and LEU at the common BBB transporter.

The primary aim of this study was to make a comparison of the new dietary depletion protocol's efficacy against that of the established ATD Moja-De, contrasting challenge conditions (ATD, $ATD_{PHE/LEU}$) and their counterbalanced control conditions (BAL, $BAL_{PHE/LEU}$) in healthy adults. We collected several blood samples over a defined time interval and calculated TRP influx rates across the BBB using Michaelis–Menten kinetics with a correction for multiple substrate inhibition.

Methods

Study design

The study employed a controlled, double-blind, between-subjects design. One of the four different AA mixtures, ATD Moja-De, BAL (a TRP-balanced AA load serving as a control condition for ATD Moja-De), $ATD_{PHE/LEU}$ (the new ATD AA mixture), or $BAL_{PHE/LEU}$ (the newly developed control condition for $ATD_{PHE/LEU}$), was administered to a sample group of healthy adult subjects. Blood samples were collected at hourly intervals for 6 h. Participants also completed questionnaires on mood, challenge tolerance, and taste evaluations.

Ethics statement

The ethics committee of the Medical Faculty of the RWTH Aachen University, Germany, evaluated and approved the study protocol. The study was carried out in accordance with the Declaration of Helsinki. All participants provided oral and written informed consent. After completion of all measurements, participants were financially compensated.

Sample

Participants were recruited through local advertisements. A total of 72 subjects (50% females) aged between 18 and 33 years (mean age 23.60 ± 3.08 years) participated in the study. All subjects were right-handed native German speakers who did not suffer from any physical (excluded by interview) or psychiatric disorder (evaluated by a standardized screening interview for psychiatric disorders, the SKIDPIT-light (39)). The exclusion criteria included the following: an IQ lower than 85; smoking; the use of regular medications excluding oral contraceptives; drug abuse; pregnancy; psychoorganic syndromes; schizophrenia; affective disorders; and neurological and somatic diseases such as migraines, asthma, diabetes, metabolic or hormonal disorders, allergies or obesity. The mean BMI of the participants was 22.4 ± 2.5 kg/m^2. Using the CFT-20R (40), the participants' IQ (mean IQ = 112 ± 13.6) was assessed. Approximately 20 individuals were excluded by these criteria during the recruitment process. Primary prescreening for inclusion/exclusion criteria was conducted by telephonic interview. Written informed consent was obtained after in-person screening and clarification by a doctor. Subjects verified by self-report that they had followed the instructions regarding beverage and food intake. Negative urine drug screens and pregnancy tests were required before the administration of the AA beverages. The complete descriptive data of the sample are given in Table 1.

Depletion procedure

Measurements began at the same time each morning in order to avoid the influence of circadian rhythms on metabolism and central nervous 5-HT synthesis. The AA beverages were administered between 9:00 and 10:00 a.m. The study duration was approximately 6 h. The participants were instructed to abstain from food high in protein beginning at 8:00 p.m. the night before each study day, and they were not allowed to drink any beverages other than water. They received a standardized low-protein breakfast (carbohydrate 68.3 g, fat 1.13 g, protein 5.1 g, and dietary fiber 2.3 g) containing two wheat rolls as well as one small pack of jam (25 g) and honey (25 g) immediately following the administration of the AA beverages with a 20-min time frame for breakfast. The particular AA mixtures were composed by a pharmacist and delivered within an aqueous suspension. In order to reduce the risk of undesired lump formation, the crystalline amino acids were solubilized as much as possible with a low sugar substitute in an amount of 200 ml of water using a milk frother. Beverage intake period was reduced to a minimum of approximately 3 min. The sample was divided into four randomized and counterbalanced groups of 18 people with equal gender distributions (9 women and 9 men). The administration of the different AA beverages was counterbalanced for sex. Participants of each group either received ATD, BAL, $ATD_{PHE/LEU}$, or $BAL_{PHE/LEU}$.

The neurodietary challenge procedure ATD Moja-De was previously used successfully with children and adolescents and had few side effects due to the administration regimen that adapted dosage to body weight (26, 36–38, 41–44). The dosage per 10 kg of body weight contained L-PHE (1.32 g), L-LEU (1.32 g), L-ILE (0.84 g), L-MET (0.5 g), L-VAL (0.96 g), L-THR (0.6 g), and L-LYS (0.96 g). TRP (0.7 g per 10 kg of body weight) was added to the corresponding control condition (BAL). The newly developed AA mixture ($ATD_{PHE/LEU}$), also dosed per

Table 1. Descriptive data of the study sample

		ATD	BAL	$ATD_{PHE/LEU}$	$BAL_{PHE/LEU}$
Age	M±SD	23.11±2.89	23.94±3.15	23.67±2.66	23.72±3.69
	Min.	18	18	18	19
	Max.	30	32	29	33
IQ	M±SD	107.67±16.36	113.22±12.10	114.61±14.97	112.89±10.27
	Min.	80	97	76	97
	Max.	138	142	142	134
BMI	M±SD	22.90±2.53	22.18±2.81	22.21±2.52	22.25±2.41
	Min.	18.8	17.9	19.4	18.8
	Max.	27.3	29.0	29.4	26.9

Descriptive data of the study sample are divided into four conditions/groups: acute tryptophan depletion mixture Moja-De (ATD), the TRP-balanced control condition for ATD Moja-De (BAL), the new ATD amino acid mixture ($ATD_{PHE/LEU}$), or the newly developed control condition for $ATD_{PHE/LEU}$ ($BAL_{PHE/LEU}$). Mean±standard deviation (M±SD), maximum (Max.), and minimum (Min.) values are listed for age, IQ, and body mass index (BMI).

10 kg of body weight, consisted only of L-PHE (3.2 g) and L-LEU (3.0 g); $BAL_{PHE/LEU}$, the new mixture's control condition, contained an additional dose of 0.7 g of TRP per 10 kg of body weight.

Blood samples

Blood samples (BS) were collected using a permanent venous catheter at baseline (T_0) and each hour (T_1, T_2, T_3, T_4, T_5, and T_6) after the intake of ATD, BAL, $ATD_{PHE/LEU}$, or $BAL_{PHE/LEU}$ (BS_0, BS_1, BS_2, BS_3, BS_4, BS_5, and BS_6), resulting in seven blood samples per subject. A 9-ml Ethylenediaminetetraacetic acid (EDTA-Tube) (EDTA S-Monovette®, Sarstedt, Germany) and one 7.5-ml Serum-Tube (Serum S-Monovette®, Sarstedt, Germany) were used for sample collection each hour. To avoid falsification of the blood values, the first 4.5 ml of every sample was rejected. The collected blood samples were kept at room temperature for 20 min and centrifuged at 2,500 g for 10 min. The resulting clear supernatant was removed with a pipette and kept in 2-ml Eppendorf Tubes® at $-80°C$ until transportation to the laboratory.

For the TRP influx calculations, plasma levels of PHE, Tyrosine (TYR), and TRP were measured using enzyme-linked immunosorbent assay (ELISA) kits (Immundiagnostik AG, Bensheim, Germany) in accordance with the manufacturer's instructions. The detection of the branched-chained AAs (BCAA: LEU, ILE and VAL) concentration using a BCAA test kit (Immundiagnostik AG, Bensheim, Germany) for photometric analyses of enzyme levels in plasma and serum was carried out according to the manufacturer's instructions. Information regarding sensitivity and specificity of the employed test kits is provided in Supplementary Table 1.

Influx calculation into the brain for TRP, TYR, and PHE

We calculated the influx of TRP across the BBB using Michaelis–Menten kinetics with a correction for multiple substrate competition, which is an established procedure in ATD-related research (16, 45). As the competitive substrate inhibition of TRP and the LNAAs at the common transporting enzyme L-1 determines the uptake of TRP into the brain, this equation provides a valid mathematical model for calculating the unidirectional TRP influx rates into the central nervous system (26, 36, 46). The equation (see Supplementary file) includes both components influencing TRP uptake: the facilitated diffusion of AAs at L-1 and passive diffusion (36). Influx rates of the competing LNAAs PHE, TYR, as well as BCAA influx were calculated using the same equation. In addition to the abovementioned influx calculations, we also provided the following ratios to ensure comparability with previous ATD studies: [TRP]/[CAA], [TYR]/[CAA], [PHE]/[CAA], and [PHE+TYR]/[BCAA+TRP] (CAA = competing amino acids). These ratios predict the entry rates of the involved amino acids into the brain and present another possible approach for evaluating ATD protocols.

Questionnaires

Mood

The German version of the Positive and Negative Affect Schedule (PANAS) (47) containing 10 items for positive (PA) and 10 items for negative (NA) affect was used to measure the extent to which depletion influenced the subjects' mood state. Participants rated the intensity of each item on a five-point Likert scale (from 1 = not at all to 5 = very much) at baseline and every hour before the collection of the blood samples.

Challenge tolerance

We developed an in-house questionnaire on the tolerance of the AA challenges to detect if the newly developed mixture caused an equal amount of side effects as the established ATD Moja-De procedure. The questionnaire contained 12 items rated from 0 (disagree) to 3 (strongly agree). For evaluation purposes, we summarized the matching items and calculated a somatic complaints score, an awakeness score, and a hunger score. The common side effects observed in previous ATD studies, namely, headache, nausea, vomiting, dizziness, and sweating (48), were included in this questionnaire (the entire questionnaire is available in the Supplementary file). Participants completed this questionnaire every hour and immediately before and after the intake of the AA beverages.

Taste

For taste evaluation, an in-house questionnaire consisting of six items was employed (see Supplementary file). The consistency, the sulfuric taste, the difficulty of intake, and revulsion were assessed using a scale of 0 (disagree) to 3 (strongly agree) immediately after the intake of the AA beverages.

Statistical analysis

As primary analysis, the influence of the four different AA mixtures on TRP influx across the BBB was investigated using repeated measures analyses of variance (rmANOVAs) with treatment as the between-subjects factor, time as the within-subjects factor, and gender as a covariate in SPSS Version 21.0 for MacOS. The degrees of freedom for the ANOVA *F*-statistics were adjusted according to the Greenhouse–Geisser correction for non-sphericity ($p < 0.05$). Similar analyses were performed on TYR and PHE influx across the BBB, on [TRP]/[CAA] ratio, on tolerance (the somatic complaints score, awakeness score, and hunger score), and on the PA- and NA-PANAS scores over time. In addition, separate ANOVAs, with the Greenhouse–Geisser correction, on the TRP influx for each group using time as a within-subjects factor were performed. One-way ANOVA was used to determine any significant differences in [TRP]/[CAA] ratio, in TRP, TYR, and PHE influx rates between the groups at baseline (T_0). The influences of the different side effects (e.g. headache, nausea, vomiting, dizziness, and sweating), part of the somatic complaints score, were assessed by rmANOVAs with time as the within-subjects factor and treatment as the between-subjects factor. One-way ANOVA with gender as a covariate was employed to analyze taste differences between the four mixtures. Gaussian distribution for all dependent variables was established with the Kolmogorov–Smirnov test for each of the four groups and for the groups formed by dividing the participants by gender. The level of statistical significance was set and kept at $p < 0.05$. Because of the explorative nature of this study, alpha-adjustment was not employed. *Post hoc* power analyses were performed using G*Power Version 3.1.9.2. for MacOS.

Results

All plasma AA concentrations of TRP, PHE, TYR, and BCAA are presented in Table 2. Table 3 includes all calculated influx values for TRP, TYR, PHE, (TYR + PHE), and BCAA across the BBB.

TRP influx into the brain

No significant differences in TRP influx were present at baseline (T_0) when comparing ATD, BAL, $ATD_{PHE/LEU}$, and $BAL_{PHE/LEU}$ ($F_{[3, 71]} = 2.005$; $p = n.s.$). An rmANOVA yielded main effects of time ($F_{[3.801, 258.437]} = 69.972$; $p < 0.001$) and group ($F_{[3, 68]} = 97.577$; $p < 0.001$) and a significant time by group interaction ($F_{[11.402, 258.437]} = 25.875$; $p < 0.001$). Bonferroni *post hoc* analyses indicated significant differences between each of the four groups (mean TRP influx BAL > $BAL_{PHE/LEU}$ > ATD > $ATD_{PHE/LEU}$; see Supplementary Tables 2 and 3 for detailed results). The comparison of the influx curves for all groups is given in Fig. 1a. Separate rmANOVAs with time as the within-subjects factor indicated a main effect of time for each group. Table 4 summarizes the degrees of freedom (df) and *F*- and *p*-values of these analyses. Time points of maximum TRP influx decline (T_{max}), maximum decline in TRP influx in relation to baseline ($Decline_{max}$), and overall TRP influx declines from baseline to time point T_6 for each group are given in Table 5. Maximum decrease in TRP influx 4 h after intake was 11.9% higher for $ATD_{PHE/LEU}$ compared with the decrease found for ATD. In contrast to ATD, $ATD_{PHE/LEU}$, and $BAL_{PHE/LEU}$ administration, a significant increase in TRP influx was detected in the BAL condition control group during the first 60 min after beverage administration ($p = 0.002$), while no significant changes in influx rates were detected over the entire period from T_0 to T_6. No effect of gender was detected ($F_{[1, 67]} = 2.537$; $p = $ n.s.). *Post hoc* power analysis showed that our study was adequately powered (power of 0.95) to detect effect sizes of 0.25 with an alpha level of 0.05 using a between-subjects repeated measures approach (ANOVA). In addition, we calculated Cohen's *d*-values as an estimate for effect sizes (*d*-value of $d = 0.24$ for the comparison of TRP-influx after ATD versus BAL administration; $d = 0.14$ for the comparison of $ATD_{PHE/LEU}$ and $BAL_{PHE/LEU}$).

TYR and PHE influx into the brain

An rmANOVA on TYR influx rates indicated main effects of time ($F_{[2.122, 144.270]} = 226.885$; $p < 0.001$) and group ($F_{[3, 68]} = 11.191$; $p < 0.001$) and a significant time by group interaction ($F_{[6.365, 144.270]} = 2.255$; $p = 0.038$). Bonferroni *post hoc* analyses indicated that only ATD showed significant difference from the other three treatment conditions, while no significant difference could be found between the three of them. With regard to TYR influx, the curve progression for all treatment conditions was overall comparable with a strong decrease in TYR influx during the first hour (see Fig. 1b). While TYR influx after ATD administration was maximally decreased by 48% of the baseline value, influx after $ATD_{PHE/LEU}$ displayed a decrease of 71%. Similar analyses for PHE influx values also showed main effects of time ($F_{[3.849, 261.745]} = 204.575$; $p < 0.001$) and group ($F_{[3, 68]} = 77.348$;

Table 2. Blood concentrations of tryptophan, phenylalanine, tyrosine, and BCAA

Parameter	Mixture	Baseline (T_0)	T_1	T_2	T_3	T_4	T_5	T_6
[TRP] in µmol/l	ATD	70±3	117±22	111±23	95±22	83±22	75±23	69±17
	BAL	68±3	418±22	437±23	393±22	372±22	261±23	178±17
	ATD$_{PHE/LEU}$	66±3	107±22	110±23	111±22	108±22	105±23	97±17
	BAL$_{PHE/LEU}$	68±3	460±22	407±23	422±22	409±22	397±23	308±17
[PHE]	ATD	51±24	376±53	484±92	393±96	419±117	313±118	242±115
	BAL	55±24	329±53	400±92	330±96	310±117	284±118	192±115
	ATD$_{PHE/LEU}$	112±24	972±53	1236±92	1457±96	1571±117	1427±118	1182±115
	BAL$_{PHE/LEU}$	86±24	977±53	1474±92	1816±96	1926±117	1683±118	1416±115
[TYR]	ATD	59±4	108±8	120±13	109±14	100±14	94±15	88±12
	BAL	55±4	97±8	97±13	85±14	79±14	71±15	60±12
	ATD$_{PHE/LEU}$	59±4	132±8	170±13	193±14	204±14	197±15	189±12
	BAL$_{PHE/LEU}$	62±4	130±8	169±13	195±14	207±14	206±15	196±12
[BCAA]	ATD	416±20	1444±53	1458±56	1374±61	1251±57	1040±64	819±47
	BAL	412±20	1278±53	1297±56	1249±61	1137±57	905±64	744±47
	ATD$_{PHE/LEU}$	405±20	1078±53	971±56	953±61	822±57	628±64	485±47
	BAL$_{PHE/LEU}$	400±20	1024±53	945±56	973±61	827±57	604±64	446±47

Plasma amino acid concentrations (in µmol/l) of tryptophan, phenylalanine, tyrosine, and branched-chain amino acids (BCAA; including valine, leucine, and isoleucine) after the administration of four different amino acid mixtures: ATD (acute tryptophan depletion; challenge condition), BAL (control condition for ATD), ATD$_{PHE/LEU}$ (newly developed challenge condition), and BAL$_{PHE/LEU}$ (control condition for ATD$_{PHE/LEU}$). Mean values ± standard error are given for the different groups (each including 18 subjects) at the seven time points of blood withdrawal (T0–T6).

$p<0.001$) and a significant time by group interaction ($F_{[11.548,\ 261.745]}=2.255$; $p<0.001$). Bonferroni *post hoc* analyses indicated significant differences between all groups, except of ATD$_{PHE/LEU}$ versus BAL$_{PHE/LEU}$ that did not present any significant results. PHE influx curves for all groups can be found in Fig. 1c. For ATD$_{PHE/LEU}$ and BAL$_{PHE/LEU}$, PHE influx values showed an increase during the first 4 h, followed by only a small decrease until T_6 (ATD$_{PHE/LEU}$: maximum increase by 159% of baseline; BAL$_{PHE/LEU}$: maximum increase by 179% of

Table 3. Calculated influx values of particular amino acids across the BBB

Parameter	Mixture	Baseline (T_0)	T_1	T_2	T_3	T_4	T_5	T_6
TRP-influx	ATD	13.573±0.479	6.912±0.603	6.004±0.609	5.715±0.645	4.897±0.637	5.485±0.752	6.452±0.552
	BAL	13.313±0.479	17.190±0.603	16.533±0.609	16.821±0.645	16.864±0.637	14.122±0.752	14.236±0.552
	ATD$_{PHE/LEU}$	12.135±0.479	3.969±0.603	3.434±0.609	3.125±0.645	2.934±0.637	3.155±0.752	3.557±0.552
	BAL$_{PHE/LEU}$	12.483±0.479	12.449±0.603	9.483±0.609	8.828±0.645	8.435±0.637	8.939±0.752	8.191±0.552
TYR-influx	ATD	5.647±0.297	2.997±0.167	3.002±0.173	3.139±0.173	2.911±0.189	3.514±0.266	4.078±0.311
	BAL	5.338±0.297	2.054±0.167	1.866±0.173	1.877±0.173	1.921±0.189	1.959±0.266	2.523±0.311
	ATD$_{PHE/LEU}$	5.213±0.297	1.905±0.167	2.038±0.173	1.964±0.173	2.022±0.189	2.285±0.266	2.765±0.311
	BAL$_{PHE/LEU}$	5.464±0.297	1.515±0.167	1.530±0.173	1.501±0.173	1.582±0.189	1.859±0.266	2.348±0.311
PHE-influx	ATD	10.391±0.630	18.342±0.628	19.733±0.918	18.719±0.981	19.493±1.120	18.008±1.219	16.975±1.119
	BAL	10.819±0.630	14.706±0.628	16.091±0.918	14.764±0.981	14.540±1.120	14.522±1.219	14.088±1.119
	ATD$_{PHE/LEU}$	12.234±0.630	26.229±0.628	28.661±0.918	30.627±0.981	31.642±1.120	30.493±1.219	28.378±1.119
	BAL$_{PHE/LEU}$	11.978±0.630	24.250±0.628	29.411±0.918	32.387±0.981	33.428±1.120	31.321±1.219	29.325±1.119
BCAA-influx	ATD	11.968±0.453	15.582±0.448	15.112±0.501	15.502±0.570	14.340±0.544	14.018±0.612	12.901±0.435
	BAL	11.736±0.453	12.198±0.448	11.692±0.501	12.092±0.570	11.570±0.544	10.245±0.612	10.809±0.435
	ATD$_{PHE/LEU}$	10.937±0.453	8.505±0.448	7.131±0.501	6.524±0.570	5.587±0.544	4.464±0.612	3.872±0.435
	BAL$_{PHE/LEU}$	10.814±0.453	7.352±0.448	6.171±0.501	5.968±0.570	5.044±0.544	3.958±0.612	3.164±0.435

Calculated influx values (in nmol/min/g brain tissue) for tryptophan (TRP), tyrosine (TYR), phenylalanine (PHE), and branched-chain amino acids (BCAA; including valine, leucine, and isoleucine) across the blood-brain barrier after the administration of four different amino acid mixtures: ATD (acute tryptophan depletion; challenge condition), BAL (control condition for ATD), ATD$_{PHE/LEU}$ (newly developed challenge condition), and BAL$_{PHE/LEU}$ (control condition for ATD$_{PHE/LEU}$). Mean values ± standard error are presented for the different groups (each including 18 subjects) at the seven time points of blood withdrawal (T_0–T_6).

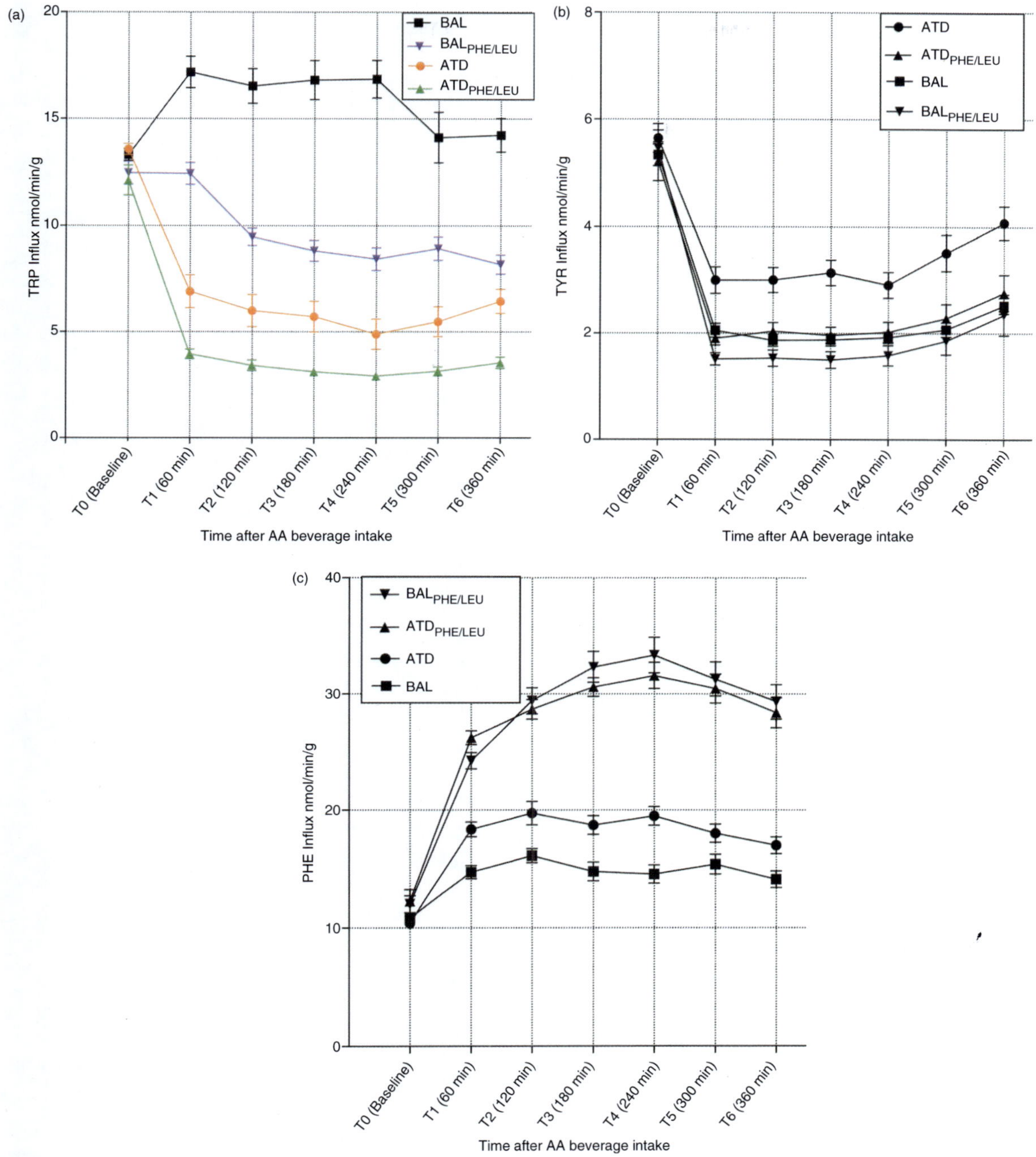

Fig. 1. (a, b, c) Influx curves (nmol/min/g brain tissue) of tryptophan (TRP), tyrosine, and phenylalanine across the blood-brain barrier at baseline (T0) and time points T1–T6 after the intake of the ATD Moja-De amino acid (AA) mixture, its balanced control condition (BAL), the newly developed tryptophan depletion protocol $ATD_{PHE/LEU}$, and the corresponding control condition ($BAL_{PHE/LEU}$). Data are given as the mean values, with bars representing the standard errors.

baseline). In comparison, a much smaller increase of PHE influx appeared after ATD (maximum increase by 89% of baseline) and BAL (increase by 49% of baseline) administration.

[TRP]/[CAA]

Figure 2 shows the time course of [TRP]/[CAA] ratios for the four treatment conditions, which offers a comparable development with regard to TRP influx calculations, but with a focus on plasma concentrations. No significant differences in the ratios were present at baseline (T_0) when comparing ATD, BAL, $ATD_{PHE/LEU}$, and $BAL_{PHE/LEU}$ ($F_{[3,\ 71]} = 0.898$; $p =$ n.s.). An rmANOVA yielded main effects of time ($F_{[4.213,\ 286.489]} = 5.447$; $p < 0.001$) and group ($F_{[3,\ 68]} = 73.368$; $p < 0.001$) and a significant time by group interaction ($F_{[12.639,\ 286.489]} = 17.960$; $p < 0.001$). Bonferroni *post hoc* analyses indicated significant differences between each of the four groups except of no significant result for

Table 4. Results of rmANOVA on tryptophan influx values

	ATD	BAL	$ATD_{PHE/LEU}$	$BAL_{PHE/LEU}$
df	2.130, 36.206	3.136, 53.314	1.269, 21.579	4.057, 68.962
F	86.110	7.646	120.067	20.645
p	<0.001	<0.001	<0.001	<0.001

Results of separate repeated measurements analyses of variance (rmANOVAs) on tryptophan (TRP) influx across the blood-brain barrier for ATD (challenge condition), BAL (control condition for ATD), $ATD_{PHE/LEU}$ (newly developed challenge condition), and $BAL_{PHE/LEU}$ (control condition for $ATD_{PHE/LEU}$), with time as the within-subjects factor. df, degrees of freedom; *F*, *F* values; *p*, statistical significance.

ATD and $ATD_{PHE/LEU}$. Maximum decrease in [TRP]/[CAA] ratio is reached 4 h after intake (T_4) for both protocols. ATD and $ATD_{PHE/LEU}$ reduced the ratio by 66 and 65%, respectively, when compared with baseline. Values of all calculated ratios are given in Table 6, and additional graphs for [TYR]/[CAA] and [PHE]/[CAA] ratios of all groups are presented in Supplementary Fig. S1a and S1b.

Taste

One-way ANOVA of the taste evaluation scores with gender as a covariate yielded no significant difference in taste perceptions between the groups ($F_{[3,\ 67]} = 0.997$; $p =$ n.s.) and no effect of gender ($F_{[1,\ 67]} = 0.102$; $p =$ n.s.).

Challenge tolerance

An rmANOVA evaluation of challenge tolerance indicated a main effect of time for the analysis of the hunger score ($F_{[4.760,\ 314.190]} = 4.457$; $p = 0.001$); *post hoc* testing indicated a significant increase in hunger from baseline (T_0) to T_6 ($p = 0.001$). Similar analyses of the awakeness score also yielded a main effect of time ($F_{[4.182,\ 275.991]} = 9.741$; $p < 0.001$). Within the 6 h from baseline (T_0) to T_6, the awakeness score decreased significantly ($p = 0.001$), but participants felt most tired at T_2. The main effects of time ($F_{[4.018,\ 265.208]} = 5.077$; $p = 0.001$) and group ($F_{[3,\ 66]} = 3.939$; $p = 0.012$) were detected for the somatic complaints score and indicated an increase in somatic complaints over time. Bonferroni *post hoc* analyses showed a significant difference between $BAL_{PHE/LEU}$ and BAL administration ($p = 0.012$). The average somatic complaints score related to $BAL_{PHE/LEU}$ administration (average score 0.708 ± 0.117) was four times greater than the values reported by the BAL condition group (average score 0.169 ± 0.121). While the participants overall felt more unwell 2 h (T_2) after the intake of the AA mixtures ($p = 0.022$), the somatic complaints scores decreased from T_2 to T_4 ($p = 0.002$), with only a slight, non-significant increase observed at T_6 compared with the baseline score. At baseline, there were no significant differences in somatic complaints scores between the groups ($F_{[3,\ 68]} = 0.169$; $p =$ n.s.). Analyses of each individual item in the somatic complaints score showed a comparable development of nausea. The report of nausea significantly increased from T_0 to T_2 ($p = 0.046$) and then significantly decreased from T_2 to T_4 ($p = 0.014$). No gender effects were detected in the hunger ($F_{[1,\ 65]} = 0.192$; $p =$ n.s.), awakeness ($F_{[1,\ 65]} = 0.769$; $p =$ n.s.), or somatic complaints scores ($F_{[1,\ 65]} = 0.179$; $p =$ n.s.).

Table 5. Descriptive data of tryptophan depletion graphs

	ATD	BAL	$ATD_{PHE/LEU}$	$BAL_{PHE/LEU}$
T_{max} (min)	240	60	240	360
$Decline_{max}$ (%)	63.9	29.1 (increase)	75.8	34.4
$Decline_{T0\text{-}T6}$ (%)	52.5	6.9 (increase)	70.7	34.4

Time points of maximum tryptophan (TRP) influx decline (T_{max}), maximum declines of TRP influx in relation to baseline (T_0) ($Decline_{max}$), and overall TRP influx declines from baseline (T_0) to time point T_6 (time point of last blood sample) for the groups ATD (challenge condition), BAL (control condition for ATD), $ATD_{PHE/LEU}$ (newly developed challenge condition), and $BAL_{PHE/LEU}$ (control condition for $ATD_{PHE/LEU}$).

Mood assessment (PANAS)

An rmANOVA of the PA score showed a main effect of time ($F_{[3.335,\ 220.091]} = 54.110$; $p < 0.001$), but no significant effect of group ($F_{[3,\ 65]} = 0.215$; $p =$ n.s.) or gender ($F_{[1,\ 65]} = 0.933$; $p =$ n.s.). Compared with the baseline score, a decrease in the PA score of 28.5% at T_6 was observed ($p < 0.001$). The NA score also decreased (11.4% from baseline to T6; $F_{[3.198,\ 211.086]} = 12.502$; $p < 0.001$, rmANOVA) regardless of gender ($F_{[1,\ 65]} = 0.268$; $p =$ n.s.).

Discussion

The results of this pilot study indicate that dietary administration of $ATD_{PHE/LEU}$ led to a greater depletion magnitude with regard to the TRP influx across the BBB compared with the depletion observed when using the ATD Moja-De protocol, but not with regard to plasma TRP concentrations because of an unintended initial short increase in plasma TRP concentrations that was observed after $ATD_{PHE/LEU}$ intake (see further below in this section for a discussion). The found effect on TRP influx across the BBB was observed even though $ATD_{PHE/LEU}$, which consisted of only two AAs (PHE and LEU), was administered in a lower overall AA dose. Participants evaluated the tolerance level of the new AA challenge beverage as acceptable. No situations or events necessitating premature termination of the study occurred (such as participants vomiting during measurements or other incidents affecting ratings). Thus, several criteria for a potentially valid and effective ATD-test protocol were already achieved, while other aspects such as the observed unexpected increase in plasma TRP levels

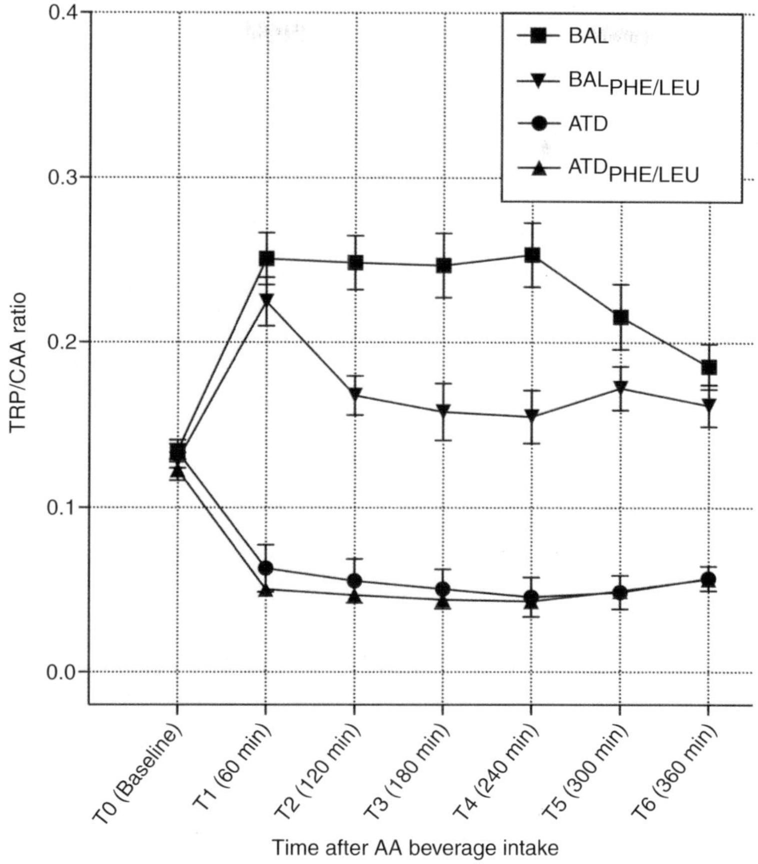

Fig. 2. Curve progression for calculated TRP/CAA ratios from baseline (T0) to time point T6 after the intake of the ATD Moja-De amino acid (AA) mixture, its balanced control condition (BAL), the newly developed tryptophan depletion protocol $ATD_{PHE/LEU}$, and the corresponding control condition ($BAL_{PHE/LEU}$). Data are given as the mean values, with bars representing the standard errors.

require further improvements and future studies in order to validate the findings of the current pilot study.

The altered composition of $ATD_{PHE/LEU}$, including only two AAs, in contrast to the ATD Moja-De that includes seven different AAs, should lead to a greatly simplified production of the AA beverage. Moreover, it also enables facilitated monitoring of relevant blood parameters (i.e. AA concentrations) as their number was consequently reduced. Such monitoring was further simplified by the development and use of ELISA and BCAA test kits (Immundiagnostik AG, Bensheim, Germany). $ATD_{PHE/LEU}$ uses the same body weight-adapted dosing regimen of the ATD AA mixtures that was first successfully applied in the ATD Moja-De protocol (36, 37). This well-tolerated dosing regimen is based on the assumption of a positive correlation between body weight and plasma TRP levels (36, 37) and, as a significant advantage, leads to a possible application for children and adolescents with fewer side effects (42–44, 49, 50).

The greater effectiveness of $ATD_{PHE/LEU}$ in terms of a greater reduction in TRP influx across the BBB when compared with ATD Moja-De could be seen as an advantage, whereas the found effects on plasma TRP concentrations require further investigation. The reason for the detected effects on TRP influx into the brain may lie in the different affinities of the LNAAs to the common L-1 transporter. The Michaelis constant (K_M) represents a measurement of these particular affinities. Precisely, it is indicative of the specific substrate concentration needed to achieve the half-maximal rate of turnover of an enzyme. Thus, a lower K_M value of a substrate is associated with its higher affinity to the related enzyme. Smith et al. (16) determined the values of transport constants for seven LNAAs, including PHE (0.011 $\mu mol \cdot ml^{-1}$) and LEU (0.029 $\mu mol \cdot ml^{-1}$), in anesthetized rats. It must be acknowledged that transferring findings from rodent research to humans is subject to limitations. However, these values for the respective transport constants can serve as a first rough estimate, and the high and significant positive correlations between TRP influx and the TRP/CAA ratio (a previous measure for the effects of ATD) are consistent with the theoretical considerations for using Michaelis–Menten kinetics to characterize TRP influx across the BBB. The high affinity of PHE and LEU to L-1, compared

Table 6. Amino acid ratios

Parameter	Mixture	Baseline (T_0)	T_1	T_2	T_3	T_4	T_5	T_6
[TRP]/[CAA]	ATD	0.134 ± 0.006	0.063 ± 0.013	0.055 ± 0.012	0.051 ± 0.014	0.046 ± 0.014	0.049 ± 0.014	0.057 ± 0.010
	BAL	0.135 ± 0.006	0.251 ± 0.013	0.248 ± 0.012	0.247 ± 0.014	0.253 ± 0.014	0.204 ± 0.014	0.186 ± 0.010
	ATD$_{PHE/LEU}$	0.123 ± 0.006	0.050 ± 0.013	0.047 ± 0.012	0.044 ± 0.014	0.043 ± 0.014	0.0493 ± 0.014	0.057 ± 0.010
	BAL$_{PHE/LEU}$	0.129 ± 0.006	0.225 ± 0.013	0.168 ± 0.012	0.158 ± 0.014	0.155 ± 0.014	0.172 ± 0.014	0.162 ± 0.010
[PHE]/[CAA]	ATD	0.094 ± 0.043	0.232 ± 0.037	0.320 ± 0.078	0.293 ± 0.077	0.329 ± 0.087	0.308 ± 0.117	0.254 ± 0.139
	BAL	0.102 ± 0.043	0.182 ± 0.037	0.220 ± 0.078	0.193 ± 0.077	0.193 ± 0.087	0.213 ± 0.117	0.191 ± 0.139
	ATD$_{PHE/LEU}$	0.206 ± 0.043	0.759 ± 0.037	1.039 ± 0.078	1.183 ± 0.077	1.399 ± 0.087	1.548 ± 0.117	1.561 ± 0.139
	BAL$_{PHE/LEU}$	0.163 ± 0.043	0.610 ± 0.037	0.952 ± 0.078	1.155 ± 0.077	1.334 ± 0.087	1.403 ± 0.117	1.462 ± 0.139
[TYR]/[CAA]	ATD	0.108 ± 0.006	0.056 ± 0.004	0.059 ± 0.004	0.059 ± 0.005	0.059 ± 0.006	0.068 ± 0.009	0.081 ± 0.012
	BAL	0.103 ± 0.006	0.048 ± 0.004	0.046 ± 0.004	0.043 ± 0.005	0.045 ± 0.006	0.047 ± 0.009	0.056 ± 0.012
	ATD$_{PHE/LEU}$	0.105 ± 0.006	0.063 ± 0.004	0.075 ± 0.004	0.079 ± 0.005	0.086 ± 0.006	0.103 ± 0.009	0.124 ± 0.012
	BAL$_{PHE/LEU}$	0.112 ± 0.006	0.054 ± 0.004	0.062 ± 0.004	0.063 ± 0.005	0.070 ± 0.006	0.085 ± 0.009	0.112 ± 0.012
[PHE + TYR]/	ATD	0.226 ± 0.051	0.318 ± 0.043	0.428 ± 0.093	0.405 ± 0.093	0.447 ± 0.103	0.451 ± 0.145	0.395 ± 0.194
[BCAA + TRP]	BAL	0.229 ± 0.051	0.250 ± 0.043	0.289 ± 0.093	0.255 ± 0.093	0.257 ± 0.103	0.285 ± 0.145	0.270 ± 0.194
	ATD$_{PHE/LEU}$	0.359 ± 0.051	0.963 ± 0.043	1.373 ± 0.093	1.594 ± 0.093	1.927 ± 0.103	2.268 ± 0.145	2.450 ± 0.194
	BAL$_{PHE/LEU}$	0.313 ± 0.051	0.756 ± 0.043	1.188 ± 0.093	1.452 ± 0.093	1.723 ± 0.103	1.882 ± 0.145	2.096 ± 0.194

Ratios of tryptophan, phenylalanine, tyrosine, and branched-chain amino acids (BCAA; including valine, leucine, and isoleucine) and their competing amino acids (CAA) after the administration of four different amino acid mixtures: ATD (acute tryptophan depletion; challenge condition), BAL (control condition for ATD), ATD$_{PHE/LEU}$ (newly developed challenge condition), and BAL$_{PHE/LEU}$ (control condition for ATD$_{PHE/LEU}$). Mean values ± standard error are given for the different groups (each including 18 subjects) at the seven time points of blood withdrawal (T0–T6).

with all other LNAAs, may have caused the best displacement of TRP at the common transporter and therefore was possibly associated with a greater reduction of TRP influx across the BBB. By contrast, the ATD Moja-De, containing a mixture of seven different AAs with partly lower K_M values, was less effective with regard to the competition of the AAs against TRP, resulting in a smaller TRP depletion magnitude in terms of TRP influx across the BBB compared with the ATD$_{PHE/LEU}$ depletion magnitude. It is possible that the use of this competitive mechanism in the respective AAs enables the potential effectiveness of TRP depletion after ATD$_{PHE/LEU}$ administration, despite the simultaneous reduction in the overall AA dose and thus a possibly decreased stimulation of protein synthesis in the liver when compared to other ATD protocols. This could have impacted the observed findings with regard to changes in plasma TRP concentrations and a possible redistribution between free and protein-bound TRP. The observed TRP influx curves of the old and new challenge protocols over the entire study duration resulted in maximum depletion in terms of decreased TRP influx across the BBB at 4 h after intake for both challenge procedures. In particular, TRP influx correlated highly and significantly with the TRP/CAA ratio for both ATD challenge conditions used (see Supplementary Tables S5 and S6 and Fig. S2a and S2b), but the influx rates are likely to be a more adequate reflection of TRP availability in the brain as they also take the individual affinities of the different amino acids to the L-1 transport system at the BBB into account.

It is important to keep in mind that this work only claims to be a first pilot study. Therefore, the assessment of brain TRP and 5-HT concentrations after ATD$_{PHE/LEU}$ application in rodents has to be an essential part of future research as well as PET-studies and the measurement of 5-hydroxyindoleacetic acid (5-HIAA) concentrations (the primary metabolite of 5-HT) in human cerebrospinal fluid in order to validate the effectiveness of ATD$_{PHE/LEU}$ revealed by this study. A recent study by Sánchez et al. (12) has provided preliminary evidence for the effectiveness of simplified ATD protocols using a three-AA-formulation (PHE, LEU, and ILE); however, future studies in humans assessing cerebrospinal fluid (CSF) 5-HIAA concentrations after intake of the challenge procedure are needed.

The absence of any gender effects in the blood parameters was an expected outcome. Although central nervous 5-HT synthesis is known to significantly differ in males and females (51), we monitored peripheral TRP and LNAA plasma levels for TRP influx calculations; these parameters are not influenced by gender-specific alterations in TRP influx and related central nervous 5-HT synthesis. The performed power analyses confirmed that this study was adequately powered to detect small effects, and Cohen's d calculations indicated small estimates for effect sizes for the analyses conducted.

Specificity for depleting central nervous 5-HT synthesis (in particular with regard to possible effects on dopamine and other neurotransmitters) is always an important point to be considered with regard to all available ATD-related amino acid formulations. Previous research from our group indicated that the Moja-De protocol does not affect central nervous dopamine synthesis in mice (38). As such evidence is currently missing for the newly developed protocol $ATD_{PHE/LEU}$, we looked at TYR and PHE plasma values and their calculated influx into the brain. The strong decrease in TYR influx after challenge application, as described above, questions the specificity of the newly developed $ATD_{PHE/LEU}$ condition. The phenomenon of highly increasing PHE influx values in the $ATD_{PHE/LEU}$ protocol group can be explained by its high PHE concentrations. As the strong decrease in TYR influx indicates, the high PHE dose does not mitigate the decrease in TYR influx (calculated from peripheral blood values). Whether the high PHE amount in the $ATD_{PHE/LEU}$ mixture directly affects central nervous concentrations of TYR formation can only be answered using future neurochemical challenge studies. However, specificity for respective neurotransmitters is always a critical issue when dealing with different TRP depletion protocols. This is a general problem in ATD-related research in humans and affects all currently available ATD amino acid formulations. Badawy et al. (52) provided an approach to enhance ATD formulations' specificity by decreasing the amount of BCAAs. In accordance with this, the reduction of the LEU amount in our newly developed $ATD_{PHE/LEU}$ protocol might be a potential avenue for future research. An unintended rather substantial increase in plasma TRP was observed after $ATD_{PHE/LEU}$ intake besides the fact that no TRP was ingested, and future studies are needed to investigate and replicate this unknown effect. Protein synthesis can be stimulated by the ingested amino acids, which in turn might have led to a possible redistribution between free and protein-bound TRP. Following this train of thought, the amount of free TRP possibly was slightly higher while the overall balance remained unaffected. It also needs to be outlined that TRP-related metabolites, such as quinolinic acid, kynurenic acid, and tryptamine that can be changed due to administration of the balanced mixture, can influence brain function. This stands in line with the issue of the specificity of all ATD/BAL paradigms currently available. Finally, the reason why the fasting TRP levels (T0) were higher than those mentioned in the literature is not clear but worth noting and might be specific to the investigated sample.

Another issue regarding our new ATD challenge protocol is the absence of an appropriate control condition that 'maintains baseline values without altering the biochemical or behavioral parameters' (52). The observed rise in TRP influx approximately 1 h after administration of the BAL control condition seems to be a logical consequence of the enhanced TRP availability because the BAL mixture contained TRP. For this particular reason, the decline in TRP influx of 34.4% after $BAL_{PHE/LEU}$ administration over the 6-h period appears to be counterintuitive. When comparing $BAL_{PHE/LEU}$ with its challenge condition $ATD_{PHE/LEU}$, the administration of $BAL_{PHE/LEU}$ led to a depletion of approximately 50% in magnitude of the depletion observed following $ATD_{PHE/LEU}$ administration. The large amount of PHE in the $BAL_{PHE/LEU}$ mixture may be a possible explanation for this particular phenomenon, which in turn could lead to an unexpected increase in displacement of TRP at the BBB in this control condition. To address this particular problem, either an increase in TRP or decreased levels of PHE or LEU in the control condition could be evaluated in future research in order to establish a valid control condition for $ATD_{PHE/LEU}$.

Both protocols that were applied in this study, ATD and BAL on the one hand and $ATD_{PHE/LEU}$ and $BAL_{PHE/LEU}$ on the other hand, were well tolerated by the subjects. In particular, we did not observe any headaches, vomiting, dizziness, or sweating as indicated by the itemizing analyses of our somatic complaints score (see Supplementary Table S3). There were no dropouts caused by side effects. Hence, this requirement of a valid test protocol was met. Although we could not observe a significant group effect for the somatic complaints score between ATD and $ATD_{PHE/LEU}$ indicating a reduction of side effects in the new challenge condition, we achieved the goal of maintaining the high-grade safety of the established ATD Moja-De.

The monitored increase in hunger throughout the study day most likely resulted from the 6-h abstinence from food and a breakfast overall low in nutrition. The lack of any group effect in hunger ratings supports the previous assumption. This observation justifies the necessity of the low-protein breakfast at the beginning of the study day. However, although its carbohydrate content can, to some extent, affect plasma TRP concentration and binding and levels of BCAA, it would not be justifiable to demand fasting beginning at 8 p.m. the night before the study day till 3 p.m. on the study day. Furthermore, the collection of additional behavioral, cognitive, and emotional data during this study for future analysis would have been likely to be skewed by significant fasting effects if no breakfast had been given. In this context, a variety of ATD-using studies also administer low-protein meals during the depletion procedure (53–56). In the present sample, we attribute the occurrence of increasing tiredness during the study day to external circumstances, such as the study environment and the long testing period, as opposed to a side effect of the protocol. The missing group effect can be seen as somewhat indicative for this phenomenon. Moreover, breakfast intake could also have impacted side effect ratings as assessed within the present study.

As stated above, we found an effect of group and time for the somatic complaints score. In the separated item analyses, nausea is the only side effect showing a main effect of time and displays an equal development.

Although few ATD studies focused on the examination of side effects, nausea appears to be a frequent problem in these particular studies (31, 48). It is very likely that the ingestion of a substantial amount of crystalline AAs (Moja-De: 6.5 g/10 kg body weight, $ATD_{PHE/LEU}$ 6.2 g/10 kg body weight) that remain in the stomach until dissolution in the acidic environment contributed to the reports of nausea (57). The missing group effect in somatic complaint investigations partially supports this assumption because all groups were equally affected. Moreover, *post hoc* analyses of the somatic complaints scores revealed a significant difference between BAL and $BAL_{PHE/LEU}$ administration as a group effect with an average somatic complaints score four times greater after $BAL_{PHE/LEU}$ intake. However, with a maximal somatic complaints score of 24 and a minimal score of 0, the very low mean value observed in this study was not indicative of the intolerability of the new control condition. A modification of the $BAL_{PHE/LEU}$ control condition, as mentioned above, might help improve the side effect profile of $BAL_{PHE/LEU}$.

Presently, there is no ATD-specific validated questionnaire available for somatic complaint or taste assessment. This study provides first questionnaire-based pilot data and certainly requests validation in future ATD studies. In particular, further refinement is needed regarding the gradual and sensible detection of symptom nuances.

Both positive (PA) and negative (NA) PANAS assessments decreased over the 6-h study duration. In addition to these controversial findings, no group effect was detected, which suggests that the ratings were influenced by the situation during measurements and, perhaps, not a direct consequence of altered brain 5-HT function. This is in agreement with previous findings which suggested that ATD's influence on mood was largely dependent on the susceptibility of the study sample, and this variability led to a lack of clear mood effects in many cases (58, 59). However, the assessment of mood only served as an ancillary controlling variable in this study, and these results do not significantly impact or question its major findings.

Although subjects took the amino acid mixtures without any major problems and the new mixture was well tolerated in our study, the uncomfortable palatability seen in all groups certainly requests further modification to ensure trouble-free utilization. Bitterness in general is a problematic issue in all ATD studies as it arises from the specific biochemical structure of polar and hydrophobic groups in some amino acids (60). The reduction of the overall amount and dose as well as the absence of the worst tasting AAs (i.e. MET, cysteine, and arginine) might have contributed to an easier administration of $ATD_{PHE/LEU}$; however, improvements are still required. For this particular purpose, we suggest to add some of the conventional flavoring supplements, such as vanilla, peppermint, raspberry, and lemonade, with low sugar substitutes to our challenge procedure.

The between-subjects design is a limitation of this study. Behavioral paradigms conducted as a part of this study (the findings will be the subject of further publications) did not allow for a within-subject repeated measures design due to possible learning effects; a within-subjects design could be used in further investigations.

Regarding the use of $ATD_{PHE/LEU}$ in behavioral studies, the high amount of LEU might present a problem, in particular as LEU is known to alter glutamate formation within the leucine-glutamate cycle (61, 62). Since LEU might also affect various other parameters, a separate analysis of LEU blood values would be essential to achieve better knowledge of $ATD_{PHE/LEU}$'s metabolic consequences. In this study, we chose the assessment of the BCAAs within a sum parameter for initial investigations as it provides a cost-saving alternative. Moreover, a further aspect that should be considered in future studies would be to add caffeine withdrawal as an additional exclusion criterion since caffeine has been shown to induce alterations in serotonergic neurotransmission (63, 64).

The ATD method as a serotonergic challenge tool was criticized by Van Donkelaar et al. in a review article (65). Specifically, the authors advised caution in interpreting the selective serotonergic effect of ATD-related results, postulating a contribution by various other non-serotonergic mechanisms to diminished 5-HT metabolism (e.g. alterations in cerebrovascular blood flow, stress influence, and metabolic effects). Furthermore, the missing possibility of direct attribution of ATD-induced behavioral alterations to changes in 5-HT neuronal activity was noted. However, many of the suggested mechanisms and the related hypotheses were based on limited data and primarily indirect conclusions. Overall, there is sufficient and convincing evidence that ATD leads to diminished central nervous 5-HT synthesis. In a rodent model, Biskup et al. (38) demonstrated substantially impaired brain 5-HT synthesis after ATD Moja-De administration. Furthermore, they found a lowered content of 5-HIAA, which is the primary metabolite of 5-HT, and a consequently reduced 5-HT release. As summarized and outlined by Crockett et al. (66), all of the alternative mechanisms suggested in the aforementioned review would lead to broad attentional and executive impairments that have not been found in any ATD study involving humans. In general, we support the need for further research to gain a solidly grounded understanding of the underlying mechanisms of ATD because the extent of contributions of additional mechanisms cannot be reliably estimated.

In conclusion, the greater decline in TRP influx rates across the BBB in healthy adults after the dietary administration of the newly developed simplified ATD protocol, $ATD_{PHE/LEU}$, relative to the established ATD Moja-De mixture, was the major finding of this study. The altered composition of $ATD_{PHE/LEU}$, composed of only two LNAAs (PHE and LEU), enabled the reduction in the overall AA amount, had acceptable tolerance, and ensured simplified blood value monitoring due to the reduced components. Nevertheless, this work only represents a first pilot study. Future research is warranted not only to replicate the present findings (optimally a within-subject repeated measures design) but also to improve beverage palatability, its specificity for central nervous 5-HT depletion, and to develop a more suitable balanced control condition ($BAL_{PHE/LEU}$) without significant TRP-related depletion effects. The direct proof of reduced brain 5-HT synthesis in a rodent model (i.e. 5-HT concentrations in brain tissue) would be beneficial, as well as investigations of 5-HIAA levels in human cerebrospinal fluid in order to further validate the newly developed $ATD_{PHE/LEU}$ mixture. Moreover, as an additional step, $ATD_{PHE/LEU}$ requires further study before administering this mixture to children and adolescents can be considered. If the remaining questions with regard to changes in plasma TRP levels, aspects of specificity, and the respective control condition are clarified, the simplified composition of $ATD_{PHE/LEU}$ might have the potential to become an advantageous alternative to the currently available ATD Moja-De protocol for the investigation of the physiological and behavioral effects of reduced central nervous 5-HT synthesis in translational research. However, at this stage, the newly developed $ATD_{PHE-LEU}$ mixture needs further validation and is currently not suitable to specifically study central nervous 5-HT function in humans, and at this point in time it cannot replace the ATD Moja-De ATD protocol.

Acknowledgements

This study was funded by the German Federal Ministry of Economics and Technology (Bundesministerium für Wirtschaft und Technologie, BMWi) with a grant to the senior author of this article (FDZ). The lead author (ML) was supported by the German Research Council (Deutsche Forschungsgemeinschaft DFG, IRTG 1328).

Conflict of interest and funding

FDZ was the recipient of an unrestricted award donated by the American Psychiatric Association (APA), the American Psychiatric Institute for Research and Education (APIRE), and AstraZeneca (Young Minds in Psychiatry Award). He has also received research support from the German Federal Ministry for Economics and Technology, the European Union (EU), the German Society for Social Pediatrics and Adolescent Medicine, the Paul and Ursula Klein Foundation, the Dr. August Scheidel Foundation, the IZKF fund of the University Hospital of RWTH Aachen University, the Telethon Perth Childrens' Hospital Research Fund (TPCHRF), the Princess Margaret Hospital Foundation, the Telethon Kids Institute, and a travel stipend donated by the GlaxoSmithKline Foundation. He is the recipient of an unrestricted educational grant, travel support, and speaker honoraria by Shire Pharmaceuticals, Germany. In addition, he has received support from the Raine Foundation for Medical Research (Raine Visiting Professorship) and editorial fees from Co-Action Publishing (Sweden). All authors report no conflicts of interest.

References

1. Zepf FD, Hood S, Guillemin GJ. Food and your mood: nutritional psychiatry. Lancet Psychiatry 2015; 2(7): e19.
2. Delgado PL, Charney DS, Price LH, Aghajanian GK, Landis H, Heninger GR. Serotonin function and the mechanism of antidepressant action. Reversal of antidepressant-induced remission by rapid depletion of plasma tryptophan. Arch Gen Psychiatr 1990; 47(5): 411–18.
3. Kishi T, Yoshimura R, Fukuo Y, Okochi T, Matsunaga S, Umene-Nakano W, et al. The serotonin 1A receptor gene confer susceptibility to mood disorders: results from an extended meta-analysis of patients with major depression and bipolar disorder. Eur Arch Psychiatr Clin Neurosci 2013; 263(2): 105–18.
4. Kotting WF, Bubenzer S, Helmbold K, Eisert A, Gaber TJ, Zepf FD. Effects of tryptophan depletion on reactive aggression and aggressive decision-making in young people with ADHD. Acta Psychiatr Scand 2013; 128(2): 114–23.
5. Mette C, Zimmermann M, Grabemann M, Abdel-Hamid M, Uekermann J, Biskup CS, et al. The impact of acute tryptophan depletion on attentional performance in adult patients with ADHD. Acta Psychiatr Scand 2013; 128(2): 124–32.
6. Smith KA, Fairburn CG, Cowen PJ. Symptomatic relapse in bulimia nervosa following acute tryptophan depletion. Arch Gen Psychiatr 1999; 56(2): 171–6.
7. Zimmermann M, Grabemann M, Mette C, Abdel-Hamid M, Uekermann J, Kraemer M, et al. The effects of acute tryptophan depletion on reactive aggression in adults with attention-deficit/ hyperactivity disorder (ADHD) and healthy controls. PLoS One 2012; 7(3): e32023.
8. Biskup CS, Gaber T, Helmbold K, Bubenzer-Busch S, Zepf FD. Amino acid challenge and depletion techniques in human functional neuroimaging studies: an overview. Amino Acids 2015; 47(4): 651–83.
9. Helmbold K, Zvyagintsev M, Dahmen B, Bubenzer-Busch S, Gaber TJ, Crockett MJ, et al. Effects of serotonin depletion on punishment processing in the orbitofrontal and anterior cingulate cortices of healthy women. Eur Neuropsychopharmacol 2015; 25(6): 846–56.
10. Hildebrand P, Königschulte W, Gaber TJ, Bubenzer-Busch S, Helmbold K, Biskup CS, et al. Effects of dietary tryptophan and phenylalanine–tyrosine depletion on phasic alertness in healthy adults–a pilot study. Food Nutr Res 2015; 59: 26407.
11. Sanchez CL, Biskup CS, Herpertz S, Gaber TJ, Kuhn CM, Hood SH, et al. The role of serotonin (5-HT) in behavioral control: findings from animal research and clinical implications. Int J Neuropsychopharmacol 2015; 18(10): pyv050.
12. Sánchez CL, Van Swearingen AE, Arrant AE, Biskup CS, Kuhn CM, Zepf FD. Simplified dietary acute tryptophan

depletion: effects of a novel amino acid mixture on the neurochemistry of C57BL/6J mice. Food Nutr Res 2015; 59: 27424.
13. Gaber TJ, Dingerkus VL, Crockett MJ, Bubenzer-Busch S, Helmbold K, Sánchez CL, et al. Studying the effects of dietary body weight adjusted acute tryptophan depletion on punishment-related behavioral inhibition. Food Nutr Res 2015; 59: 28443.
14. Pardridge WM, Oldendorf WH. Kinetic analysis of blood-brain barrier transport of amino acids. Biochim Biophys Acta 1975; 401(1): 128–36.
15. Oldendorf WH, Szabo J. Amino acid assignment to one of three blood-brain barrier amino acid carriers. Am J Physiol 1976; 230(1): 94–8.
16. Smith QR, Momma S, Aoyagi M, Rapoport SI. Kinetics of neutral amino acid transport across the blood-brain barrier. J Neurochem 1987; 49(5): 1651–8.
17. Smith QR, Takasato Y. Kinetics of amino acid transport at the blood-brain barrier studied using an in situ brain perfusion technique. Ann N Y Acad Sci 1986; 481: 186–201.
18. Moja EA, Restani P, Corsini E, Stacchezzini MC, Assereto R, Galli CL. Cycloheximide blocks the fall of plasma and tissue tryptophan levels after tryptophan-free amino acid mixtures. Life Sci 1991; 49(15): 1121–8.
19. Wurtman RJ, Hefti F, Melamed E. Precursor control of neurotransmitter synthesis. Pharmacol Rev 1980; 32(4): 315–35.
20. Marsh DM, Dougherty DM, Moeller FG, Swann AC, Spiga R. Laboratory-measured aggressive behavior of women: acute tryptophan depletion and augmentation. Neuropsychopharmacology 2002; 26(5): 660–71.
21. Dougherty DM, Marsh-Richard DM, Mathias CW, Hood AJ, Addicott MA, Moeller FG, et al. Comparison of 50- and 100-g L-tryptophan depletion and loading formulations for altering 5-HT synthesis: pharmacokinetics, side effects, and mood states. Psychopharmacology (Berl) 2008; 198(3): 431–45.
22. Fernstrom JD. Role of precursor availability in control of monoamine biosynthesis in brain. Physiol Rev 1983; 63(2): 484–546.
23. Chanut E, Zini R, Trouvin JH, Riant P, Tillement JP, Jacquot C. Albumin binding and brain uptake of 6-fluoro-DL-tryptophan: competition with L-tryptophan. Biochem Pharmacol 1992; 44(10): 2082–5.
24. Frazer A, Hensler JG. Serotonin. In: Siegel GJ, Agranoff BW, Albers RW, Molinoff PB, eds. Basic neurochemistry: molecular, cellular and medical aspects. New York: Raven Press; 1994, pp. 283–308.
25. Marsden CA. The neuropharmacology of serotonin in the central nervous system. In: Feighner JP, Boyer WF, eds. Selective serotonin re-uptake inhibitors. Chichester: Wiley; 1996, pp. 1–34.
26. Dingerkus VL, Gaber TJ, Helmbold K, Bubenzer S, Eisert A, Sanchez CL, et al. Acute tryptophan depletion in accordance with body weight: influx of amino acids across the blood-brain barrier. J Neural Transm (Vienna) 2012; 119(9): 1037–45.
27. Zepf F. Principles of rapid tryptophan depletion and its use in research on neuropsychiatric disorders. In: D'Mello J, ed. Amino acids in human nutrition and health. Oxfordshire: Cabi; 2012, pp. 418–26.
28. Concu A, Fadda F, Blanco S, Congia S, Lostia M. Mental changes induced by the oral administration of tryptophan-free amino acid mixtures in man. IRCS Med Sci 1977; 5: 520.
29. Fadda F. Tryptophan-free diets: a physiological tool to study brain serotonin function. News Physiol Sci 2000; 15: 260–4.
30. Moja EA, Stoff DM, Gessa GL, Castoldi D, Assereto R, Tofanetti O. Decrease in plasma tryptophan after tryptophan-free amino acid mixtures in man. Life Sci 1988; 42(16): 1551–6.
31. Young SN, Smith SE, Pihl RO, Ervin FR. Tryptophan depletion causes a rapid lowering of mood in normal males. Psychopharmacology 1985; 87(2): 173–7.
32. Booij L, Van der Does AJ, Haffmans PM, Spinhoven P, McNally RJ. Acute tryptophan depletion as a model of depressive relapse: behavioural specificity and ethical considerations. Br J Psychiatr 2005; 187: 148–54.
33. Allen PP, Cleare AJ, Lee F, Fusar-Poli P, Tunstall N, Fu CH, et al. Effect of acute tryptophan depletion on pre-frontal engagement. Psychopharmacology 2006; 187(4): 486–97.
34. Klaassen T, Riedel WJ, Deutz NE, Van Someren A, Van Praag HM. Specificity of the tryptophan depletion method. Psychopharmacology 1999; 141(3): 279–86.
35. Moeller FG, Dougherty DM, Swann AC, Collins D, Davis CM, Cherek DR. Tryptophan depletion and aggressive responding in healthy males. Psychopharmacology 1996; 126(2): 97–103.
36. Kewitz A. Biochemische Untersuchungen zur Optimierung des 'Rapid Tryptophan Depletion-Test' (RTD): Eine physiologische Methode zur akuten Verminderung der zentrainervösen Serotonin-Synthese in der psychobiologischen Forschung. Johann Wolfgang Goethe-Universität zu Frankfurt am Main; 2002.
37. Demisch L, Kewitz A, Schmeck K, Sadigorsky S, Barta S, Dierks T, et al. Methodology of rapid tryptophan depletion (RTD): impact of gender and body weight. Eur Arch Psychiatry Clin Neurosci 2002; 252(2): 1.
38. Biskup CS, Sanchez CL, Arrant A, Van Swearingen AE, Kuhn C, Zepf FD. Effects of acute tryptophan depletion on brain serotonin function and concentrations of dopamine and norepinephrine in C57BL/6J and BALB/cJ mice. PLoS One 2012; 7(5): e35916.
39. Demal U. SKIDPIT-light Screeningbogen. Universität Wien; 1999.
40. Weiß R. Grundintelligenztest skala 2 – revision CFT 20-R [Culture fair intelligence test scale 2 – revision]. Göttingen: Hogrefe; 2006.
41. Zepf FD, Poustka F. 5-HT functioning and aggression in children with ADHD and disruptive behaviour disorders. Hum Psychopharmacol 2008; 23(5): 438.
42. Zepf FD, Wockel L, Poustka F, Holtmann M. Dietary tryptophan depletion according to body weight – a new treatment option in acute mania? Med Hypotheses 2009; 72(1): 47–8.
43. Zepf FD, Stadler C, Demisch L, Schmitt M, Landgraf M, Poustka F. Serotonergic functioning and trait-impulsivity in attention-deficit/hyperactivity-disordered boys (ADHD): influence of rapid tryptophan depletion. Hum Psychopharmacol 2008; 23(1): 43–51.
44. Zepf F, Holtmann M, Stadler C, Demisch L, Schmitt M, Wöckel L, et al. Diminished serotonergic functioning in hostile children with ADHD: tryptophan depletion increases behavioural inhibition. Pharmacopsychiatry 2008; 41(2): 60–5.
45. Pardridge WM. Brain metabolism: a perspective from the blood-brain barrier. Physiol Rev 1983; 63(4): 1481–535.
46. Helmbold K, Bubenzer S, Dahmen B, Eisert A, Gaber TJ, Habel U, et al. Influence of acute tryptophan depletion on verbal declarative episodic memory in young adult females. Amino Acids 2013; 45(5): 1207–19.
47. Watson D, Clark LA, Tellegen A. Development and validation of brief measures of positive and negative affect: the PANAS scales. J Pers Soc Psychol 1988; 54(6): 1063–70.
48. aan het Rot M, Benkelfat C, Boivin DB, Young SN. Bright light exposure during acute tryptophan depletion prevents a lowering of mood in mildly seasonal women. Eur Neuropsychopharmacol 2008; 18(1): 14–23.
49. Stadler C, Zepf FD, Demisch L, Schmitt M, Landgraf M, Poustka F. Influence of rapid tryptophan depletion on

laboratory-provoked aggression in children with ADHD. Neuropsychobiology 2007; 56(2–3): 104–10.
50. Zepf FD, Wockel L, Poustka F, Holtmann M. Diminished 5-HT functioning in CBCL pediatric bipolar disorder-profiled ADHD patients versus normal ADHD: susceptibility to rapid tryptophan depletion influences reaction time performance. Hum Psychopharmacol 2008; 23(4): 291–9.
51. Nishizawa S, Benkelfat C, Young SN, Leyton M, Mzengeza S, de Montigny C, et al. Differences between males and females in rates of serotonin synthesis in human brain. Proc Natl Acad Sci USA 1997; 94(10): 5308–13.
52. Badawy AA, Dougherty DM, Richard DM. Specificity of the acute tryptophan and tyrosine plus phenylalanine depletion and loading tests part II: normalisation of the tryptophan and the tyrosine plus phenylalanine to competing amino acid ratios in a new control formulation. Int J Tryptophan Res 2010; 3: 35–47.
53. Riedel WJ, Klaassen T, Deutz NE, Van Someren A, Van Praag HM. Tryptophan depletion in normal volunteers produces selective impairment in memory consolidation. Psychopharmacology 1999; 141(4): 362–9.
54. Schmitt JA, Jorissen BL, Sobczak S, Van Boxtel MP, Hogervorst E, Deutz NE, et al. Tryptophan depletion impairs memory consolidation but improves focussed attention in healthy young volunteers. J Psychopharmacol 2000; 14(1): 21–9.
55. Sobczak S, Riedel WJ, Booij I, Aan Het Rot M, Deutz NE, Honig A. Cognition following acute tryptophan depletion: difference between first-degree relatives of bipolar disorder patients and matched healthy control volunteers. Psychol Med 2002; 32(3): 503–15.
56. Evers EA, Sambeth A, Ramaekers JG, Riedel WJ, Van der Veen FM. The effects of acute tryptophan depletion on brain activation during cognition and emotional processing in healthy volunteers. Curr Pharm Des 2010; 16(18): 1998–2011.
57. Young SN. Acute tryptophan depletion in humans: a review of theoretical, practical and ethical aspects. J Psychiatry Neurosci 2013; 38(5): 294–305.
58. Young SN, Leyton M. The role of serotonin in human mood and social interaction. Insight from altered tryptophan levels. Pharmacol Biochem Behav 2002; 71(4): 857–65.
59. Booij L, Van der Does W, Benkelfat C, Bremner JD, Cowen PJ, Fava M, et al. Predictors of mood response to acute tryptophan depletion. A reanalysis. Neuropsychopharmacology 2002; 27(5): 852–61.
60. Wieser H, Belitz HD. Relations between structure and bitter taste of amino acids and peptides. I. Amino acids and related compounds]. Z Lebensm Unters Forsch 1975; 159(2): 65–72.
61. Yudkoff M. Brain metabolism of branched-chain amino acids. Glia 1997; 21(1): 92–8.
62. Hutson SM, Lieth E, LaNoue KF. Function of leucine in excitatory neurotransmitter metabolism in the central nervous system. J Nutr 2001; 131(3): 846s–50s.
63. Khaliq S, Haider S, Naqvi F, Perveen T, Saleem S, Haleem DJ. Altered brain serotonergic neurotransmission following caffeine withdrawal produces behavioral deficits in rats. Pak J Pharm Sci 2012; 25(1): 21–5.
64. Haleem DJ, Yasmeen A, Haleem M, Zafar A. 24h withdrawal following repeated administration of caffeine attenuates brain serotonin but not tryptophan in rat brain: implications for caffeine-induced depression. Life Sci 1995; 57(19): PL285–92.
65. Van Donkelaar EL, Blokland A, Ferrington L, Kelly PA, Steinbusch HW, Prickaerts J. Mechanism of acute tryptophan depletion: is it only serotonin? Mol Psychiatry 2011; 16(7): 695–713.
66. Crockett MJ, Clark L, Roiser JP, Robinson OJ, Cools R, Chase HW, et al. Converging evidence for central 5-HT effects in acute tryptophan depletion. Mol Psychiatry 2012; 17(2): 121–3.

*Florian Daniel Zepf
Centre and Discipline of Child and Adolescent Psychiatry, Psychosomatics and Psychotherapy
University of Western Australia
35 Stirling Highway (M561)
Crawley WA 6009, Perth
Australia
Email: florian.zepf@uwa.edu.au

Enhanced nutrition improves growth and increases blood adiponectin concentrations in very low birth weight infants

Elin W. Blakstad[1,2,3]*, Sissel J. Moltu[3,4], Britt Nakstad[1,2], Marit B. Veierød[3,5], Kenneth Strømmen[3,6], Pétur B. Júlíusson[7], Astrid N. Almaas[1,2,3], Arild E. Rønnestad[6], Kristin Brække[4], Christian A. Drevon[3] and Per O. Iversen[3]

[1]Department of Pediatric and Adolescent Medicine, Akershus University Hospital, Lørenskog, Norway; [2]Institute of Clinical Medicine, Campus Ahus, University of Oslo, Oslo, Norway; [3]Department of Nutrition, Institute of Basic Medical Sciences, Faculty of Medicine, University of Oslo, Oslo, Norway; [4]Department of Neonatal Intensive Care, Women and Children's Division, Oslo University Hospital, Ullevål, Oslo, Norway; [5]Oslo Centre of Biostatistics and Epidemiology, Department of Biostatistics, Institute of Basic Medical Sciences, Faculty of Medicine, University of Oslo, Oslo, Norway; [6]Department of Neonatal Intensive Care, Division of Paediatric and Adolescent Medicine, Oslo University Hospital, Rikshospitalet, Oslo, Norway; [7]Department of Clinical Science, University of Bergen, Bergen, Norway

Abstract

Background: Adequate nutrient supply is essential for optimal postnatal growth in very low birth weight (VLBW, birth weight < 1,500 g) infants. Early growth may influence the risk of metabolic syndrome later in life.
Objective: To evaluate growth and blood metabolic markers (adiponectin, leptin, and insulin-like growth factor-1 (IGF-1)) in VLBW infants participating in a randomized nutritional intervention study.
Design: Fifty VLBW infants were randomized to an enhanced nutrient supply or a standard nutrient supply. Thirty-seven infants were evaluated with growth measurements until 2 years corrected age (CA). Metabolic markers were measured at birth and 5 months CA.
Results: Weight gain and head growth were different in the two groups from birth to 2 years CA (weight gain: $p_{\text{interaction}} = 0.006$; head growth: $p_{\text{interaction}} = 0.002$). The intervention group improved their growth *z*-scores after birth, whereas the control group had a pronounced decline, followed by an increase and caught up with the intervention group after discharge. At 5 months CA, adiponectin concentrations were higher in the intervention group and correlated with weight gain before term ($r = 0.35$) and nutrient supply ($0.35 \leq r \leq 0.45$). Leptin concentrations correlated with weight gain after term and IGF-1 concentrations with length growth before and after term and head growth after term ($0.36 \leq r \leq 0.53$).
Conclusion: Enhanced nutrient supply improved early postnatal growth and may have prevented rapid catch-up growth later in infancy. Adiponectin concentration at 5 months CA was higher in the intervention group and correlated positively with early weight gain and nutrient supply. Early nutrition and growth may affect metabolic markers in infancy.
Clinical Trial Registration (ClinicalTrials.gov) no.: NCT01103219

Keywords: *premature*; *metabolic syndrome*; *leptin*; *adiponectin*; *IGF-1*

Early supply of adequate nutrient supply to premature infants is essential for optimal postnatal growth and development (1). Increased nutritional support reduces the incidence of growth failure (2–4) and improves neurodevelopmental outcomes (5, 6). Despite improvements in nutritional care, with evidence of increased growth velocity among very low birth weight (VLBW, birth weight (BW) < 1,500 g) infants, a recent study showed that 50% of VLBW infants still exhibit postnatal growth failure (7). Moreover, it has been reported that premature infants have higher fat mass and increased risk of adverse cardiovascular and metabolic outcomes later in life as compared to full-term infants (8–10). How and when postnatal nutrition and growth may affect these outcomes are not fully understood (11). Few have studied the associations between growth and metabolic markers in VLBW infants fed according to recent nutritional recommendations.

Adiponectin and leptin, secreted by adipose tissues, are examples of relevant metabolic markers that can be measured in blood (12, 13). In adults, adiponectin concentrations are bell shaped: low with very small adipose depots, increasing with enhancing adipose tissues, and decreasing with obesity (14). Adiponectin levels in newborns are higher than in adults and correlate positively with BW (15, 16). During the first weeks of life, adiponectin levels increase before they decrease to lower values at 1 year of age (17). Premature infants have lower adiponectin levels as compared to term infants, but the levels increase markedly postnatally (18, 19). Reduced adiponectin levels are associated with increased risk of obesity and metabolic syndrome in children (20).

Leptin levels correlate positively with body fat mass, and leptin is important in the regulation of food intake and energy expenditure (12). In term infants, leptin levels correlate positively with birth weight, gain in fat mass, and body mass index (BMI) (17, 21). Leptin levels increase after birth until 6 months, but showed a trend to return to birth levels by 1 year of age (17).

Insulin-like growth factor-1 (IGF-1) promotes cell growth, inhibits apoptosis, and stimulates glucose uptake and protein synthesis (22). This polypeptide is related to nutritional status (22) and associated with postnatal growth in term and preterm infants (23–25).

In a randomized controlled trial (RCT), we investigated the effects of enhanced versus standard nutrient supply to VLBW infants (3). Enhanced nutrition resulted in improved growth during the first weeks of life (3). In this study, we evaluated growth during the first 2 years of life and blood concentrations of adiponectin, leptin, and IGF-1 at birth and at 5 months corrected age (CA). We hypothesized that enhanced nutrition has an effect on metabolic markers and promotes steady growth patterns.

Methods

The original RCT

This is a follow-up of an open RCT conducted at Akershus and Oslo University Hospitals in 2010. The study was approved by the Regional Committee for Medical and Health Research Ethics (3). VLBW infants were included after informed parental consent was obtained. Exclusion criteria, estimation of sample size, and the randomization procedure have been described previously (3). The primary endpoint of the RCT was to reduce the proportion of infants discharged as growth restricted from 60 to 40%. After inclusion of 50 infants, a pre-planned safety analysis revealed increased occurrence of late-onset septicemia in the intervention group and further enrollment was stopped (26). Thus, the original study included 50 infants (hereby referred to as the PreNu cohort). Thirty-seven infants (hereby referred to as the PreNu follow-up cohort) were followed up with anthropometric measurements during the first 2 years of life (Fig. 1a).

Nutrition intervention

The nutrition protocol has previously been described in detail (3, 26). Fifty infants were randomized to either an intervention group (enhanced nutrient supply) or a control group (standard nutrient supply). The intervention group started with 3.5 g/kg/d of amino acids and 2.0 g/kg/d of fish oil-containing lipid emulsion (SMOF; Fresenius Kabi, Norway), and the control group started with 2.0 g/kg/d of amino acids and 0.5 g/kg/d of lipid emulsion (Clinoleic; Baxter, Norway). Enteral feeding was given from the first day of life, mother's milk or banked human donor milk, increased equally with time and fortified with Nutriprem® (Nutricia, Norway) in both groups. Additional supplements for the intervention group were amino acids (0.6 g Complete Amino Acid Mix®, Nutricia, Norway/100 mL human milk), long-chain polyunsaturated fatty acids (PUFA), 60 mg/kg/d each of docosahexaenoic acid (DHA) and arachidonic acid (AA) (Formulaic, Martek, USA), and 1,500 µg/kg/d of vitamin A (Aas Laboratory, Norway). The total amount of energy and protein on full enteral feeding was estimated to be 166 kcal/kg/d and 4.4 g/kg/d to the intervention group and 146 kcal/kg/d and 3.6 g/kg/d to the control group.

When breastfeeding, the intervention group infants received additional 'protein-shots' (1.6 g Complete Amino Acid Mix/20 mL human milk) per kg (maximum of 3/day). If they were not breastfed, the infants got a special preterm formula (Enfalac Premature, 81 kcal/100 mL, Mead Johnson, Norway). The intervention ended at 52 weeks postmenstrual age (PMA) and/or when the body weight reached 5.5 kg. Parenteral and enteral nutrient intakes were registered daily and calculated during the first 4 weeks of life.

Assessments of growth

Small for gestational age (SGA) was defined as weight <10th percentile. Length, weight, and head circumference (HC) were monitored until 2 years CA. From birth to discharge, growth data were collected from the hospital growth charts. After discharge, the infants were followed at local health care centers where trained nurses monitored their growth. At 5 months CA, body weights were registered at a follow-up visit at the hospital. We used the weights collected at the 5 month follow-up. For the remaining growth data we used the measurements closest to selected time points during the first 2 years of life. Non-sex-specific z-scores for length and HC were calculated by Fenton growth charts until 36 weeks PMA (www.ucalgary.ca/fenton). Sex-specific weight z-scores were obtained by Skjærven's growth charts until 36 weeks (27). Norwegian growth data were used as a reference to calculate z-scores from term (minimum gestational age [GA] 38 weeks + 6 days) until 2 years CA (28).

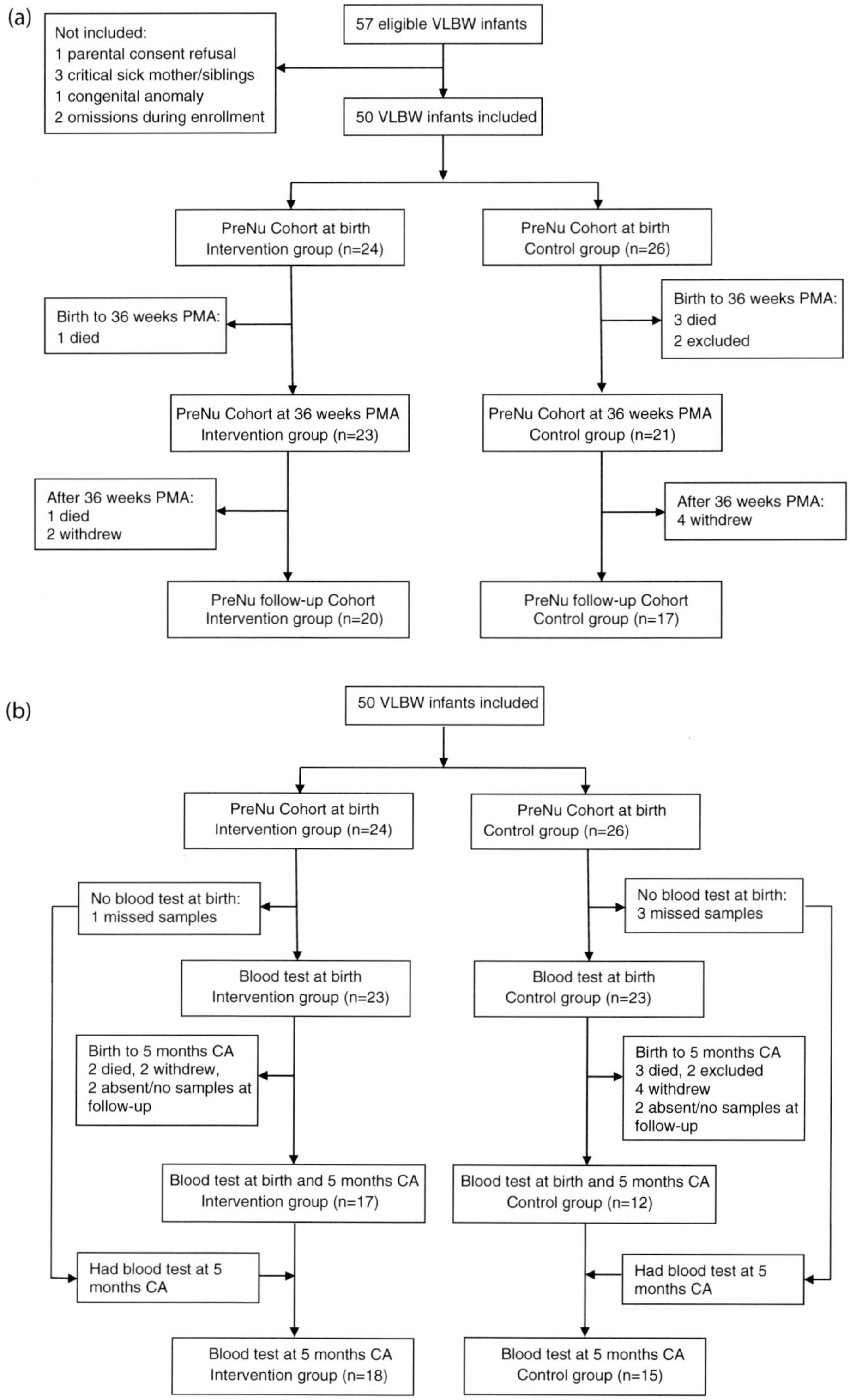

Fig. 1. (a) Flowchart of study participants with anthropometric data. During the first weeks of life, four infants died and two infants were excluded due to critical illness and congenital heart disease. After discharge, one infant died and six withdrew from the study. (b) Flowchart of study participants with blood tests sampled. Four infants did not have blood samples at birth. During the first weeks of life, four infants died and two infants were excluded due to critical illness and congenital heart disease. After discharge, one infant died and six withdrew. Four infants did not attend/did not have samples collected at follow-up. The four infants without blood tests at birth had tests at 5 months CA. CA = corrected age, PMA = post menstrual age, VLBW = very low birth weight.

Measurements of metabolic markers

The blood concentrations of adiponectin, leptin, and IGF-1 were assessed within the first 2 days of life (hereafter referred to as at birth) and at approximately 5 months CA using dried blood spots (DBS; Vitas Analytical Services, Oslo, Norway). At both sampling points, whole blood was collected from central/peripheral catheters or from a heel/finger prick, added to a special filter card, and stored at −80°C until analyses. Analyses of metabolic markers were performed with AM-296, AM-263, and AM-248 quantification for adiponectin, leptin, and IGF-1, respectively, in DBS using ELISA (www.vitas.no).

Statistics

Analyses of clinical characteristics and nutrient intake

To study group differences in clinical characteristics and nutritional intakes, we used a Student's *t*-test or a Mann–Whitney's U test for continuous variables and a chi-square or Fisher's exact test for categorical variables. Results are presented as means (ranges), percentages, or medians (interquartile ranges, IQRs).

Analyses of growth

To assess growth and growth differences between the two groups from birth to 2 years of age, we used a linear mixed model procedure (covariance structured model for repeated observations with unstructured variance). The dependent variables were *z*-scores for weight, length, or HC, and fixed factors were group and time. We tested for interaction between group and time (i.e. whether the two groups changed over time in different ways).

Analyses of metabolic markers

To study blood concentrations of adiponectin, leptin, and IGF-1, the results were $\log_e$ (ln) transformed to normalize data. Statistical analyses were performed on transformed data, and the back-transformed means (geometric means) with confidence intervals are presented. Group differences in metabolic markers at birth were evaluated with Student's *t*-test. Analysis of covariance (29) was used to study differences in change in metabolic markers from birth to 5 months CA. Infants without data of metabolic markers at birth were excluded from the analysis at 5 months CA. Due to a strong correlation between birth adiponectin concentrations and BW (i.e. the problem of collinearity), we did not adjust for BW when comparing adiponectin concentrations between the groups. For leptin and IGF-1, adjusting for BW did not change the conclusions of the analyses (data not shown).

Pearson's correlation coefficient (*r*) was calculated to study associations between metabolic markers and clinical characteristic at birth, between metabolic markers and parameters of growth, and between metabolic markers and specific nutrients. All test results at birth ($n = 46$) and at 5 months CA ($n = 33$) were used in the correlation analyses. Significance was assumed for $p < 0.05$. Statistical analyses were performed by SPSS, version 22 (SPSS, Chicago, IL, USA).

Results

Study sample

Forty-four infants (PreNu cohort) had anthropometric data at 36 weeks GA, and 37 infants (the PreNu follow-up cohort) were followed with anthropometric measurements throughout the first 2 years of life (Fig. 1a). Forty-six infants (23 in each group) had blood samples collected at birth (Fig. 1b). Thirty-three infants had blood samples at 5 months CA, but 4 of these infants did not have blood samples at birth, leaving 29 infants with samples at both birth and 5 months CA (Fig. 1b). Clinical characteristics were similar between the two groups, except in the PreNu follow-up cohort where mean BW was significantly lower in the intervention group compared to the controls (Table 1).

Weight, length and HC z-scores

There was a significant difference between the groups in weight gain from birth to 24 months CA ($p_{\text{interaction}} = 0.006$) (Fig. 2a). However, the difference was most evident from birth to 40 weeks GA, when the control group had a pronounced decline in weight *z*-scores followed by an increase in growth and subsequent catch-up with the intervention group (Fig. 2a and b) after discharge. Mean weight *z*-scores remained negative for both groups, and 27% of the infants were growth restricted (weight <10th percentile [28]) at 2 years CA (intervention group 30%, control group 24%; $p = 0.73$).

There was no significant difference between the groups in length growth over time ($p_{\text{interaction}} = 0.35$) (Fig. 2c), but length *z*-scores changed significantly in both groups over time ($p < 0.001$), and the change was most evident between birth and 36 weeks CA ($p = 0.001$) (Fig. 2c and d). Mean *z*-scores remained negative and 25% of the infants had length *z*-scores below the 10th percentile (28) at 2 years CA (intervention 25%, control group 25%; $p = 1.00$).

We observed a significant difference between the groups in HC growth over time ($p_{\text{interaction}} = 0.002$) (Fig. 2e). The intervention group had a positive change in *z*-scores between birth and 36 weeks PMA, whereas the control group had a marked decline. From 36 weeks PMA, mean HC *z*-scores in the control group also increased (Fig. 2e and f). Mean *z*-scores remained positive for both groups. However, at 13 months CA, 22% of the infants had *z*-scores under the 10th percentile (28) (intervention group 25%, control group 18%; $p = 0.70$).

Additional adjustment for SGA did not change the conclusions for weight, length, and HC growth (data not shown). One infant in the control group was diagnosed

Table 1. Clinical characteristics at birth and calculated daily nutrient intakes during the first 4 weeks of life

	PreNu cohort			PreNu follow-up cohort		
	Intervention ($n=24$)	Control ($n=26$)	p	Intervention ($n=20$)	Control ($n=17$)	p
GA at birth (weeks), mean (range)	28.1 (25.0–33.6)	28.1 (23.0–32.6)	0.94	28.0 (25.0–33.6)	28.6 (24.0–32.6)	0.54
Sex, boys, n (%)	15 (63%)	15 (58%)	0.73	12 (60%)	12 (71%)	0.51
SGA, n (%)	11 (46%)	6 (23%)	0.09	10 (50%)	3 (18%)	0.08
Birth weight (g), mean (range)	940 (460–1311)	1,035 (426–1414)	0.19	912 (460–1244)	1,122 (571–1,414)	<0.01
Birth weight z-score, mean (range)	−1.29 (−3.51–0.70)	−0.95 (−2.64–0.03)	0.22	−1.34 (−3.51–0.70)	−0.87 (−1.90– −0.15)	0.14
Energy, kcal/kg/d, median (IQR)	139 (128–145)^{a}	126 (121–128)^{b}	<0.001	139 (129–145)	126 (121–127)	<0.001
Protein, g/kg/d, median (IQR)	4.0 (3.9–4.2)^{a}	3.2 (3.1–3.3)^{b}	<0.001	4.1 (3.9–4.2)	3.2 (3.1–3.3)	<0.001
AA, mg/kg/d, median (IQR)	68 (57–73)^{a}	24 (23–25)^{b}	<0.001	68 (58–72)	24 (23–24)	<0.001
DHA, mg/kg/d, median (IQR)	87 (81–91)^{a}	36 (34–38)^{b}	<0.001	87 (81–91)	36 (34–37)	<0.001

Data are presented as mean (range), median (interquartile range, IQR), or frequency (%). AA = arachidonic acid, DHA = docosahexaenoic acid, GA = gestational age, SGA = small for gestational age. $^{a}n=23$, $^{b}n=21$.

with a congenital heart defect causing heart failure and poor growth. Analysis without this infant did not change the conclusions for weight, length, or HC (data not shown). Individual growth profiles are presented in Fig. 3.

Metabolic markers at birth and at 5 months CA

The two groups had similar mean (SD) age at blood sampling at birth (intervention group vs. control group: 0.2 [0.5] days vs. 0.4 [0.5] days chronological age [$p=$ 0.23]), and at 5 months CA (intervention group vs. control group: 155 (11) and 159 (13) days CA; $p=0.25$)).

There were no significant differences between the two groups in blood concentrations of adiponectin, leptin and IGF-1 at birth (Table 2). A few outliers were identified with higher blood concentrations of metabolic markers. Excluding these infants from the analysis did not change the results (data not shown).

At 5 months CA, the intervention group had significantly higher adiponectin concentrations compared to controls ($p=0.03$), while no significant differences were observed for leptin and IGF-1 (Table 2). One infant in the control group had a very high leptin value at 5 months CA. After excluding this outlier, there was still no significant difference between the groups ($p=0.46$).

There were no differences in any of the metabolic markers at birth or at 5 months CA when comparing infants born SGA to infants born appropriate for gestational age (AGA) (Table 3).

Correlations between metabolic markers and birth characteristics, growth and nutrient supply

Strong positive correlations were observed between blood concentrations of adiponectin at birth and weight, length, HC, and GA at birth ($0.63 \le r \le 0.76$) (Table 4). No significant correlations were found between leptin and IGF-1 concentrations at birth and anthropometric measures or GA ($0.04 \le r \le 0.20$), or between any of the metabolic markers and birth z-scores ($-0.01 \le r \le 0.18$).

Blood concentration of adiponectin at 5 months CA correlated positively with weight gain from birth to 40 weeks PMA ($r=0.35$) (Table 5). Leptin concentrations correlated positively with weight gain from 40 weeks PMA to 5 months CA ($r=0.53$). IGF-1 concentration correlated positively with length growth from birth to 43 weeks PMA ($r=0.50$) and from 43 weeks PMA to 6 months CA ($r=0.36$) and HC growth from 42 weeks PMA until 6 months CA ($r=0.51$). Adiponectin correlated positively with the first 4 weeks mean supply of protein, DHA, and AA and with first week mean supply of energy, protein, DHA, and AA ($0.35 \le r \le 0.45$) (Table 5).

Discussion

Our data demonstrate that enhanced nutrient supply improves growth in VLBW infants. After the initial physiological weight loss, the intervention group infants

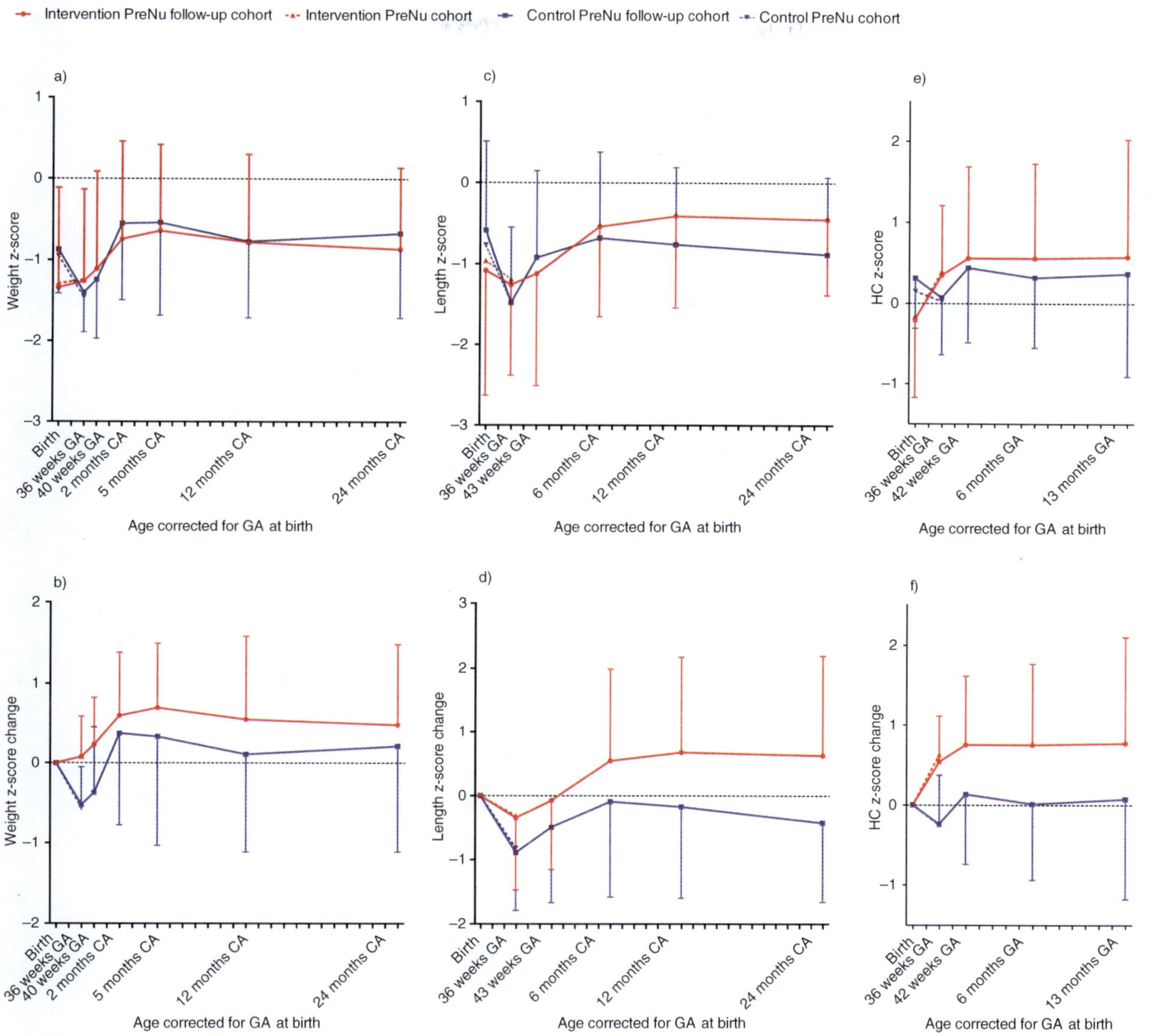

Fig. 2. Anthropometric data from birth to 2 years corrected age. *z*-scores and *z*-score changes for weight, length and head circumference (HC). Panel a, c, e: mean (SD) *z*-scores for each group at selected time points; panel b, d, f: change in *z*-scores from birth, estimated from means from each group at specific time points. Error bars represents standard deviations. Whole lines represent the PreNu follow-up cohort ($n = 35–37$). Red and blue dotted lines represent the PreNu cohort ($n = 49–50$ at birth and $n = 40–44$ at 36 weeks). GA = gestational age.

showed early catch-up growth followed by a more steady growth pattern up to 2 years CA. The control group infants had a pronounced initial decline in *z*-scores followed by catch-up growth mainly after neonatal hospitalization. As far as we are aware, this is the first RCT to examine whether enhanced nutrient supply and improved early growth have an effect on metabolic markers in VLBW infants. Blood adiponectin concentrations correlated positively with anthropometric measures at birth, weight gain from birth to term, and supply of nutrients. At 5 months CA, adiponectin concentrations were higher in the intervention group compared to the controls.

Enhanced nutrient supply limited the prolonged and severe decline in postnatal growth, which was observed in the control group. This is in line with Senterre and Rigo's (4) study, which also demonstrated that postnatal weight loss can be limited by reducing postnatal nutrient deficiencies. For premature infants, early growth failure appears to be especially harmful in certain periods of organ development. The brain is extremely vulnerable to deprivation of specific nutrients between 24 and 42 weeks PMA (30). Impaired postnatal growth has negative effects on neurodevelopment in premature infants (31), and increased early protein and energy supply has been associated with higher cognitive scores (5). Belfort et al. (6) reported a positive association between increased BMI and weight gain before term and improved neurodevelopment in preterm infants. After term weight gain,

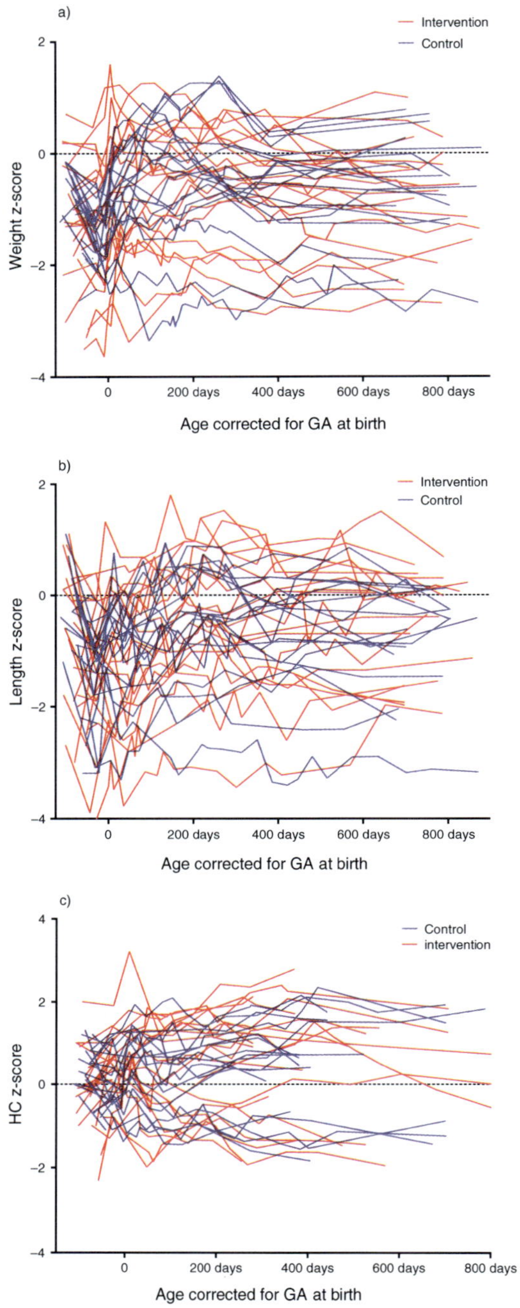

Fig. 3. Individual growth profiles. Individual *z*-scores for weight (a), length (b), and head circumference (HC) (c). GA = gestational age.

but not weight gain out of proportion to length, was beneficial for neurodevelopment (6).

In our study, growth restriction (< 10th percentile) was still prevalent through the first years of life in almost a quarter of the infants. Mean *z*-scores for weight and length remained negative throughout the first 2 years, whereas mean HC *z*-scores were positive for both groups at 13 months CA, suggesting that head growth was prioritized before weight and length growth. Others also report that head growth recovers before weight and length growth. Westerberg et al. (32) identified that VLBW children were smaller and lighter than their peers, but that head growth normalized after 2 months. Ramel et al. (33) demonstrated that head growth recovered by 4 months CA, whereas linear growth continued to be suppressed at 24 months.

We observed that blood adiponectin concentrations increased from birth to 5 months CA in both groups, supporting what has previously been reported by others (19, 34, 35). Moreover, we found that infants on enhanced nutrient supply had a greater increase in adiponectin concentrations as compared to the infants on standard nutrient supply. This is the first study to report a difference in adiponectin concentrations between two groups of premature infants with different nutrient supplies. Other studies of premature infants have described positive associations between adiponectin and postnatal growth. Hansen-Pupp et al. (19) demonstrated a positive correlation between adiponectin concentrations during the first 3 weeks of life and growth variables at 35 weeks GA. Saito et al. (35) observed a positive correlation between weight gain and change in adiponectin concentrations. Siahanidou et al. (36) reported that adiponectin concentration at discharge correlated positively with the last week weight gain.

We found that the first week supply of protein, energy, and essential fatty acids correlated positively with adiponectin concentrations at 5 months CA. The correlations remained positive for the first 4 weeks' mean values of protein and PUFAs, but not for energy. Hansen-Pupp et al. (19) reported that adiponectin concentrations correlated positively with energy intake, but the correlation disappeared after adjusting for GA at birth. Yoshida et al. (34) reported that adiponectin concentration at term correlated inversely with age to regain birth weight, but not with energy supply. Notably, the nutrient supply in these two studies was much lower than in our intervention. Siahanidou et al. (36) found higher levels of adiponectin concentrations in infants fed formula containing long-chain PUFAs, but did not observe an effect of last week energy supply.

In line with other studies (19, 35, 37, 38), we found that adiponectin concentrations at birth had a strong positive correlation with anthropometric measures and GA at birth. We did not observe differences in adiponectin concentrations at birth or at 5 months CA between infants born SGA or AGA. In contrast to this, one study of term and preterm infants reported lower adiponectin concentrations 3–13 days postnatally in infants born SGA compared with AGA (38). Saito et al. (35) found no effect of SGA status on adiponectin concentrations at birth, but demonstrated lower adiponectin concentrations at term-equivalent age in SGA born infants. Other studies also report that preterm SGA born infants have consistently lower adiponectin concentrations postnatally

Table 2. Concentrations of metabolic markers in the intervention and the control group at birth and at 5 months corrected age

	PreNu cohort at birth			PreNu follow-up cohort at birth			PreNu follow-up cohort at months CA		
	Intervention ($n = 23$)	Control ($n = 23$)	p*	Intervention ($n = 17$)	Control ($n = 12$)	p*	Intervention ($n = 17$)	Control ($n = 12$)	p**
Adiponectin (µg/mL)	3.9 (2.9–5.4)	4.7 (3.3–6.5)	0.44	3.8 (2.6–5.5)	5.4 (3.8–7.6)	0.17	16.5 (14.2–19.1)	13.7 (11.8–15.9)	0.03
Leptin (pg/mL)	2.0 (1.9–2.2)	2.1 (1.9–2.3)	0.64	2.1 (1.9–2.3)	2.0 (1.8–2.3)	0.79	2.3 (2.1–2.6)	2.8 (2.1–3.9)	0.19
IGF-1 (nmol/L)	27.1 (26.0–28.2)	27.7 (26.2–29.2)	0.54	27.0 (25.6–28.4)	28.8 (26.6–31.1)	0.13	29.8 (28.6–31.0)	28.7 (26.8–30.8)	0.12

Data are presented as geometric mean (95% CI). *Student's t-test. **Analysis of covariance. CA = corrected age, IGF-1 = insulin-like growth factor 1.

until term (19) and at discharge (36). Even though it was not significant, the majority of the SGA born infants in our study was randomized to the intervention group. It is possible that enhanced nutrient supply and subsequent improved early growth had a positive impact on adiponectin concentrations in the SGA infants, promoting similar concentrations as the AGA infants.

We demonstrated a positive correlation between blood leptin concentrations at 5 months and weight gain from term to 5 months CA. This is supported by van Poelje et al. (21) who identified that weight z-scores gain from term to 6 months CA resulted in higher fat mass and higher leptin concentrations at 6 months CA, indicating that leptin is a marker of body fat mass during the first 6 months after term. Bozzola et al. (17) identified higher leptin concentrations in AGA versus SGA term born infants at birth and comparable levels at 1st, 6th and 12th month of age. The authors suggested the increased leptin levels were due to increased adipose tissue.

In this study, we observed positive correlations between IGF-1 concentrations and length growth (birth to 6 months) and head growth (birth to 43 weeks). A recent review pointed out that IGF-1 concentrations correlate differently with growth before and after term-equivalent age in preterm infants (22). Hansen-Pupp et al. (24) reported that IGF-1 concentrations correlated positively with weight gain at an early postnatal age in preterm infants. Brain volumes in preterm infants at term age were positively associated with postnatal IGF-1 concentrations (39). Van de Lagemaat et al. (25) reported that both preceding length and weight growth were positively associated with IGF-1 at term, 3 and 6 months CA. After term age, studies show contradictive results in relation to IGF-1 concentrations and correlations with subsequent growth (22).

There have been concerns that enhanced nutrient supply and excessive postnatal growth increase the risk of developing adiposity and metabolic syndrome later in life in preterm infants (8–10). Metabolic markers measured in children have been associated with adiposity and adverse metabolic outcomes (20, 40). The association between metabolic markers in infancy and later risk of obesity and metabolic syndrome is, however, not clear. Increase in leptin concentrations between term and birth may mirror an increase in fat deposition. The increase in fat depositions could be a result of rapid catch-up growth after the period of growth retardation similar to what we observed in our control group. Furthermore, excessive fat deposition is a possible risk factor for metabolic syndrome. The infants in the intervention group did not experience the prominent growth retardation and avoided the subsequent period of rapid catch-up growth. We speculate that the higher adiponectin concentration in the intervention group could be an indication of a healthier growth pattern. However, this needs to be investigated further.

Our study has limitations. The sample size is small (3) and differences may not have been detected due to low statistical power. Despite randomization, the intervention group had a significantly lower BW than the

Table 3. Concentrations of metabolic markers in infants born appropriate for gestational age (AGA) and small for gestational age (SGA)

	PreNu cohort at birth			PreNu follow-up cohort at birth			PreNu follow-up cohort at months CA		
	AGA ($n = 31$)	SGA ($n = 15$)	p*	AGA ($n = 19$)	SGA ($n = 10$)	p*	AGA ($n = 19$)	SGA ($n = 10$)	p**
Adiponectin (µg/mL)	4.4 (3.5–5.5)	4.1 (2.3–7.2)	0.82	4.8 (3.8–6.1)	3.7 (2.0–7.1)	0.43	15.0 (13.1–17.2)	15.7 (12.8–19.3)	0.51
Leptin (pg/mL)	2.1 (1.9–2.3)	2.0 (1.8–2.3)	0.79	2.0 (1.9–2.2)	2.2 (1.8–2.5)	0.39	2.5 (2.1–3.1)	2.5 (2.1–3.1)	0.99
IGF-1 (nmol/L)	27.7 (26.5–28.9)	26.8 (25.2–28.4)	0.34	27.8 (26.3–29.4)	27.4 (25.3–29.8)	0.77	29.0 (27.7–30.5)	29.9 (28.4–31.5)	0.36

Data are presented as geometric mean (95% CI). *Student's t-test. **Analysis of covariance. CA = corrected age, IGF-1 = insulin-like growth factor 1.

Table 4. Correlations between metabolic markers and anthropometric data and gestational age at birth

	Adiponectin ($n=46$)		Leptin ($n=46$)		IGF-1 ($n=46$)	
	r	p	r	p	r	p
BW	0.76	<0.001	0.05	0.77	0.14	0.36
BW z-scores	0.06	0.69	−0.01	0.91	0.04	0.80
Birth length[a]	0.64	<0.001	0.20	0.19	0.15	0.32
Birth length z-scores[a]	−0.01	0.93	0.14	0.37	0.05	0.73
Birth HC	0.74	<0.001	0.13	0.39	0.20	0.19
Birth HC z-scores	0.17	0.26	0.09	0.56	0.18	0.24
GA birth	0.63	<0.001	0.04	0.78	0.11	0.46

BW = birth weight, GA = gestational age, HC = head circumference, IGF-1 = insulin-like growth factor 1, r = Pearson's correlation coefficient, Δz-score = z-score change, [a]$n=45$.

control group (3). BW *z*-scores were non-significantly lower in the intervention group. *Z*-scores were used when comparing growth over time. The lower BW in the intervention group may have had an undetected impact on the potential of growth and changes in metabolic markers. Also, we did not fully adjust for confounding factors because of low power. However, the sample size is similar to other studies examining metabolic markers in premature infants (17, 19, 24, 34, 35). Another limitation was the variety in number of anthropometric measurers for each participant. This was due to differences in lengths of hospital stay and number of visits to the local health care institutions. The anthropometric measurement closest to each selected time points was used to calculate mean values. Also, we would have preferred to use one growth chart, but there are no common Norwegian growth charts for weight, length, and HC for premature infants from birth through early childhood. We justify the use of different growth charts, because we compared differences between two groups and not to the general population. In this study, we did not include information about maternal nutrition, BMI, smoking habits, and morbidities. These factors might influence nutrition and growth. We used DBS in our analysis to reduce blood volumes and still keep the sensitivity of the assays (38, 41). Most other studies have used plasma or serum. This makes it difficult to directly compare our values of the metabolic markers with levels reported by others.

Conclusions

Enhanced nutrient supply improved postnatal growth with a marked reduction in infants subjected to postnatal growth restriction. The correction of early growth might have prevented the need for catch-up growth close to term age, where excessive growth often is dominated by increase in adipose tissue and a subsequent increase in the risk of metabolic syndrome. We observed a higher adiponectin concentration in the intervention group at 5 months CA and a positive correlation between adiponectin concentrations and growth before term. Early nutrition and growth may affect metabolic markers in infancy. We did not demonstrate any changes in the metabolic markers suggesting elevated risk of metabolic syndrome among the infants receiving enhanced nutrient supply.

Table 5. Correlations between metabolic markers at 5 months corrected age and growth and nutrient supply

	Adiponectin ($n=33$)		Leptin ($n=33$)		IGF-1 ($n=33$)	
	r	p	r	p	r	p
Δz-score weight, birth to term (40 weeks PMA)	0.35	0.04	−0.11	0.55	0.19	0.29
Δz-score weight, term (40 weeks PMA) to 5 months CA	−0.25	0.17	0.53	0.001	0.32	0.07
Δz-score length, birth to term (43 weeks PMA)[a]	0.09	0.65	−0.10	0.61	0.50	0.004
Δz-score length, term (43 weeks PMA) to 6 months CA[a]	−0.14	0.46	0.26	0.16	0.36	0.05
Δz-score HC, birth to term (42 weeks PMA)	−0.01	0.95	−0.23	0.21	0.10	0.58
Δz-score HC, term (42 weeks PMA) to 6 months CA	−0.02	0.92	0.15	0.40	0.51	0.002
First 4 weeks mean protein supply	0.35	0.05	−0.26	0.15	0.10	0.59
First 4 weeks mean energy supply	0.28	0.11	−0.28	0.12	0.28	0.12
First 4 weeks mean DHA supply	0.37	0.03	−0.28	0.11	0.16	0.37
First 4 weeks mean AA supply	0.35	0.05	−0.26	0.15	0.18	0.31
First week mean protein supply	0.41	0.02	−0.33	0.06	0.18	0.32
First week mean energy supply	0.45	0.008	−0.28	0.11	0.34	0.05
First week mean DHA supply	0.39	0.03	−0.28	0.12	0.19	0.29
First week mean AA supply	0.41	0.02	−0.20	0.27	0.27	0.13

AA = arachidonic acid, CA = corrected age, DHA = docosahexaenoic acid, HC = head circumference, IGF-1 = insulin-like growth factor 1, PMA = post menstrual age, r = Pearson's correlation coefficient, Δz-score = z-score change, [a]$n=31$.

Acknowledgements

We thank Martek Biosciences Corporation for providing essential fatty acid oils free of charge.

Conflict of interest and funding

Funding was obtained from the Research Council of Norway, the Norwegian Foundation for Health and Rehabilitation, South-Eastern Norway Regional Health Authority, Johan Throne Holst Foundation for Nutrition Research, and Freia Medisinske Fond. Christian A. Drevon is a stock owner, board member, and consultant for contract laboratory Vitas AS.

References

1. Lafeber HN, van de Lagemaat M, Rotteveel J, van Weissenbruch M. Timing of nutritional interventions in very-low-birth-weight infants: optimal neurodevelopment compared with the onset of the metabolic syndrome. Am J Clin Nutr 2013; 98(2): 556S–60.
2. Maas C, Poets CF, Franz AR. Avoiding postnatal undernutrition of VLBW infants during neonatal intensive care: evidence and personal view in the absence of evidence. Arch Dis Child Fetal Neonatal Ed 2015; 100(1): F76–81.
3. Moltu SJ, Blakstad EW, Strommen K, Almaas AN, Nakstad B, Ronnestad A, et al. Enhanced feeding and diminished postnatal growth failure in very-low-birth-weight infants. J Paediatr Gastroenterol Nutr 2014; 58(3): 344–51.
4. Senterre T, Rigo J. Reduction in postnatal cumulative nutritional deficit and improvement of growth in extremely preterm infants. Acta Paediatr 2012; 101(2): e64–70.
5. Stephens BE, Walden RV, Gargus RA, Tucker R, McKinley L, Mance M, et al. First-week protein and energy intakes are associated with 18-month developmental outcomes in extremely low birth weight infants. Pediatrics 2009; 123(5): 1337–43.
6. Belfort MB, Rifas-Shiman SL, Sullivan T, Collins CT, McPhee AJ, Ryan P, et al. Infant growth before and after term: effects on neurodevelopment in preterm infants. Pediatrics 2011; 128(4): 899–906.
7. Horbar JD, Ehrenkranz RA, Badger GJ, Edwards EM, Morrow KA, Soll RF, et al. Weight growth velocity and postnatal growth failure in infants 501 to 1500 grams: 2000–2013. Pediatrics 2015; 136(1): 84–92.
8. Doyle LW, Faber B, Callanan C, Ford GW, Davis NM. Extremely low birth weight and body size in early adulthood. Arch Dis Child 2004; 89(4): 347–50.
9. Sipola-Leppanen M, Vaarasmaki M, Tikanmaki M, Hovi P, Miettola S, Ruokonen A, et al. Cardiovascular risk factors in adolescents born preterm. Pediatrics 2014; 134(4): e1072–81.
10. Sipola-Leppanen M, Vaarasmaki M, Tikanmaki M, Matinolli HM, Miettola S, Hovi P, et al. Cardiometabolic risk factors in young adults who were born preterm. Am J Epidemiol 2015; 181(11): 861–73.
11. Lapillonne A, Griffin IJ. Feeding preterm infants today for later metabolic and cardiovascular outcomes. J Paediatr 2013; 162(3 Suppl): S7–S16.
12. Drevon CA. Fatty acids and expression of adipokines. Biochim Biophys Acta 2005; 1740(2): 287–92.
13. Okada T, Takahashi S, Nagano N, Yoshikawa K, Usukura Y, Hosono S. Early postnatal alteration of body composition in preterm and small-for-gestational-age infants: implications of catch-up fat. Paediatr Res 2015; 77(1–2): 136–42.
14. Haugen F, Drevon CA. The interplay between nutrients and the adipose tissue. Proc Nutr Soc 2007; 66(2): 171–82.
15. Kotani Y, Yokota I, Kitamura S, Matsuda J, Naito E, Kuroda Y. Plasma adiponectin levels in newborns are higher than those in adults and positively correlated with birth weight. Clin Endocrinol (Oxf) 2004; 61(4): 418–23.
16. Tsai PJ, Yu CH, Hsu SP, Lee YH, Chiou CH, Hsu YW, et al. Cord plasma concentrations of adiponectin and leptin in healthy term neonates: positive correlation with birthweight and neonatal adiposity. Clin Endocrinol (Oxf) 2004; 61(1): 88–93.
17. Bozzola E, Meazza C, Arvigo M, Travaglino P, Pagani S, Stronati M, et al. Role of adiponectin and leptin on body development in infants during the first year of life. Ital J Pediatr 2010; 36: 26.
18. Nakano Y, Itabashi K, Sakurai M, Aizawa M, Dobashi K, Mizuno K. Preterm infants have altered adiponectin levels at term-equivalent age even if they do not present with extra-uterine growth restriction. Horm Res Paediatr 2013; 80(3): 147–53.
19. Hansen-Pupp I, Hellgren G, Hard AL, Smith L, Hellstrom A, Lofqvist C. Early surge in circulatory adiponectin is associated with improved growth at near term in very preterm infants. J Clin Endocrinol Metab 2015; 100(6): 2380–7.
20. Korner A, Kratzsch J, Gausche R, Schaab M, Erbs S, Kiess W. New predictors of the metabolic syndrome in children – role of adipocytokines. Pediatr Res 2007; 61(6): 640–5.
21. van Poelje MW, van de Lagemaat M, Lafeber HN, Van Weissenbruch MM, Rotteveel J. Relationship between fat mass measured by dual-energy X-ray absorptiometry and leptin in preterm infants between term age and 6 months' corrected age. Horm Res Paediatr 2014; 82(6): 405–10.
22. Yumani DF, Lafeber HN, van Weissenbruch MM. Dietary proteins and IGF I levels in preterm infants: determinants of growth, body composition, and neurodevelopment. Pediatr Res 2015; 77(1–2): 156–63.
23. Ong KK, Langkamp M, Ranke MB, Whitehead K, Hughes IA, Acerini CL, et al. Insulin-like growth factor I concentrations in infancy predict differential gains in body length and adiposity: the Cambridge Baby Growth Study. Am J Clin Nutr 2009; 90(1): 156–61.
24. Hansen-Pupp I, Lofqvist C, Polberger S, Niklasson A, Fellman V, Hellstrom A, et al. Influence of insulin-like growth factor I and nutrition during phases of postnatal growth in very preterm infants. Pediatr Res 2011; 69(15 Pt 1): 448–53.
25. van de Lagemaat M, Rotteveel J, Heijboer AC, Lafeber HN, van Weissenbruch MM. Growth in preterm infants until six months postterm: the role of insulin and IGF-I. Horm Res Paediatr 2013; 80(2): 92–9.
26. Moltu SJ, Strommen K, Blakstad EW, Almaas AN, Westerberg AC, Braekke K, et al. Enhanced feeding in very-low-birth-weight infants may cause electrolyte disturbances and septicemia – a randomized, controlled trial. Clin Nutr 2013; 32(2): 207–12.
27. Skjaerven R, Gjessing HK, Bakketeig LS. Birthweight by gestational age in Norway. Acta Obstet Gynecol Scand 2000; 79(6): 440–9.
28. Juliusson PB, Roelants M, Nordal E, Furevik L, Eide GE, Moster D, et al. Growth references for 0–19 year-old Norwegian children for length/height, weight, body mass index and head circumference. Ann Hum Biol 2013; 40(3): 220–7.
29. Vickers AJ, Altman DG. Statistics notes: analysing controlled trials with baseline and follow up measurements. BMJ 2001; 323(7321): 1123–4.

30. Georgieff MK. Nutrition and the developing brain: nutrient priorities and measurement. Am J Clin Nutr 2007; 85(2): 614S–20.
31. Franz AR, Pohlandt F, Bode H, Mihatsch WA, Sander S, Kron M, et al. Intrauterine, early neonatal, and postdischarge growth and neurodevelopmental outcome at 5.4 years in extremely preterm infants after intensive neonatal nutritional support. Pediatrics 2009; 123(1): 101–9.
32. Westerberg AC, Henriksen C, Ellingvag A, Veierod MB, Juliusson PB, Nakstad B, et al. First year growth among very low birth weight infants. Acta Paediatr 2010; 99(4): 556–62.
33. Ramel SE, Demerath EW, Gray HL, Younge N, Boys C, Georgieff MK. The relationship of poor linear growth velocity with neonatal illness and two-year neurodevelopment in preterm infants. Neonatology 2012; 102(1): 19–24.
34. Yoshida T, Nagasaki H, Asato Y, Ohta T. Early weight changes after birth and serum high-molecular-weight adiponectin level in preterm infants. Pediatr Int 2011; 53(6): 926–9.
35. Saito M, Nishimura K, Nozue H, Miyazono Y, Kamoda T. Changes in serum adiponectin levels from birth to term-equivalent age are associated with postnatal weight gain in preterm infants. Neonatology 2011; 100(1): 93–8.
36. Siahanidou T, Mandyla H, Papassotiriou GP, Papassotiriou I, Chrousos G. Circulating levels of adiponectin in preterm infants. Arch Dis Child Fetal Neonatal Ed 2007; 92(4): F286–90.
37. Kajantie E, Hytinantti T, Hovi P, Andersson S. Cord plasma adiponectin: a 20-fold rise between 24 weeks gestation and term. J Clin Endocrinol Metab 2004; 89(8): 4031–6.
38. Klamer A, Skogstrand K, Hougaard DM, Norgaard-Petersen B, Juul A, Greisen G. Adiponectin levels measured in dried blood spot samples from neonates born small and appropriate for gestational age. Eur J Endocrinol 2007; 157(2): 189–94.
39. Hansen-Pupp I, Hovel H, Hellstrom A, Hellstrom-Westas L, Lofqvist C, Larsson EM, et al. Postnatal decrease in circulating insulin-like growth factor-I and low brain volumes in very preterm infants. J Clin Endocrinol Metab 2011; 96(4): 1129–35.
40. Panagopoulou P, Galli-Tsinopoulou A, Fleva A, Pavlitou-Tsiontsi E, Vavatsi-Christaki N, Nousia-Arvanitakis S. Adiponectin and insulin resistance in childhood obesity. J Pediatr Gastroenterol Nutr 2008; 47(3): 356–62.
41. Yeung EH, McLain AC, Anderson N, Lawrence D, Boghossian NS, Druschel C, et al. Newborn adipokines and birth outcomes. Paediatr Perinat Epidemiol 2015; 29(4): 317–25.

*Elin W. Blakstad
Department of Pediatric and Adolescent Medicine
Akershus University Hospital
P.O. Box 1000
NO-1478 Lørenskog, Norway
Email: e.w.blakstad@medisin.uio.no

5

Fish consumption pattern among adults of different ethnics in Peninsular Malaysia

Nurul Izzah Ahmad[1]*, Wan Rozita Wan Mahiyuddin[1], Tengku Rozaina Tengku Mohamad[2], Cheong Yoon Ling[1], Siti Fatimah Daud[1], Nasriyah Che Hussein[1], Nor Aini Abdullah[1], Rafiza Shaharudin[1] and Lokman Hakim Sulaiman[3]

[1]Institute for Medical Research, Kuala Lumpur, Malaysia; [2]School of Food Science and Technology, Universiti Malaysia Terengganu, Kuala Terengganu, Malaysia; [3]Ministry of Health Malaysia, Federal Government Administration Centre, Putrajaya, Malaysia

Abstract

Background: Understanding different patterns of fish consumption is an important component for risk assessment of contaminants in fish. A few studies on food consumption had been conducted in Malaysia, but none of them focused specifically on fish consumption. The objectives of this study were to document the meal pattern among three major ethnics in Malaysia with respect to fish/seafood consumption, identify most frequently consumed fish and cooking method, and examine the influence of demographic factors on pattern of fish consumption among study subjects.

Methods: A cross-sectional survey was conducted between February 2008 and May 2009 to investigate patterns of fish consumption among Malaysian adults in Peninsular Malaysia. Adults aged 18 years and above were randomly selected and fish consumption data were collected using a 3-day prospective food diary.

Results: A total of 2,675 subjects, comprising male (44.2%) and female (55.7%) participants from major ethnics (Malays, 76.9%; Chinese, 14.7%; Indians, 8.3%) with a mean age of 43.4 ± 16.2 years, were involved in this study. The results revealed 10 most frequently consumed marine fish in descending order: Indian mackerel, anchovy, yellowtail and yellow-stripe scads, tuna, sardines, torpedo scad, Indian and short-fin scads, pomfret, red snapper, and king mackerel. Prawn and squid were also among the most preferred seafood by study subjects. The most frequently consumed freshwater fish were freshwater catfish and snakehead. The most preferred cooking style by Malaysians was deep-fried fish, followed by fish cooked in thick and/or thin chili gravy, fish curry, and fish cooked with coconut milk mixed with other spices and flavorings. Overall, Malaysians consumed 168 g/day fish, with Malay ethnics' (175 ± 143 g/day) consumption of fish significantly ($p < 0.001$) higher compared with the other two ethnic groups (Chinese = 152 ± 133 g/day, Indians = 136 ± 141 g/day).

Conclusion: Fish consumption was significantly associated with ethnicity, age, marital status, residential area, and years of education of adults in Peninsular Malaysia, and the data collected are beneficial for the purpose of health risk assessment on the intake of contaminants through fish/seafood consumption.

Keywords: *seafood*; *fish*; *consumption pattern*; *Malaysian*; *ethnicity*

Populations in eastern Asia consumed fish with cooked rice daily, or as part of rice dishes or as side dishes (1). Malaysians, in particular, consumed fish at least once a day in the amounts of one and one-half medium fish per day (2). In fact, the annual per capita fish consumption of Malaysian was the second highest after Japan, among Asian nations, or ranked number fifth throughout the world (3). The consumption of fish is an essential part of a healthy and well-balanced diet (4). Potential health benefits related to fish consumption are due to the presence of protein, unsaturated essential fatty acids, minerals, and vitamins (5). Additional health benefits from the consumption of fish or fish oil may relate to polyunsaturated fatty acids (PUFAs), especially eicosapentaenoic acid (EPA) and docosahexaenoic acid (DHA) (5, 6). Fish provide omega-3 fatty acids that could reduce cholesterol levels and the incidence of heart disease, stroke, and preterm delivery (7). It also acts as a mood stabilizer (8), especially among females (9).

In contrast to the potential health benefits of dietary fish intake, fish could be contaminated with environmental toxicants that may pose health risk to human

(6, 10, 11). Major chemical contaminants in fish were methyl mercury and polychlorinated biphenyls, while other potential toxic contaminants were polychlorinated dibenzo-*p*-dioxins, dibenzofurans, and polycyclic aromatic hydrocarbons or pollutants such as polybrominated diphenyl ethers, polychlorinated diphenyl ethers, and polychlorinated naphthalenes (PCNs) (6, 12, 13). These contaminants were the highest contributors to the human daily intake through fish consumption (6). Other possible hazard contributors were cadmium and hexachlorobenzene (6, 12, 14).

Understanding the patterns of fish consumption is the key factor for assessing exposure to harmful chemicals from the ingestion of contaminated fish. Fish consumption is one item that forms the basis of food consumption patterns that are defined as the consumption of specific food items and their combination in dishes and meals (15). Many factors affect fish consumption patterns, which vary widely between countries, and among different cultures as a result of the availability of commodities and economic factors (3, 4, 15–18). The most prominent measures of food consumption behavior are income and price elasticity (19). Other than evaluating the intake and exposure of various contaminants, fish consumption pattern is also important for exploring the difference in patterns, assessing the adequacy of nutrient intake, plus establishing policies in agriculture, production, trade, and health (2, 16, 19).

The objectives of this study were to document the meal patterns among three major ethnics in Malaysia with respect to fish/seafood consumption, and identify the most frequently consumed fish and cooking method. It is also aimed to examine the influence of demographic factors on the pattern of fish consumption among study subjects. The results of this study can be used as a baseline for estimating and assessing the risk of contaminated the seafood consumed by Malaysians.

Material and methods

Study design and subjects

A house-to-house survey was conducted and data were collected through face-to-face interviews using pre-design questionnaires in Peninsular Malaysia, between February 2008 and May 2009. The sampling frame used for the selection of study subjects' household addresses was based on the National Household Sampling Frame (NHSF), Department of Statistics, Malaysia (20). This sampling frame was made up of enumeration blocks (EBs) created for the 2,000 Population and Housing Census. EBs are geographical contiguous areas of land with identifiable boundaries. On average, each EB contains about 80 to 120 living quarters. Generally, all EBs were formed within gazetted boundaries, particularly administrative districts, mukim, or local authority areas.

In order to obtain a representative sample, a two-stage proportionate stratified sampling technique was applied with states as the primary sampling units and urban or rural status as the secondary sampling units. Interviews were done with the head of the household or adult males and females aged 18 years and above residing in the house. The only exclusion criterion was pregnant women.

The sample size (N) calculation was as below:

$$\text{Formulation } N = (Z_{\alpha}^{2}\text{P}(1-\text{P}))/\text{E}^{2} \approx 208\times$$
$$\text{factors of different areas, ethnicity, and age}$$

where:

$Z = 1.96$ (based on 95% CI)

$P =$ Prevalence of seafood consumption in grams per person per day. Based on consumption survey data for the Selangor population (16.2%)

$E =$ Maximum tolerance error (5%)

$\alpha = 0.05$ at 95% CI

Sample size calculated includes 20% expected drop – out

The calculation was based on consumption survey data for the Selangor population, in which the adult population of Selangor consumed fish at 16.2% (153 g/person/day compared with 944 g/person/day total food) (21). In addition, factors of the two different areas (urban and rural), three major ethnics (Malays, Chinese, and Indian), and two different age groups were used at the final stage. The number, 2,496 subjects, was required in order to obtain 95% confidence interval and a 5% margin of error. Taking into account a 20% dropped-off rate, 2,996 subjects were identified. A minimum count of two adults in each household was selected in this survey, and 1,500 household addresses were identified from the NHSF.

At the end of the survey, only 2,704 participated, and a final count of 2,675 subjects completed the questionnaire. Figure 1 showed the household addresses of study subjects plotted throughout Peninsular Malaysia using Quantum GIS 2.8.1. The response rate was 89.2%, and the sample characteristics are given in Table 1.

Questionnaire

The study instrument used was a set of questionnaires that had been validated prior to the study by distributing the questionnaires to other researchers who were not involved in the study. The questionnaires consisted of two parts. The first part comprised nine pages of self-administered questions, which consisted of a socio-demographic information section as well as questions on the pattern of fish consumption, frequency of fish consumption, and a final section on knowledge, perception, and practices toward fish consumption. The second part was three

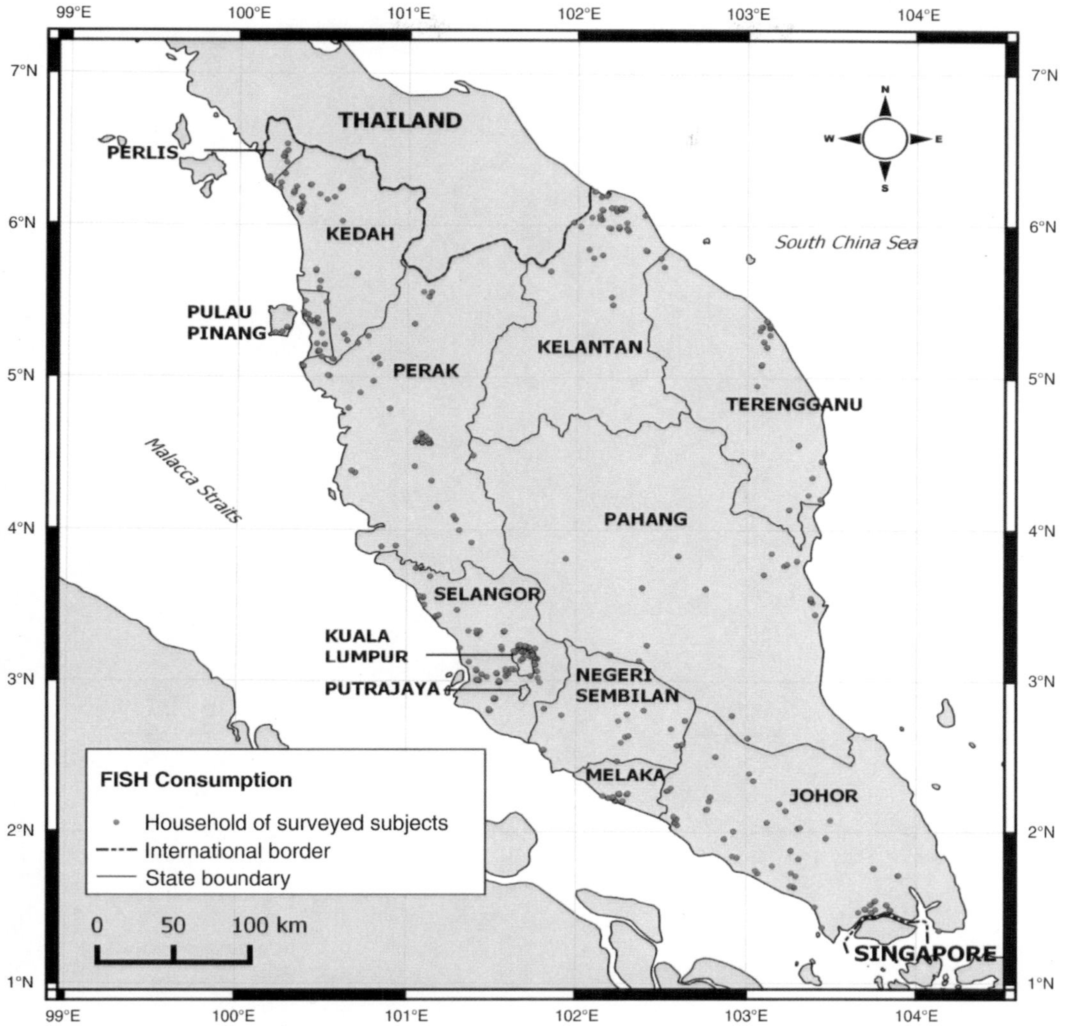

Fig. 1. The household addresses of study subjects plotted throughout Peninsular Malaysia using Quantum GIS 2.8.1.

copies of 24-h dietary diary forms. In this part, subjects were asked to record food and drinks they consumed at every meal of the day. The form was divided into six meal sections (breakfast, morning tea, lunch, afternoon tea, dinner, and supper) that required recording the time, place, and with whom the subjects took each meal. They were also required to record types of food and drinks, the portion size, and cooking style.

The interviewers were trained to review and understand the questionnaires. During training, they were taught how to give instructions to subjects. They were equipped with a set of questionnaire tools to help the subjects record the type of foods they consumed. The questionnaire tools included pictures of serving dishes; fish commonly found in Malaysia; and common household measures, such as standard measuring cups, bowls, ladles, and spoons. The self-administrated questionnaire was given between 9.00 a.m. and 6.00 p.m. but sometimes interviewers had to visit at night because subjects were not home during the day. Interviewers assisted by reading the questionnaires to some of the elderly or illiterate respondents. They also rechecked all food recorded in dietary diary forms to verify the types and amounts of food consumed by subjects.

The portion weight of food was referred to the local food atlas 'Atlas Makanan: Saiz pertukaran dan Porsi' (22, 23) and the nutrient and composition of Malaysian foods (24). If the food consumed was not listed in all these references, at least five different sources were obtained and mean values were calculated as the weight of that particular food. The collection of the 3-day dietary diary was conducted during weekdays and weekends.

The height and weight of study subjects were measured using a calibrated SECA digital weighing machine. The body mass index (BMI) was calculated using the formula of body weight (kg) divided by square roots of height (m^2). The WHO criteria for obesity based on the BMI guidelines (25) was a reference in this study that used the following range: underweight (BMI <18.5 Kg/m^2), normal (BMI 18.5–24.9 Kg/m^2), overweight (BMI 25.0–29.9 Kg/m^2), and obese (BMI ≥ 30 Kg/m^2).

Table 1. Socio-demographic characteristics of the subjects

Socio-demographic Variables	Malaysian ($n = 2,058$)	Chinese ($n = 394$)	Indian ($n = 223$)	Overall Total ($n = 2,675$)	$^{*}p$
Age (year ± SD)	42.7 ± 16.2[a]	48.1 ± 16.3[b]	41.5 ± 15.1[a]	43.4 ± 16.2	0.000
Gender (%)					
Male	44.5	45.9	37.4	44.2	–
Female	55.4	54.1	62.6	55.7	
Body weight (kg ± IQR)	62.0 ± 17.9	60.5 ± 16.8	63.9 ± 20.0	62.0 ± 17.5	**0.001
Height (cm ± SD)	158.0 ± 8.7[a]	160.2 ± 9.1[b]	160.3 ± 9.5[b]	158.5 ± 8.8	0.000
BMI (± SD)	25.6 ± 5.5[a]	24.4 ± 4.9[b]	26.4 ± 6.1[c]	25.4 ± 5.5	0.000
Household number (± SD)	5.2 ± 2.3[a]	4.6 ± 2.4[b]	4.9 ± 2.1[c]	5.1 ± 2.3	0.000
Marital status (%)					
Single	21.1	19.1	19.5	20.6	
Married	71.5	73.4	71.4	71.9	–
Widowed/divorced	7.4	7.5	9.1	7.5	
Residential region (%)					
North	30.4	36.9	50.7	33.0	
Middle	25.1	17.0	39.5	25.2	
South	16.0	36.6	6.3	18.2	
East	28.6	9.4	3.6	23.7	–
Years of education (year ± SD)	9.1 ± 3.9[a]	8.4 ± 4.1[b]	9.1 ± 3.7[a]	9.0 ± 3.9	0.004

IQR is the interquartile range. SD is the standard deviation.

*Significant difference ($p < 0.05$) between different ethnics was evaluated using a one-way ANOVA. Equal variance was assumed using LSD.

**KW A Kruskal–Wallis U test was applied ($\chi^2 = 13.956$).

Different alphabets within the same row indicate significant difference ($p < 0.05$).

Ethical approval

The project was funded by the National Institutes of Health Malaysia, and the proposal was priorly reviewed and approved by the Medical Research and Ethics Committee, Ministry of Health Malaysia. The inform consent and confidentiality was obtained from the subjects beforehand.

Data analysis

Data analyses were conducted using SPSS for Windows version 16.0 (SPSS Inc). The data included demographic characteristics and different categories of the group, and the cooking style of the seafood consumption data. After data entry, a check was made for any discrepancies, including coding numbers, typographical errors, and so on. At the initial stage, descriptive statistics were conducted to assess data normality using a one-sample Kolmogorov–Smirnov test and/or the skewness of descriptive statistics was controlled between −1 and +1, whichever is true. Normally distributed numerical results were expressed as mean ± SD, and the categorical results were expressed in percentage. However, numerical data, which were not normally distributed, were expressed as median ± IQR (interquartile range). Differences between groups were assessed using a Student's *t*-test, and one-way ANOVA with equal variances was assumed using LSD, for normally distributed data. Conversely, for non-normal distributed data, the differences between groups were assessed using the Mann–Whitney *U* and Kruskal–Wallis *H* test. A $p \leq 0.05$ was considered statistically significant.

Results

Subjects characteristics

Table 1 shows the socio-demographic characteristic of the study subjects. The mean age of study subjects was 43.4 ± 16.2 years. The Chinese had significantly ($p < 0.001$) the highest mean age of 48.1 ± 16.3 years compared with the other two ethnics. A gender proportion among subjects was about equal such that the percentages ratio was 44:55 for males and females, respectively. The body weight (kg) and height (cm) measurements for different ethnics showed significantly difference ($p < 0.001$) leading toward significant differences ($p < 0.001$) of the overall BMI as well. The mean BMI was at the overweight range (25.4 ± 5.5), and this is true among Malays and Indians. However, the BMI for the Chinese is at the normal range (24.4 ± 4.9). The mean number of household was five and most of the subjects were married (71.9%), 20.6% of them were single, and only 7.5% were either widowed or divorced. The distribution of subjects throughout the regions was highest at the northern region of Peninsular Malaysia (33%), followed by the middle region (25.2%), the east region

(23.7%), and finally the southern region of the Peninsular Malaysia (18.2%). The mean education years for all ethnics were 9 ± 3.9 years. This shows that most of the subjects completed at least lower secondary school. The Chinese, significantly ($p = 0.004$), had the lowest mean education years (8.4 ± 4.1 years) compared with other ethnics.

Fish/seafood preferences

Generally, the result from this study showed that 33% of the study subjects consumed fish every day from the 3 days of the food survey records (Fig. 2). Another 30.1 and 15% consumed 2 and 1 day, respectively. The remainder of 21.2% subjects did not consume any fish during the 3-day survey. Of the Malays, 38% consumed fish every day during this 3-day records compared with the Chinese (19.8%) and the Indians (13.8%). Conversely, high percentages of Chinese subjects (38.1%) did not consume any fish during the 3-day survey, followed by the Indians (23.2%) and the Malays (17.9%) (Fig. 2). The results also showed that more than half (55–57%) of these study subjects consumed seafood at least one to two meals per day during the 3-day study records.

Table 2 shows fish frequencies captured from the 3-day records of food consumption survey conducted among adults of study subjects. The most consumed fish by adults of Peninsular Malaysia was Indian mackerel. The second most consumed marine fish was anchovy,

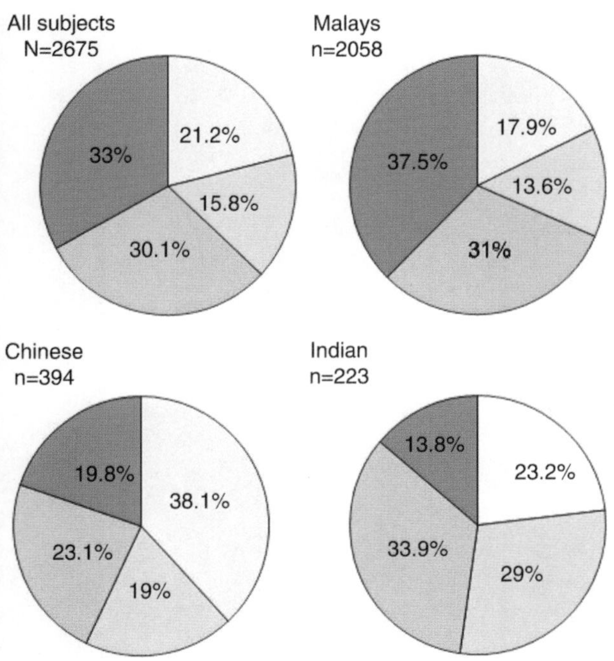

Fig. 2. Number of days (in percentages) in which fish was consumed among the adults of different ethnicities from Peninsular Malaysia, using 3-day records of food consumption as a survey method.

followed by yellowtail and yellow-stripe scads, tuna, sardines, torpedo scads, Indian and short-fin scads, pomfret, red snapper, and king mackerel. Other fish such as threadfin bream, croaker, marine catfish, stingray, and barramundi were also among highly preferred marine fish by study subjects. The following descending orders were another nine types of marine fish that were fairly consumed by study subjects: eel-tailed catfish, John's snapper, toli shad, big eye scads, wolf-herring, queen fish, Indian salmon, bigeye trevally, and mullet. Another 15 types of marine fish were only consumed by less than 10 times, which showed less preference by study subjects.

On the contrary, out of 12 types of freshwater fish consumed during the 3-day diaries, freshwater catfish acquired the highest preference by study subjects, followed by the snakehead fish. Other freshwater fish that were fairly consumed were gourami, iridescent shark, and tilapia. Another seven types of freshwater fish (climbing perch, hampala, mahseer, hoven's carp, Java barb, bagrid catfishes, and pacu) were less consumed by study subjects.

Cephalopods and mollusk were among highly preferred seafood by Malaysian and these preferences fall within the most preferred five groups of marine seafood by Malaysian adults.

Fish cooking style preferences

The most common cooking styles obtained from the 3-day records of food consumption survey conducted among adults of Peninsular Malaysia are shown in Table 3. Deep-fried fish is the cooking style for fish/seafood that was most preferred by study subjects. This was followed by fish cooked in thick chili gravy (*masak sambal*), fish curry, fish cooked in coconut milk with other spices and flavoring (*masak lemak*), and fish cooked in thin chili gravy and other additional spices and flavorings (*Masak asam pedas*). Other cooking styles that were also highly preferred were fish boiled with asam gelugur and lemongrass (*masak singgang*), grilled fish, and deep-fried fish cooked with soy sauce and spices (*masak kicap*). Moderately preferred fish cooking styles were boiled fish, steamed, sweet sour and *masak sos.* Less preferred cooking styles for fish were soup, *masak merah, masak taucu, masak gulai tempoyak,* and *ikan sumbat sambal.* The least preferred cooking styles were *masak tiga rasa, tomyam, masak kurma, masak rendang,* and *paprik*.

Fish consumption among different ethnicity

Table 4 showed the fish consumption among different ethnicities in Peninsular Malaysia. There were no significant differences ($p > 0.05$) for each category of fish/seafood across different ethnics. However, the consumption of marine fish showed marginal significant differences ($\chi^2 = 5.7$; $p = 0.058$), such that the Indians consumed less of this category (81 ± 89 g/day) compared with the other two ethnic groups (Malays $= 100 \pm 88$ g/day; Chinese $= 110 \pm 88$ g/day). Subjects consumed more fish

Table 2. Fish frequencies from 3-day records of food consumption survey conducted among adults of Peninsular Malaysia ($n = 2{,}675$)

No.	Local name	English name	[a]Species	[b]F
Marine fish				
1	Kembung/pelaling/ mabung/temenung	Indian mackerel	*Rastrelliger brachysoma, Rastrelliger faughni, Rastrelliger kanagurta*	1,397
2	Ikan bilis	Anchovy	*Encrasicholina heteroloba, E. punctifer, S. tri, Stolephorus andhraensis, S. baganensis, S. waitei, S. chinensis, S. commersonnii, S. indicus, S. dubiosus, S. insularis, Lycothrissa crocodile*	320
3	Selar kuning/pelata	Scad (yellowtail, yellowstripe, smallmouth)	*Selar crumenopthalmus, Selaroides leptolepis, Seriola dumerili, S. leptolepis, Alepes djedaba, A. melanoptera, A. vari, Atule mate, A. apercna*	280
4	Tongkol	Kawakawa/Tuna/Bonito	*Auxis thazard, Gymnosarda unicolor, Sarda orientalis, Thunnus tonggol, Euthynnus affinis, Katsuwonus pelamis, T. obesus, T. albacares*	236
5	Sardine/tamban	Sardines/pilchards	*Amblygaster sirm, Spratelloides delicatulus, Sardinella fimbriata, S. gibbosa, Dussumieria acuta, S. albella, S. brachysoma, S. jussieui, S. lemuru, S. melanura, Spratelloides gracilis, S. delicatulus*	229
6	Cencaru	Torpedo scad	*Megalaspis cordyla*	190
7	Selayang	Scad (Indian, shortfin, and mackerel)	*Decapterus akaadsi, D. macrosoma, D. maruadsi, D. russelli, D. tabl, D. macarellus, D. kurroides, D. lajang*	172
8	Bawal (hitam and putih)	Pomfret (black and silver)	*Parastromateus niger, Pampus argenteus, P. chinensis*	168
9	Merah	Red Snapper	*Lutjanus lemniscatus, L. malabaricus, L. sanguineus, L. sebae, L. argentimaculatus, L. bohar, L. erythropterus, L. bengalensis, L. boutton, L. decussate, L. dodecacantboides*	105
10	Tenggiri	King Mackerel	*Scomberomorus commerson, S. guttatus, S. lineolatus*	105
11	Kerisi	Threadfin bream	*Nemipterus virgatus, N. peronii, N. nematophorus, N. japonicus, N. bathybius, N. hexodon, N. marginatus, N. mesoprion, N. nemurus, N. thosaporni, N. nematopus, N. furcosus, N. tambuloides, N. isacanthus, N. bipunctatus, N. vitiensis, N. zysron, N. aurora, N. balinensoides*	95
12	Gelama	Croaker	*Johnius amblycephalus, J. goldmani, J. weberi, Chrysochir aureu, Nibea soldado, O. cuvieri, Panna microdon, P. anea, J. borneensis, J. coitor, Paranibea semiluctuosa, J. carouna, Pennahia macrocephalus, J. glaucus, P. pawa, J. macrorhynus, Pterotolithus lateoides, P. maculatus, N. albiflora, J. macropterus, J. trachycephalus, Aspericorvina jubata, Kathala axillaris, Daysciaena albida, Otolithoides pama, Atrobucca kyushini, Bahaba polykladiskos, Boesemania microlepis, J. heterolepis*	90
13	Mayong/seludu/duri/ pelotan	Marine catfish	*Nemapteryx caelata, Plicofollis platystomus, Osteogeneiosus militaris, Arius oetik, A. maculates, N. macronotacantha, Arius jella, Picofollis tenuispinis, P. tonggo, A. venosus, N. macronotacantha, Netuma thalassina, P. tenuispinis, A. platystomus, A. subrostratus, Hemarius sona*	63
14	Pari	Stingray	*Himantura walga, H. lobistoma, Gymnura poecilura, H. bleekeri, Dasyatis kuhlii*	60
15	Siakap	Barramundi	*Lates calcarifer*	46
16	Sembilang	Eel-tailed catfish	*Tandanus tandanus, Plotosus canius*	29
17	Jenahak	John's snapper	*Lutjanus russelli, L. johnii*	29
18	Terubuk	Toli shad	*Tenualosa toli*	20
19	Lolong	Bigeye scad	*Selar crumenophthalmus*	19
20	Parang	Wolf-Herring	*Chirocentrus dorab*	19
21	Talang	Queenfish	*Scomberoides commersonnianus, S. lysan, S. tala*	19
22	Senangin	Indian Salmon	*Eleutheronema tetradactylum*	18
23	Nyok-nyok	Bigeye trevally	*Caranx sexfasciatus*	13
24	Belanak	Mullet	*Moolgarda cunnesius, Mugil cephalus, Chelon planiceps, C. macrolepis, Valamugil buchanani, C. subviridis, C. melanopterus, Moolgarda, M. seheli engeli, Ellochelon vaigiensis, V. speigleri, Liza subviridis, L. vaigiensis, L. macrolepis, Paramugil parmatus*	10
25	Gerut-gerut	Silver Grunter	*Pomadasys argenteus, P. argyreus, P. kaakan, P. olivaceus, P. commersonnii, P. maculatus, P. unimaculatus, P. guoraca, P. hasta, P. multimaculatum*	8
26	Kurau	Atlantic threadfin	*Polydactylus octonemus*	7

Table 2. (Continued)

No.	Local name	English name	[a]Species	[b]F
27	Kekek	Ponyfish	*Photopectoralis bindus, Equulites elongates, Leiognathus equulus, Aurigequula fasciata, E. leuciscus, Eubleekeria splendens, L. berbis, S. indicus, Secutor insidiator, Gazza minuta, L. lineolatus, Karalla daura, N. blochii, E. rivulatus, Nuchequula nuchalis, N. gerreoides, L. brevirostris, S. ruconius, G. achlamys, E. stercorarius, L. longispinis*	6
28	Selangat	Gizzard shad	*Nematalosa come, N. galatheae, N. nasus, Anodontostoma chacunda, A. thailandiae*	6
29	Putih, ebek	Diamond trevally	*Alectis indica, A. ciliaris*	5
30	Yu	Shark	*Nebrius ferrugineus, Carcharhinus leucas*	5
31	Kerapu	Grouper	*Epinephelus sexfasciatus, E. coioides, E. morrhua, Plectropomus maculatus, Grammistes sexlineatus, E. fasciatus, E. cyanopodus, E. ongus, Variola louti, E. areolatus, P. areolatus, E. malabaricus, E. coeruleopunctatus, E. corallicola, Aethaloperca rogaa, Cephalopholis miniata, C. sonnerati, Cromileptes altivelis, E. amblycephalus, E. fasciatomaculosus, E. lanceolatus, E. magniscuttis, E. polyphekadion, E. quoyanus, E. undulosus, V. albimarginata Gracila albomarginata*	5
32	Puput	Chinese herring/slender shad	*Ilisha elongata*	5
33	Sebelah	Halibut	*Psettodes erumei, Pseudorhombus malayanus*	4
34	Biji Nangka	Yellow goatfish	*Upeneus sulphureus*	3
35	Belut	Eel	*Congresox talabonoides*	1
36	Tongsan	Bighead carp	*Hypophthalmichthys nobilis*	1
37	Salmon	Atlantic Salmon	*Salmo salar*	1
38	Kacang-kacang	Barracuda	*Sphyraena jello*	1
39	Jolong	Halfbeaks	*Dermogenys pusilla, Hemiramphus achipelagicus, H. far, H. lutkei, N. marginatus, Hyporhamphus dussumieri, H. limbatus, H. quoyi, H. xanthopterus, Rhynchorhamphus georgi, Zenarchopterus dispar, Z. ectuntio, Z. gilli*	1
Freshwater fish				
1	Keli	Freshwater catfish	*Clarias batrachus*	77
2	Haruan	Snakehead fish	*Channa micropeltes*	31
3	Sepat	Gourami	*Trichogaster trichopterus, Trichopodus pectoralis*	19
4	Patin	Iridescent shark	Pangasius hypophthalmus	17
5	Talapia	Tilapia	*Oreochromis mossambicus*	13
6	Puyu	Climbing perch	*Anabas testudineus*	9
7	Sebarau	Hampala	*Hampala macrolepidota*	7
8	Kelah	Mahseer	Tor tambroides	6
9	Jelawat	Hoven's carp	*Leptobarbus hoevenii*	3
10	Lampam	Java barb	*Barbonymus gonionotus, B. schwanenfeldii*	2
11	Baung	Bagrid catfishes	*Chrysichthys nigrodigitatus*	2
12	Pacu	Pacu	*Piaractus mesopotamicus*	1
Cephalopods and mollusk				
1	Udang	Prawn and shrimp	*Penaeus monodon, P. semisulcatus, M. affinis, P. japonicus, Parapenaeopsis sculptilis, M. ensis, Metapenaeus brevicornis, M. barbata, Parapenaeospsis hardwickii, P. merguiensis, P. indicus, Parapenaeospsis hardwickii, P. latisulcatus* Kishinouye	298
2	Sotong	Squid and octopus	*Loligo uyii, Cistopus indicus, L. chinensis, L. duvauceli, L. edulis, L. sibogue, Sepia esculenta, S. phuruonis*	263

[a]Species names were based on fish landed and/or available at the wholesale market in Peninsular Malaysia (26–28) and at the website: www.fishbase.org/ComNames/CommonNameSearchList.

[b]The frequency of fish obtained from the subjects of the food consumption survey (3-day records). Of the fish consumption records, 40% did not mentioned fish name, and therefore are not included in this list.

(marine fish 100±87 g/day; freshwater fish 106±130 g/day) compared with other types of seafood, namely cephalopod and mollusk. Although the higher frequencies of consumption of cephalopod and mollusk were observed in Table 2, the amount of consumption per person per day was much lower compared with marine

Table 3. Frequencies of cooking style obtained from 3-day records of the food consumption survey conducted among adults of Peninsular Malaysia ($n = 2{,}675$)

No	Cooking styles	Cooking description	[a]F
1	Goreng	Deep-fried seafood marinated with salt and turmeric powder.	2,021
2	Masak sambal	Deep-fried seafood cooked in chili, shrimp paste, and tamarind paste. Thick gravy.	521
3	Masak kari	Seafood curry. Cooked with curry powder and coconut milk.	401
4	Masak lemak	Seafood boiled in coconut milk, spices, and flavorings such as lemongrass, basil leaves (*Ocimum sanctum*), turmeric leaves (*Curcuma domestic*), and asam gelugur (dried *Garcinia atroviridis*).	320
5	Masam asam pedas	Seafood cooked with chili, tamarind paste, and other spices and flavorings; kesum leaves (*Polygonum minus*) and ginger flower (*Etlingera elatior*). Thin gravy.	309
6	Masak singgang	Seafood boiled with asam gelugur (dried *Garcinia atroviridis*) and lemongrass.	158
7	Bakar	Grilled (charcoal, flat pan or oven).	148
8	Masak kicap	Deep-fried seafood cook with soy sauce and spices.	144
9	Rebus	Seafood boiled with onion, salt, and asam gelugur (dried *Garcinia atroviridis*).	67
10	Stim	Fish seasoned with soy sauce, coriander, onion, and other flavorings, cook with steamer.	45
11	Masak masam manis	Deep-fried seafood cooked in a sauce containing sugar, vinegar, or lemon and pineapple (especially of Chinese-style food).	43
12	Masak sos	Deep-fried seafood cooked with chili and tomato sauce.	40
13	Sup	Seafood boiled with soup spices and some flavorings (onion, garlic, ginger, and celery).	27
14	Masak merah	Deep-fried seafood cooked in red spicy tomato sauce other spices and flavorings.	25
15	Masak taucu	Deep-fried seafood cooked with minced bean paste, onion, and vegetables	21
16	Masak Gulai tempoyak	Seafood cooked with fermented durian, chili, and coconut milk.	19
17	Sumbat sambal	Completely dressed fish, which is stuffed with sambal belacan (chili and shrimp paste) and grated coconut before being deep-fried or grilled.	11
18	Masak tiga rasa	Deep-fried fish vinaigrette with sweet, hot and sour gravy, and mixed vegetables.	4
19	Tomyam	Seafood cooked in Thai hot and sour soup. The basic broth is made of stock and fresh ingredients such as lemongrass, kaffir lime leaves, galangal, lime juice, fish sauce, and crushed chili peppers.	2
20	Masak kurma	Seafood cooked with korma powder, coconut milk, yogurt, and other spices and flavorings.	2
21	Masak rendang	Seafood cooked with coconut milk and a paste of mixed ground spices, which includes ginger, galangal, turmeric leaves, lemon grass, garlic, shallot, chilies, and other spices.	1
22	Paprik	Deep-fried seafood cooked in chili paste, oyster sauce, mixed vegetables, spices, and flavorings.	1

[a]The frequency of cooking styles obtained from the subjects of the food consumption survey (3-day records).

fish and freshwater fish. No significant differences ($p > 0.05$) among different ethnics were shown for the consumption of seafood from different habitats. However, the results showed that study subjects consumed more demersal fish (112 ± 109 g/day) compared with fish from other habitats.

The Indians consumed more Indian mackerels compared with the other ethnicities, as shown by marginal significant differences ($\chi^2 = 5.32$; $p = 0.070$) between different ethnic groups. On the contrary, the Malays and Chinese consumed significantly ($\chi^2 = 7.89$; $p = 0.019$) higher amounts of black and silver pomfret compared with the Indians. None of the consumption patterns for the other types of fish showed significant differences ($p > 0.05$) between ethnicities. However, the total consumption of different seafood categories indicated that the subjects consumed more yellow tail and yellow-stripe scads (108 ± 74 g/day) and torpedo scads (100 ± 73 g/day) compared with other fish/seafood categories. Details on the consumption data disclosed that none of the Indians consumed torpedo scads, Indian scads, and short-fin scads within the 3-day survey. Only one Chinese subject consumed tuna, sardines, Indian, and short-fin scads captured during this study.

There were significant differences between consumption of deep-fried fish ($\chi^2 = 6.57$; $p = 0.037$) and boiled fish ($\chi^2 = 7.39$; $p = 0.025$) among different ethnicities. The Malaysians preferred ($p = 0.037$) deep-fried fish, while the Chinese were in favor ($p = 0.025$) of boiled fish. The total consumption of each cooking category showed approximately similar amounts for the different ethnicities, with grilled and steamed fish consumed least.

The Chinese consumed significantly ($p = 0.036$) more seafood during breakfast, while the Malays consumed more during lunchtime ($p < 0.001$). No significant differences were shown for the consumption of seafood in dinner meals ($p > 0.05$) by different ethnics. The results showed that more seafood were consumed during dinner (91 g/day) compared with lunchtime (88 g/day), but the least was consumed during breakfast (60 g/day).

Table 4. Seafood consumption (g/person/day) ($\pm$IQR)[a] among adults of different ethnics in Peninsular Malaysia

Food category	Ethnicity Malaysian ($n=2{,}058$)	Chinese ($n=394$)	Indian ($n=223$)	Total ($n=2{,}675$)	χ^2 (p)[f]
Marine fish	100 ± 88	110 ± 88	81 ± 89	100 ± 87	5.70 (0.058)
Freshwater fish	105 ± 130	260 ± 374	220	106 ± 130	2.80 (0.242)
Cephalopod	90 ± 70	101 ± 48	80 ± 240	90 ± 70	0.22 (0.896)
Mollusk	41 ± 70	30 ± 96	30 ± 88	40 ± 70	0.84 (0.656)
[b]Habitat category					
Demersal fish	112 ± 110	100 ± 146	145 ± 171	112 ± 109	1.63 (0.443)
Others	97 ± 81	110 ± 83	82 ± 86	97 ± 80	4.55 (0.103)
[c]Seafood category					
Indian mackerel	80 ± 57	80 ± 66	110 ± 52	80 ± 66	5.32 (0.070)
Anchovy	22 ± 28	30 ± 33	30 ± 58	24 ± 28	3.43 (0.180)
Scad (Yellowtail, Yelowstripe, and Smallmouth)	100 ± 74	125 ± 127	100 ± 117	108 ± 74	1.04 (0.594)
Kawakawa/Tuna/Bonito,	60 ± 55	120	60	60 ± 55	2.78 (0.249)
Sardines, and Pilchards	43 ± 47	229	41 ± 62	48 ± 56	1.54 (0.463)
Torpedo scad	110 ± 73	100 ± 9	–	100 ± 73	0.08 (0.778)
Scad (Indian, shortfin, and mackerel)	90 ± 61	315	–	92 ± 66	1.49 (0.222)
Pomfret (Black and Silver)	91 ± 84	95 ± 35	60 ± 14	90 ± 60	7.89 (0.019)
Cooking category					
Deep fried[d]	100 ± 79	85 ± 66	80 ± 72	97 ± 77	6.57 (0.037)
Boiled[e]	101 ± 94	110 ± 122	80 ± 77	99 ± 93	7.39 (0.025)
Grilled and Steamed	81 ± 66	68 ± 65	89	80 ± 59	1.99 (0.369)
Intake of seafood per meal					
Breakfast	60 ± 50	177 ± 154	75 ± 117	60 ± 51	6.67 (0.036)
Lunch	90 ± 66	80 ± 55	78 ± 50	88 ± 62	15.35 (0.000)
Dinner	93 ± 67	89 ± 87	85 ± 78	91 ± 68	2.91 (0.234)
Total consumption	175 ± 143	152 ± 133	136 ± 141	168 ± 140	16.25 (0.000)

IQR is the interquartile range.
[a]The calculations were based on the 3-day records from Food Consumption Survey conducted throughout Peninsular Malaysia. The portion size of seafood was based on published local data (22–24).
[b]Classifications were referred to the publication by the Department of Fisheries Malaysia (27). Others included pelagic, reef-associated, benthopelagic, and bathypelagic.
[c]The list of seafood was based on the most frequently consumed (frequent count >150) (Table 2).
[d]Deep-fried fish and any cooking styles that involved the deep-frying of seafood before the addition of gravy and other spices. Examples are masak sambal, masak kicap, masak masam manis, masak sos, masak merah, masak taucu, sumbat sambal, masak tiga rasa and paprik (Table 3).
[e]Seafood cooked with various other ingredients, such as spices and flavorings and often containing clear or thick liquid/gravy, with onion, garlic, or other spices stir-fried. Examples are masak kari, masak lemak, masak asam pedas, masak singgang, rebus, sup, masak gulai tempoyak, tomyam, masak kurma, and masak rendang (Table 3).
[f]Significant differences ($p<0.05$) between different ethnics were evaluated using the Kruskal–Wallis H test.

Total consumption of seafood by adult of different ethnicity from Peninsular Malaysia was 168 ± 140 g/day. The results from this study showed that the amount of seafood consumed by different ethnics were significantly different ($p<0.001$). The Malays consumed the highest amount (175 ± 143 g/person/day), followed by the Chinese (152 ± 133 g/person/day) and the least amount by the Indians (136 ± 141 g/person/day).

Fish consumption by different factors

Table 5 showed the differences of seafood consumption by the adults of Peninsular Malaysia with different factors. Amount of seafood consumed showed significant difference ($p<0.01$) between age groups. The results showed that older people consumed significantly more fish ($p=0.02$) compared with the younger ones. No significant differences ($p>0.05$) were shown between seafood consumption and different gender, as well as BMI status. Married subjects consumed significantly more seafood ($p<0.001$) compared with those who were single, widowed, or divorced. Subjects resided around the northern and eastern coastal regions, consumed significantly ($p<0.001$) more seafood compared with other areas. Subjects with higher years of education consumed significantly less

Table 5. Comparison of seafood consumptions in Peninsular Malaysia with different factors ($n = 2{,}675$)

No	Factors	n	Median ± IQR	χ^2 (p)
1	Ethnic			
	Malay	1,694	175 ± 143	KW16.253 (0.000)
	Chinese	244	153 ± 134	
	Indian	172	138 ± 139	
2	Age			
	18–40 years old	905	160 ± 141	KW12.17 (0.002)
	41–59 years old	859	174 ± 141	
	≥60 years old	368	176 ± 139	
3	Gender			
	Male	932	174 ± 140	MW538955 (0.180)
	Female	1,197	164 ± 142	
4	BMI			
	Normal	881	172 ± 140	MW365744 (0.588)
	Others	843	167 ± 144	
5	Marital status			
	Married	1,568	176 ± 142	MW361617 (0.000)
	Others	539	148 ± 133	
6	Residential area by state			
	North (Perlis, P. Pinang, Kedah, and Perak)	742	186 ± 145	KW75.903 (0.000)
	Middle (Selangor, WP Kuala Lumpur, and N. Sembilan)	527	147 ± 126	
	South (Melaka and Johor)	325	154 ± 119	
	East (Pahang, Terengganu, and Kelantan)	538	182 ± 155	
7	Years of Education			
	≤6years	636	172 ± 133	KW19.436 (0.000)
	7–11 years	965	170 ± 142	
	≥12 years	299	136 ± 135	

KWThe Kruskal–Wallis and MWMann–Whitney U tests were applied.

seafood ($p < 0.001$), compared with the other groups with less educational years.

Discussion

The present study explored a cross-cultural difference for patterns of fish/seafood consumption among adults of the three major ethnicities in Peninsular Malaysia. This study had several advantages whereby fish/seafood consumption patterns were collected using successive 3-day record surveys (dietary diaries) throughout both rural and urban areas of Peninsular Malaysia. This study also involved all adults from selected households and covered both the weekdays and weekends. A good cooperation obtained from study subjects resulted in high response rates (89.2%) of the survey demonstrating obliging Malaysians, a supportive and mature society.

Malaysia is a multiracial and multi-religion community in which all populations accept fish and seafood compared with meat-based protein foods, such as pork and beef, which are prohibited among Muslims and Hindus, respectively. Malaysians consume fish and seafood not only because of these concerns but also because it is the cheapest meat protein available in this country (29). This is because a long coastal line of 4,800 km facing both the South China Sea and the Straits of Malacca covers Peninsular Malaysia, where coastal and deep-sea fisheries activities are prime sectors (30). Results from this study verified these scenarios by showing that many Malaysians (33%)—especially the Malays—consumed fish/seafood every day or at least 4 to 5 days a week (30%). Another group (15%) consumed fish and seafood twice a week. These results, in summary, show that about 78% of Malaysians consumed fish at least twice per week. In addition, the results also showed that many subjects consumed seafood every day or at least twice a day. These findings are summarized in Fig. 2. Findings from our study were in agreement with another study (31) that reported that many of the study subjects, farmers in Muda Irrigation Area in Kedah, consumed fish (22.7%) and other seafood (22.2%) one to three times per week. Similar findings were also reported in Singapore, another South East Asian country, where people consumed fish and seafood every day and sometimes twice a day. In addition, people consumed more than one meat or fish and seafood for most of their meals per day (1).

The frequent intake of fish and seafood could also be explained by way of the traditional eating cultures practiced in this country and countries with similar eating pattern, especially around Southeast Asia. It is common for Malaysians to eat at least four times a day (breakfast, lunch, tea, and dinner) and the multiracial Malaysians consumed cooked rice or 'nasi putih' with side dishes of variable cooking styles of the fish and seafood, meat or chicken, and vegetables twice a day (32). These foods were served, especially during lunch and dinner. Meanwhile, most Malaysians enjoyed 'nasi lemak' (rice cooked in coconut milk), fried rice, fried noodle, and 'roti canai' (circular flatbread) for breakfast. These dishes were served either together with a variety of cooking styles of meat-based protein or added as an ingredient in the main dishes. For example, 'nasi lemak' is usually consumed with anchovy or other seafood, such as prawn, squid, or cockles cooked in chilies. Fish/seafood was also used as an ingredient in many other Malaysian traditional snacks/kuih (cakes), such as prawn fritters, spring rolls, curry puff, 'cucur badak' (deep-fried round mashed sweet potato with wheat flour and prawn and coconut fillings), 'pulut udang' (glutinous rice cooked with coconut milk and prawn and coconut fillings), prawn/fish crackers, and the immensely popular 'keropok lekor' (deep-fried fish sausages), which are popular dishes during tea.

A nation-wide study, the Malaysian Adults Nutrition Survey (MANS), carried out between October 2002 and December 2003, revealed that an average of two and a half plates of cooked rice was consumed by 97% of population twice daily with one medium marine fish per day. Examples of preferred marine fish consumed in this study were 'ikan kembung' (Indian mackerel), 'ikan tenggiri' (Spanish mackerel), and 'ikan merah' (red snapper) (2). The findings from this current study were also in agreement with this nation-wide study in which 'ikan kembung' that mainly included three species caught in this country, *Rastrelliger brachysoma*, *Rastrelliger faughni,* and *Rastrelliger kanagurta*, were among the most preferred fish by the study subjects, while Spanish mackerel and red snapper were among 10 most preferred fish. Another important finding from the nation-wide study was that the daily intake of marine fish, including anchovy, was significantly higher among rural adults (51%) compared with urban adults (34%) (2). On the contrary, in this current study, anchovy was the second most preferred fish by study subjects, notwithstanding its mean consumption per day (24 ± 28 g/person/day), which was not significantly different among ethnicities. This pattern was similar to other types of fish as well, except for black and silver pomfret, for which the consumption was significantly less by the Indians when compared with the other two ethnicities.

A study on food intake conducted among the young generation in Malaysia (aged less than 30 years) revealed that Malays and others ate rice more frequently than the Chinese and Indians (33). On the intake of side dishes, the preferences went to chicken, followed by fish but among different ethnicities, the Chinese preferred chicken and meat, the Indians like shrimp and squid, while the Malays like to take fish (33). These results contradicted the findings from our study that Malays and the Chinese consumed more marine fish compared with Indians, and the differences were at the borderline of statistical significance ($p = 0.058$). There were no significant ethnic differences for the consumption of cephalopods, mollusks, and freshwater fish as well. The differences may be due to an age factor because our study subjects' ages ranged from 18 to 103 years, with an overall average of 43.4 ± 16.2 years old. Only 40% of subjects in our study were younger than 30 years old.

Data from the study of the household consumption, by purpose, during the period of 2000–2009, showed that expenditures on food and non-alcoholic beverages accounted for about 23% of the total household expenditure for Malaysians, the largest single component (34). Another study on the share of food and fish expenditures, out of the total budget of Asian households, concluded that, overall, fish contributed the third largest share, ranging between 5 and 21% (35). The same researchers also found that fish expenditures by Malaysians were the highest (21%) followed by Bangladeshis (20%) and Vietnamese (19%). Their results highlighted the important role of fish in the animal-protein intake of most Asian households (35). In addition, economic development has shifted the Malaysian food consumption trend away from basic staple food (i.e. rice) and other traditional food crops (sweet potatoes, cassava, pulses, and oil seeds) to non-traditional, staple, wheat-based items, and meat, fruit and vegetables (36–39). Income, actual prices, relative prices, and demographic factors (38) are the driving forces behind the changes in the Malaysian food consumption trend. Of the widening role of income growth, food demand has shifted toward high-quality-differentiated characteristics, such as freshness, safety, texture, and appearance (38). Moreover, consumers were more willing to pay for these qualitative characteristics (38). In affluent societies like Malaysia, the diversification in the food basket is more likely to be filled by more non-staple foods for the calorie intake, hence implying a stronger purchasing power of the society to demand for higher value food products mainly (meat and fish) and functional food products (mainly vegetable and fruits) (38). A study by Sheng and co-workers had estimated expenditure elasticity among Malaysians and reported that the demand for meat (1.4064), fish (1.244), vegetables (1.1729), and fruits (1.0905) are likely to grow faster than other traditional main energy sources, such as rice (0.9091) and bread and other cereals (0.3177), corresponding to the positive income effect (40). Malaysians with higher income level will seek for a better food quality in terms of nutrition, hygiene, organic, and other features. According to another study by the same group of researchers (41), Malay consumers have different food consumption patterns than the general Malaysian diets. According to them, the Malay consumers increased their consumption of rice more than higher value food (meat and fish) and functional foods (vegetable and fruits). Their findings also showed that Malay consumers are sensitive to the prices of most food products, especially rice (41).

As the Malaysian lifestyle shifts from rural to urban, diet and activity levels have changed accordingly, such that large numbers of the urban population habitually eat out (42). Eating habits have shifted to the convenience of prepared and processed meals, hence changing the food consumption pattern of Malaysian communities. Traditional diets are being replaced with diets higher in fats, salts, and animal products and often with a lower intake of fresh fruits and vegetables (37). The change from traditional to fast-food eating habits is a major factor in the rising epidemic of obesity and associated chronic diseases in this country (43). Nevertheless, meals prepared at home are still favored, especially by those in rural areas, where older Malaysians still preferred traditional meals (32, 42). The younger generation seeks convenience options, such as noodles, fried rice, and soup (32). It was reported that the practice of eating out had become a trend among urban workers, students, and even families because they could not go home to eat (42) or because there was nobody at home to prepare home-cooked meals (44). Factors such as working away from home, working mothers, and food varieties served in many premises encouraged the practice of eating out (42, 44). In this country, strong players in food services include the mamak and kopitiam restaurants, where one can enjoy traditional food such as beef rendang (dry spice coconut beef dish), Laksa (tangy fish noodle soup), char kway teow, fried noodle, roti canai, and so on (32). Food caterers were also available to serve at formal functions such as meetings, seminars, or religious and family occasions (42). This pattern of eating changes, however, may not affect the pattern of fish and seafood consumption among elder people but may affect the younger generation in Malaysia.

The trend of the per capita consumption of fish is consistent with the increase in national wealth, which shifted almost 47% in 2000, as compared with 1985 (43). The consumption of fish per person in Malaysia, in 2005, was around 57.3 kg/person/year (39). These data were equivalent to data from our study, in which the overall fish consumption by Malaysian adults was 168 ± 140 g/person/day or 54.77 kg/person/year. With this level of fish consumption, Malaysians ranked third after the Japanese (64.7 kg/person/year) and Koreans (51 kg/person/year) (39). Compared with other regional countries, the subjects in this study consumed more fish and seafood than those in Thailand (31 kg/person/year), Philippines (29.6 kg/person/year), The Republic of China (25.4 kg/person/year), Indonesia (19 kg/person/year), Bangladesh (10.9 Kg/person/year), and India (4.6 kg/person/year) (36, 39). Total consumption of fish and seafood in our study was around 40% higher when compared with Western countries such as Australia (22.7 kg/person) and the United States (23.4 kg/person) (39). The fish consumption by Spanish (range: 50.9–72 g/person/day or 18.6–26 kg/person/year) and the Norwegians (range: 42.9–63.3 g/person/day or 15.7–23.1 kg/person/year) (45) were equivalent to the intake by Australia and the United States as reported by Warr and co-workers (39). However, for other European countries, fish consumption was even lower, ranging from 4 to 23 kg/person/year or 13–72 g/person/day (45).

York and Gossard had studied the influenced of fish consumption by cultural or geographical regions and summarized that consumption trends cannot be explained by economic or ecological perspectives alone (3). They reported that for each $1,000 of per capita GDP, Asians eat 2.31 additional kilograms per year of fish, whereas Westerners eat only 0.79 additional kilograms (3). It appears that economic development spurs Asians to eat considerably more compared with other cultural regions and it is similar for non-Asian regions in the consumption of meat (3). In both Asia and Europe, the low proportion of freshwater fish in per capita fish consumption indicated the preference for marine fish (inclusive brackish-water fish). This trend is quite evident in areas where aquaculture is growing fast, such as East and Southeast Asia. Moreover, the majority of the cultured marine species are high value and depend on high-quality complete diets (46). Factors influencing fish consumption included an increment in income and urbanization among populations in developing countries, while increased consumer awareness of the health and nutritional benefits of seafood, standardization, and the availability of products and cheaper prices affected consumption in developed countries (46). The relationships between income and urbanization, and fish consumption are clearly important factors to be taken into consideration in the calculation of future fish demand and the type of fish because of the global trend toward urbanization (46).

Medical research had shown that substituting the intake of meat with a food mix in which fat fish or lean fish and fish oil, combined with vegetables, may improve the quality of fat consumption, reduce consumer's calorie intake, and prevent lifestyle diseases (47). A study of the importance of seafood as a nutrient source in the diet of Belgian adolescents concluded that increased seafood consumption would lead to a higher intake of EPA, DHA, and vitamin D. These long-chain omega-3 PUFAs can be associated with several health benefits, such as a reduction in the risk of coronary heart disease, a decrease in mild hypertension, prevention of certain cardiac arrhythmias, and sudden death (48). In line with these researches, Verbeke and Vackier had applied the theory of planned behavior for understanding the determinants of fish consumption behavior among 429 Belgians in 2003 (11). They reported that the taste and healthy image of fish are two well-appreciated characteristics, but the bones in fish and the price of fish are identified as the most likely attitudinal barriers to more frequent fish consumption. Another study conducted among Norwegian women, aged 45–69 years, addressing health and seafood consumption had revealed that seafood consumption increased with increasing belief in the idea that diet is important for health, the use of medicine for cardiovascular disease, other healthy eating habits, increasing age, increasing household size, decreasing family income, and residence in coastal areas (18, 47).

Consumption of fish and seafood can either be essential for a healthy and well-balanced diet or may pose a health risk to consumers from environmental toxicants. Many developed countries had evaluated and issued fish advisories or bans to limit the exposure to contaminants that may accumulate in fish tissue. Information on fish consumption rates is necessary in order to accurately assess exposure to harmful chemicals from the ingestion of contaminated fish (4). Therefore, the main purpose of the study in collecting these fish and seafood data is to calculate and assess the health risk of exposure to contaminants from fish consumption, which will be reported in the next article. The variables from these data were analyzed in detail in order to correctly reflect consumption rates by particular ethnicities, different age groups, socioeconomic statuses, types of fish/seafood, and sources of fish and seafood.

Conclusions

The present results were obtained by applying a successive 3-day food record survey throughout both rural and urban areas and were conducted among subjects aged 10 or more years, selected from the three major ethnic groups in Peninsular Malaysia. Many other analyses would be possible because of the large set of recorded variables. For example, a subsample of 10- to −17-year-old children and teenagers had already been analyzed with regard to food consumption patterns and obesity (49). In this paper, the main results illustrated the most relevant aspect of fish and seafood consumption patterns for the adult population. The discussion has emphasized fish consumption frequencies or most consumed fish and seafood, most preferred cooking style, the amount of fish and seafood consumed by different types and groups of fish and seafood, cooking style, and the intake of fish and seafood per meal by three major ethnicities in Malaysia.

The advantage of the study is that the results may generalize the consumption pattern of fish and seafood among Malaysian adults as all adults in a selected household unit was included as study subjects. Moreover, the applied prospective diet record implemented in this study may offer higher accuracy of fish and seafood consumption estimates. Similar methodology may be applied for future research.

The limitation of this study was the poor response to the type of fish consumed because 40% of the fish and seafood consumption records do not mention the fish by name. Therefore, the calculation for fish and seafood consumption data were only included in the total seafood consumption. This data deficiency might be due to limited knowledge and the inability of the study subjects to identify fish type or name. Despite its limitations, this study provided a necessary update of information on fish and seafood consumption in Malaysia. Although a few similar food consumption surveys have been conducted at the national level by other researchers, our study complements those studies by providing detailed information on fish and seafood consumption. The data collected is beneficial for the purpose of health risk assessment of the intake of contaminants through fish and seafood consumption. Lastly, the experience acquired while conducting this study will be very useful for refining survey tools and data-processing procedures for future studies.

Acknowledgements

The work described in this paper was carried out with financial support from the National Institute of Health (NIH), Ministry of Health Malaysia. Project number: NON CAM- JPP-IMR-07-025. The authors thank all subjects for their cooperation in this survey; the research assistants who participated in the fieldwork; and the support staff of Environmental Health Research Center, Institute for Medical Research, who directly or indirectly supported the project. We would like to thank the Director-General of Health Malaysia for his permission to publish this article.

Conflict of interest and funding

The authors declare that they have no conflict of interest.

References

1. Burger J, Fleischer J, Gochfeld M. Fish, shellfish, and meat meals of the public in Singapore. Environ Res 2003; 92: 254–61. doi: http://dx.doi.org/10.1016/S0013-9351(03)00015-X
2. Norimah AK, Safiah M, Jamal K, Haslinda S, Zuhaida H, Rohida S, et al. Food consumption patterns: findings from the Malaysian Adult Nutrition Survey (MANS). Malays J Nutr 2008; 14(1): 25–39.
3. York R, Gossard MH. Cross-national meat and fish consumption: exploring the effects of modernization and ecological context. Ecol Econ 2004; 48: 293–302. doi: http://dx.doi.org/10.1016/j.ecolecon.2003.10.009
4. Moya J, Itkin C, Selevan SG, Rogers JW, Clickner RP. Estimates of fish consumption rates for consumers of bought and self-caught fish in Connecticut, Florida, Minnesota and North Dakota. Sci Total Environ 2008; 403: 89–98. doi: http://dx.doi.org/10.1016/j.scitotenv.2008.05.023
5. Sidhu KS. Health benefits and potential risks related to consumption of fish or fish oil. Regul Toxicol Pharmacol 2003; 38: 336–44. doi: http://dx.doi.org/10.1016/j.yrtph.2003.07.002
6. Domingo JL, Bocio A, Falco G, Llobet JM. Benefit and risk of fish consumption part 1. A quantitative analysis of the intake of omega-3 fatty acids and chemical contaminants. Toxicology 2007; 230: 219–26. doi: http://dx.doi.org/10.1016/j.tox.2006.11.054
7. Burger J. Fishing, fish consumption and knowledge about advisories in college students and others in central New Jersey. Environ Res 2005; 98: 268–75. doi: http://dx.doi.org/10.1016/j.envres.2004.09.003
8. Silvers KM, Scott KM. Fish consumption and self-reported physical and mental health status. Public Health Nutr 2002; 5(3): 427–31. doi: http://dx.doi.org/10.1079/PHN2001308
9. Timonen M, Horrobin D, Jokelainen J, Laitinen J, Herva A, Räsänen P. Fish consumption and depression: the Northern Finland 1966 birth cohort study. J Affect Disord 2004; 82: 447–52. doi: http://dx.doi.org/10.1016/j.jad.2004.02.002
10. Castro-Gon(alez MI, Mendez-Armenta M. Heavy metal: implications association to fish consumption. Environ Toxicol Phar 2008; 26: 263–71. doi: http://dx.doi.org/10.1016/j.etap.2008.06.001
11. Verbeke W, Vackier I. Individual determinants of fish consumption: application of the theory of planned behavior. Appetite 2005; 4: 67–82. doi: http://dx.doi.org/10.1016/j.appet.2004.08.006

12. Domingo JL, Falco G, Llobet JM, Casas C, Teixido A, Muller L. Polycyclic naphthalenes in foods: estimated dietary intake by the population of Catalonia. Spain. Environ Sci Technol 2003; 37: 2332–5.
13. Bocio A, Llobet JM, Domingo JL, Corbella J, Teixido A, Casas C. Polybrominated diphenyl ethers (PBDEs) in food-stuffs: human exposure through the diet. J Agric Food Chem 2003; 51: 3191–5. doi: http://dx.doi.org/10.1021/jf0340916
14. Llobet JM, Falco G, Casas C, Teixido A, Domingo JL. Concentrations of arsenic, cadmium, mercury and lead in common foods and estimated daily intake by children, adolescents, adults and seniors of Catalonia, Spain. J Agric Food Chem 2003; 51: 838–42. doi: http://dx.doi.org/10.1021/jf020734q
15. Gerbens-Leenes PW, Nonhebel S, Krol MS. Food consumption patterns and economic growth. Increasing affluence and the use of natural resources. Appetite. 2010; 55: 597–608. doi: http://dx.doi.org/10.1016/j.appet.2010.09.013
16. Moomaw W, Griffin T, Kurczak K, Lomax J. The critical role of global food consumption patterns in achieving sustainable food system and food for all, p. 44. A UNEO discussion paper, United Nations Environment Programme, Division of Technology, Industry and Economics, Paris, France; 2012. p. 44. Available from: http://fletcher.tufts.edu/CIERP/ ~ /media/Fletcher/Microsites/CIERP/Publications/2012/UNEP Global Food Consumption.pdf [cited 26 May 2015].
17. Olsen SO, Scholderer J, Brunso K, Verbeke W. Exploring the relationship between convenience and fish consumption: a cross-cultural study. Appetite 2007; 49: 84–91.
18. Trondsen T, Scholderer J, Lund E, Eggen AE. Perceived barrier to consumption of fish among Norwegian women. Appetite 2003; 41: 301–14. doi: http://dx.doi.org/10.1016/j.appet.2006.12.002
19. Muhammad A, Seale JL Jr., Meade B, Regmi A. International evidence on food consumption patterns. An update using 2005 International comparison program data, p. 59. United States Department of Agriculture. Technical Bulletin no. (TB-1929); 2011. p. 59. Available from: http://www.ers.usda.gov/media/129561/tb1929.pdf [cited 26 March 2015].
20. Statistical Department of Malaysia. Press statement: Population distribution and basic demographic characteristics report population and housing census 2000. 2001. Available from: http://www.statistics.gov.my/English/pressdemo.htm [cited 10 July 2015].
21. Nurul Izzah A. Penilaian risiko pengambilan sisa racun perosak terpilih melalui pemakanan sayur-sayuran di kalangan penduduk dewasa di negeri Selangor. PhD thesis, Universiti Kebangsaan Malaysia, Malaysia; 2007.
22. Suzana S, Noor Aini MY, Nik Shanita S, Rafidah G, Roslina A. Atlas Makanan: saiz pertukaran dan Porsi. 2nd ed. Universiti Kebangsaan Malaysia. Kuala Lumpur: MDC Publishers & Printers Sdn Bhd; 2009.
23. Suzana S, Rafidah G, Noor Aini MY, Nik Shanita S, Zahara AM, Shahrul Azman MN. Atlas Makanan:Saiz pertukaran dan Porsi. Universiti Kebangsaan Malaysia. Kuala Lumpur: MDC Publishers & Printers Sdn Bhd; 2002.
24. Tee ES, Mohd Ismail N, Mohd Nasir A, Khatijah I. Nutrient composition of Malaysian foods. ASEAN Sub-Committee on protein: food habits research and development. Kuala Lumpur: Institute for Medical Research; 1997.
25. WHO (1995). Expert Committee on physical status. Physical status: the use and interpretation of anthropometry. Report of a WHO expert Committee. WHO technical report series, No. 854. Geneva: WHO.
26. Yusri A, Hamdan J, Abdul RAM. Ikan Laut Malaysia. Glosari nama sahih spesis ikan. Kuala Lumpur: Dewan Bahasa dan Pustaka; 2010.
27. Department of Fisheries Malaysia, Ministry of Agriculture and Agro-based Industry, Malaysia. Valid local name of Malaysian marine fishes. 2009, 180 pp. Available from: http://www.fishbase.org/references/FBRefSummary.php?ID=85449 [cited 26 March 2015].
28. Mansor M, Kohno H, Ida H, Nakamura HT, Aznan Z, Abdullah S. Field guide to important commercial marine fishes of the South China Sea. MFRDMD/SP/2. Kuala Terengganu: Southeast Asia Fisheries Development Center (SEAFDEC); 1998.
29. Nik MRA, Ahmad ZB. Demand for fish and its substitutes in Malaysia: evidence of habit formation and structural change. Pertanika J Soc Sci Hum 1999; 7(2): 111–19.
30. Teh L, Teh L. Reconstructing the marine fisheries catch of Peninsular Malaysia, Sarawak and Sabah, 1950–2010. Working Paper Series. Working paper 2014–16. Vancouver, BC: Sea Around Us, Fisheries Centre, The University of British Colombia; 2014.
31. Ahmad ZI, Aznita S. Food consumption patterns among paddy farmers Muda Irrigation area, Malaysia. Int J Soc Sci 2012; 18(1): 140–6.
32. Agriculture & Agri-Food Canada. The Malaysian consumer behavior, attitudes and perception towards products. International Market Bureau. Market analysis report, 2011. Available from: http://publications.gc.ca/collections/collection_2011/agr/A74-2-7-2011-eng.pdf [cited 4 September 2015].
33. Che WJWMR, Mohd HSMM, Osmsn B. Food intake in Malaysian culture and society: focus on the younger generation. Proceeding 11th APRU Doctoral Student Conference. Research for the sustainability of civilization in Pacific Rim. Past, present, future. 2010. Available from: https://umexpert.um.edu.my/file/publication/00003939_60280.pdf [cited 4 September 2015].
34. Bank Negara Malaysia. Economic developments in 2010. Annual report 2010. 2010, pp. 20–3. Available from: www.bnm.gov.my/files/publication/ar/en/2010/cp01.pdf [cited 4 September 2015].
35. Dey MM, Yolanda TG, Kumar P, Piumsombun S, Haque MS, Li L, et al. Demand for fish in Asia: a cross-country analysis. Aust J Agri Resource Econ 2008; 52: 321–38. doi: http://dx.doi.org/10.1111/j.1467-8489.2008.00418.x
36. Dey MM, Rab MA, Paraguas FJ, PiumSom BSY, Bhatta RA, Alam MF. Fish consumption and food security: a disaggregated analysis by types of fish and classes of consumers in selected Asian countries. Aquacult Econ Manag 2015; 9(1–2): 89–111. doi: http://dx.doi.org/10.1080/13657300590961537
37. Soon JM, Tee ES. Changing trends in dietary pattern and implications to food and nutrition security in association of Southeast Asian Nations (ASEAN). Int J Food Sci Nutr 2014; 3(4): 259–69. doi: http://dx.doi.org/10.11648/j.ijnfs.20140304.15
38. Shamsudin MN, Jinap S, Alias R, Abdul Ghariff R, Sheng TY, Ahmad Hanis IAH. Food consumption trend: transforming issues into opportunities. J Agribusiness Market 2010: 69–76. Available from: http://www.fama.gov.my/documents/10157/97223b48-9117-4ee8-bdb0-cfeb08edcfc5 [cited 4 September 2015].
39. Warr S, Rodriguez G, Penm J. Changing food consumption and imports in Malaysia. Opportunities for Australian agriculture exports. ABARE research report 08.6 for the Australian Government. Canberra: Department of Agriculture, Fisheries and Forestry; 2008.
40. Sheng TY, Shamsuddin MN, Mohamed Z, Abdullah AM, Radam A. Complete demand system of food in Malaysia. Agr Econ. 2008; 54(10): 467.
41. Sheng TY, Shamsuddin MN, Mohamed Z, Abdullah AM, Radam A. Food consumption behavior of the Malays in Malaysia. IIUM J Econ Manag 2008; 2: 209.
42. Ali N, Abdullah MA. The food consumption and eating behavior of Malaysia urbanites: issues and concerns. Malaysia J Soc Space 2012; 8(6): 157–65.

43. Mohamad IN. The nutrition and health transition in Malaysia. Public Health Nutr 2002; 5(1A): 191–5. doi: http://dx.doi.org/10.1079/PHN2001293
44. Ang KL, Foo S. An exploratory study of eating patterns of Singapore children and teenagers. Health Manag 2002; 102(5): 239–48.
45. Welch AA, Lund E, Amiano P, Dorronsoro M, Brustad M, Kumle M, et al. Variability of fish consumption within the 10 European countries participating in the European investigation into cancer and nutrition (EPIC) study. Publ Health Nutr 2002; 5(6B): 1273–85.
46. Rana KJ, Siriwardena S, Hasan MR. Impact of rising feed ingredient prices on aquafeeds and aquaculture production. FAO Fisheries and Aquaculture Technical Paper 541. Rome: Food and Aquaculture Organization of the United Nations; 2009.
47. Trondsen T, Braaten T, Lund E, Eggen AE. Health and seafood consumption patterns among women aged 45–69 years. A Norwegian seafood consumption study. Food Qual Prefer 2004; 15: 117–28.
48. Sioen I, Matthys C, De Backer G, Van Camp J, Henauw SD. Importance of seafood as nutrient source in the diet of Belgian adolescents. J Hum Nutr Diet 2007; 20: 580–6. doi: http://dx.doi.org/10.1111/j.1365-277X.2007.00814.x
49. Nurul Izzah A, Wan Rozita WM, Mohd Fairulnizal MN, Tengku Rozaina TM, Zarina Z, Hamdan J, et al. The prevalence of overweight and obesity and its associated factors among students aged 10–17 years old: findings from the seafood consumption survey in Peninsular Malaysia, 2008–2009. MASO 2011 Scientific Conference on Obesity- Towards healthy weight for life, Kuala Lumpur, 28–29 June 2011. pp. 84, 2011.

*Nurul Izzah Ahmad
Institute for Medical Research
Jalan Pahang, 50588 Kuala Lumpur
Malaysia
Email: nurul@imr.gov.my

6

Correlates of fruit, vegetable, soft drink, and snack intake among adolescents: the ESSENS study

Mekdes K. Gebremariam*, Sigrun Henjum, Laura Terragni and Liv Elin Torheim

Department of Nursing and Health Promotion, Faculty of Health Sciences, Oslo and Akershus University College of Applied Sciences, Oslo, Norway

Abstract

Background: Identifying modifiable correlates of dietary behaviors is of utmost importance for the promotion of healthy dietary behaviors.
Objective: This study explores individual, home, and school/neighborhood environmental correlates of dietary behaviors (intake of fruits, vegetables, soft drinks, and unhealthy snacks) among adolescents.
Methods: In total, 742 adolescents with a mean age of 13.6 (SD = 0.3) were included in this cross-sectional study conducted in 11 secondary schools located in the eastern part of Norway. A web-based questionnaire was used to collect data. Univariable and multivariable linear regression analyses were used to explore factors associated with the dietary behaviors included.
Results: A higher frequency of food/drink purchase in the school canteen was related to a higher consumption of soft drinks and snacks. A higher frequency of food/drink purchase in shops around schools during break or recess was related to a higher consumption of snacks. A higher frequency of food/drink purchase in shops around the neighborhood on the way to and from school was related to a higher consumption of soft drinks. Perceived parental modeling and perceived accessibility at home were found to be positively associated with all dietary behaviors. Perceived parental rules were inversely associated with soft drink and snack consumption; self-efficacy related to healthy eating was positively associated with fruit and vegetable consumption. Other included school and neighborhood environmental correlates were not associated with the dietary behaviors.
Conclusions: There is a need to address the food purchasing behavior of the adolescents using different approaches. The findings also highlight the important role of parents and the home environment for healthy and unhealthy dietary behaviors of adolescents.

Keywords: *correlates*; *dietary behaviors*; *home*; *school*; *neighborhood*; *environment*

One of the major public health challenges globally today is the pandemic of overweight and obesity. The problem is particularly pronounced among youth who can suffer from both short- and long-term complications (1–4) including tracking of body weight into adulthood (5). Unhealthy dietary behaviors are among the multiple interacting forces driving this pandemic (6). In this regard, favorable changes in the consumption of fruits, vegetables, soft drinks, and sweets have been documented in the past decade in Norway (7). However, the consumption of fruits and vegetables remains below what is recommended for health, and the consumption of added sugar is high (7–9). It is therefore of utmost importance to investigate the factors influencing dietary behaviors among adolescents.

Ecological models posit that health behaviors are influenced by factors at multiple levels including individual, interpersonal/social, and environmental levels (10). In this regard, individual factors such as preferences and self-efficacy have been identified as important correlates of dietary behaviors; the home environment has also been found to play a crucial role in determining children and adolescents' dietary behaviors (11–16). However, wider environmental (e.g. school and neighborhood) correlates of dietary behaviors have been less explored, although the past decade has seen an increase in studies focusing on such correlates (16). A systematic review of reviews documented that no school, neighborhood, or societal factors were consistently related to dietary behaviors among youth (12). Another systematic review concluded that there was little evidence supporting an effect of the retail environment around school on purchasing behavior or on consumption behavior (17). Many studies using multilevel modeling also found low school-level variance in dietary behaviors of children once individual-level characteristics were controlled (18–23). Such findings have at least partly been ascribed to a lack of high-quality studies (17) as well as to the fact that important environmental factors have not been explored. In addition, significant differences exist in the food environment across different settings, in particular in relation to the foods/drinks available at school, contributing to inconsistencies in results. Most studies of school-level correlates of dietary behaviors have been conducted in the USA where the school food environment is different from the European school food environment in general, and the Norwegian school food environment in particular. In Norway, there are no free school lunch programs, and it was documented that 95% of fifth to seventh graders bring their lunch from home (24). It is prohibited to have vending machines in schools; foods/drinks are offered via canteens/food booths that might have variable services and opening hours. Therefore, results regarding the influence of the school food environment from countries such as the USA cannot be directly extrapolated to the Norwegian setting. In addition, a recent umbrella review of correlates of dietary behaviors among youth concluded that groups of correlates have often been studied in isolation (16). There is therefore a need for studies that explore simultaneously multiple levels of influence.

Against this background, this study aimed to explore individual, home environmental, and school/neighborhood correlates of the consumption of fruits, vegetables, soft drinks, and unhealthy snacks among adolescents. It was hypothesized, based on existing literature, that the individual and home environmental correlates included would have the most significant contribution in explaining the dietary behaviors of the adolescents. It was also hypothesized that school and neighborhood environmental variables would independently contribute to the prediction of the dietary behaviors included. The participants in this study are young adolescents who are gradually gaining autonomy and are therefore likely to be increasingly influenced by food environment other than the home food environment.

Methods

Design and sample

The participants in this study were pupils from 11 secondary schools participating in the Environmental determinantS of dietary BehaviorS among adolescENtS (ESSENS) cross-sectional study. All 12 secondary schools in the Øvre Romerike region located in the eastern part of Norway were invited to participate in the study, and 11 accepted the invitation. In total, 1,163 adolescents in the eighth grade were invited to participate in this study and a total of 781 (67%) received parental consent for participation. In total, 742 adolescents (64% of those invited and 95% of those with parental consent) participated in the study.

Ethical clearance for the study was obtained from the Norwegian Social Science Data Service. Written informed consent was obtained from all parents of participating students.

Data collection and measures

A web-based questionnaire was used to collect data from the adolescents. The questionnaires were filled in at school and took approximately 30 to 45 min to complete. Research group members were present during data collection to answer questions and make sure adolescents responded independently from each other. The questionnaire was pretested among a group of adolescents ($n = 23$) of the same age as the study participants, prior to the main study.

Measures

Dietary behaviors

Intake of carbonated sugar-sweetened soft drinks (hereafter referred to as soft drinks) during weekdays was assessed using a frequency question with categories ranging from never/seldom to every weekday, and amount in glasses (from one to four or more). Weekend intake was assessed using a question about the amount of soft drink consumed with categories ranging from never/seldom to seven glasses or more. As soft drinks are usually sold in half liter bottles or cans, the participants were informed that ½ liter equals three glasses. Weekday and weekend intakes were summed up to create a weekly intake variable. The questions assessing the intake of soft drinks have been validated among 9- and 13-year-old Norwegians using a 4-day precoded food diary as the reference method, and moderate Spearman's correlation coefficients were obtained (25). However, separate assessment of weekday and weekend intake was not made in the validation study.

Consumption of fruits and vegetables (raw and cooked) was assessed using frequency questions with eight response categories ranging from never/seldom to three times per day or more. The questions assessing intake of fruits and vegetables were validated among 11-year-olds with a 7-day food record as the reference method and were found to have a satisfactory ability to rank subjects according to their intake of fruits and vegetables (26).

The consumption of snacks [sweet snacks (candies/chocolate), fatty snacks (e.g. potato chips), and sweet biscuits/muffins and similar] was assessed using three questions with seven response categories ranging from never/seldom to two times per day or more; frequencies of consumption of all the snacks were added to create a total snack intake variable.

Acceptable to moderate test–retest reliability was obtained for these measures of dietary behaviors in a previous Norwegian study conducted among 11-year-olds (27).

Perceived accessibility of vegetables was assessed using a scale with four items (e.g. 'we vary the types of vegetables served for dinner during a week'); perceived accessibility of fruits was assessed using a scale with three items (e.g. 'we vary the types of fruits that we have during the course of the week'); perceived accessibility of soft drinks was assessed using a scale with three items (e.g. 'we usually have soft drinks for dinner on weekend days'); and perceived accessibility of snacks was assessed using a scale with three items (e.g. 'we usually have sweet or fatty foods served for dessert or as snacks on weekdays'). A five-point Likert scale with answer categories ranging from 'totally disagree to totally agree' was used.

Perceived parental rules related to the consumption of vegetables were assessed using a scale with two items (e.g. 'I can eat vegetables whenever I want'); a similar scale was used to assess the perceived parental rule related to fruit consumption. Perceived parental rules for the consumption of soft drinks were assessed using a scale with four items (e.g. 'we have rules for when I can drink soft drinks'); perceived parental rules related to snack consumption was assessed using a single item ('when we have sweet or fatty snacks available, I can eat as much as I want'). A five-point Likert scale with answer categories ranging from 'totally disagree to totally agree' was used.

The items assessing perceived rules and accessibility of vegetables and soft drinks have previously shown evidence of validity among 14-year-olds (28).

Perceived parental modeling of fruit intake and of vegetable intake was assessed using a scale with two items. The measures were adopted from the Pro Children study and were found to have adequate test–retest reliability among 10–11-year-old European children (29). Parental modeling of soft drink consumption was assessed using the question 'How often do your parents drink soft drinks with sugar?' This question has shown evidence of test–retest reliability among 10–12-year-old European children (30). A similar scale was used to assess parental consumption of unhealthy snacks.

Self-efficacy related to the consumption of healthy foods was assessed using a scale with six items [e.g. Whenever I have a choice of the food I eat …, I find it difficult to choose low-fat foods (e.g. fruit or skimmed milk rather than 'full cream milk')]. The scale has been found to have adequate reliability and factorial validity among 13-year-olds (31).

All scales had acceptable to moderate internal consistency reliability in the present sample (ICC: 0.50–0.80).

The adolescents were asked about the presence of food sales outlets (e.g. supermarket, kiosk, and gas station) in a walking distance from their school (with answer categories 'none', 'yes, one', 'yes, two', and 'yes, more than two'). The question was adopted from a previous Norwegian study (23). They were asked how often they bought foods/drinks in these shops during breaks or recess. They were also asked how often they purchased foods or drinks from school canteens and on their way to and from school (answer categories ranging from 'never' to 'every day'). The frequency of purchase of foods/drinks was then recategorized into never, once a week, and more than once a week based on the distribution of the variables.

The perceived availability of fruits, vegetables, and unhealthy snacks in shops around school and in shops in the neighborhood was also assessed (e.g. a lot of fresh and varied fruits and vegetables that I like are available). Perceived accessibility of fruits and vegetables in these shops was asked using the question 'There are a lot of fruits and vegetables in a form that is easy to consume'. Perceived accessibility of soft drinks or snacks compared to fruits or vegetables in shops around schools or in the neighborhood was assessed using the question 'It is easier to find soft drinks and snacks in the shops than it is to find fruits or vegetables'. Perceived price of soft drinks and snacks compared to fruits and vegetables was explored using the question 'It is cheaper to buy soft drinks or snacks (e.g. biscuits, chips) than it is to buy fruits or vegetables'. Answer categories ranged from 'completely agree' to 'completely disagree'.

Information at school regarding food/nutrition was assessed using a scale with two items (e.g. 'food and nutrition is a topic that my teachers talk about often'). The internal consistency for the scale was moderate (ICC = 0.78). Perceived rules regarding foods and drinks allowed at school were assessed using the question: 'We have rules at school regarding the foods/drinks we should or should not bring to school' (answer categories ranging from 'completely agree' to 'completely disagree'). The question was adopted from a previous Norwegian study (23).

Sociodemographic correlates

Information on parental education was gathered as part of the parental informed consent for the adolescent. It was categorized into low (12 years of education or less, which corresponded to secondary education or lower) and high (13 years of education and more, which corresponded to university or college attendance). Educational status of the parent with the longest education or else the one available was used in the analyses.

Participants were divided into either ethnic Norwegian or ethnic minority. Ethnic minorities were defined as those having both parents born in a country other than Norway (32).

Statistical analyses

Because schools were the unit of measurement in this study, we checked for clustering effect through the linear mixed model procedure. Only $\leq 3\%$ of the unexplained variance in the dietary behaviors investigated was at the school level. Hence, adjustment for clustering effect was not done.

Descriptive analyses were first conducted. Univariable linear regression analyses were then used to explore factors at the individual (including sociodemographic characteristics), interpersonal, home environmental, and school/neighborhood environmental levels associated with the different dietary behaviors. Thereafter, variables significant at the 0.2 level on univariable regression were entered in multivariable regression models. Assumptions for the analyses were checked and considered acceptable. All analyses were conducted using SPSS version 22.

Results

The sociodemographic characteristics of the adolescents are described in Table 1. The mean age was 13.6 (SD = 0.3), and 53% of participants were females. Only 9% of adolescents were of an ethnic minority background and 40% had parents with a low level of education. The mean consumption of soft drinks was 700 mL/week. The frequency of fruit, vegetable, and snack consumption was 6.9, 8.8, and 4.5 times/week, respectively.

Table 2 shows the results of the descriptive analyses of the correlates included in the study. The lowest mean values were obtained for the perceived accessibility of unhealthy snacks and soft drinks at home. The highest values were obtained for permissive parental rules related to vegetable and fruit intake. The mean number of food sales outlets around schools was 2.2, and only 4% of participants reported that there were no food sales outlets in a walking distance from their school. In total, 73% of participants reported that they never purchased foods/drinks in shops around schools during breaks or recess; 11% reported doing so twice or more per week. Similarly, 66% of participants reported that they never purchased foods/drinks from neighborhood shops on their way to and from school, whereas 24% and 10% reported doing so once a week and twice or more per week, respectively. No food/drink purchase in school canteen was reported by 67% of participants; 20% reported purchasing foods/drinks once a week and 13% twice or more per week.

In the final adjusted models, the following factors were found to be associated with soft drink consumption (dl/week): gender (reference = female) B = 1.33 (confidence interval (CI): 0.48–2.17), perceived parental modeling

Table 1. Sociodemographic characteristics and dietary behaviors of the study sample ($n = 742$)

Age (years)	13.6 (0.3)
Gender (% girls)	53
Parental education (% low[a])	40
Ethnicity (% ethnic minority)	9
Soft drink consumption (dl/week)	7.0 (6.5–7.4)
Fruit intake (times/week)	6.9 (6.5–7.4)
Vegetable intake (times/week)	8.8 (8.2–9.2)
Snack intake (times/week)	4.5 (4.2–4.7)

Results are presented as mean and confidence interval or percentages.
[a]Low education is defined as having 12 years of education or less.

Table 2. Descriptive analysis of potential correlates of dietary behaviors among study participants ($n = 742$)

	Mean (SD) or %	Range
Perceived parental modeling of soft drink intake	2.71 (0.83)	1–5
Perceived accessibility of soft drinks at home	2.57 (1.14)	0–5
Perceived parental rules related to soft drinks	4.28 (1.11)	1–6
Perceived parental modeling of snack intake	2.70 (0.62)	1–5
Perceived accessibility of snacks at home	2.49 (0.79)	1–5
Perceived parental rules related to snacks	3.90 (1.23)	1–5
Perceived parental modeling of vegetable intake	3.68 (0.97)	1–5
Perceived accessibility of vegetables at home	4.09 (0.77)	1–5
Perceived parental rules related to vegetables	4.55 (0.71)	1–5
Perceived parental modeling of fruit intake	4.14 (0.87)	1–5
Perceived accessibility of fruits at home	3.89 (0.78)	1–5
Perceived parental rules related to fruits	4.56 (0.68)	1–5
Self-efficacy related to healthy eating	3.48 (0.65)	1–5
Number of food sales outlets around school[a]	2.19 (0.93)	0–3
Food/drink purchase in school canteen		
Never	67%	
Once a week	20%	
Twice or more per week	13%	
Food/drink purchase in neighborhood shops[b]		
Never	66%	
Once a week	24%	
Twice or more per week	10%	
Food/drink purchase in shops around school[c]		
Never	73%	
Once a week	16%	
Twice or more per week	11%	
Perceived FV availability in neighborhood shops	4.24 (1.02)	1–5
Perceived FV accessibility in neighborhood shops	4.09 (1.08)	1–5
Perceived accessibility of SD and snacks in neighborhood	3.03 (1.24)	1–5
Perceived availability of SD and snacks in neighborhood	3.88 (1.19)	1–5
Perceived price of SD and snacks compared to FV	3.08 (1.23)	1–5
Perceived school food rules	3.56 (1.36)	1–5
Information at school regarding food and nutrition	2.68 (1.05)	1–5

SD, soft drinks; FV, fruits and vegetables.
[a]In a walking distance from school, [b]on the way to and from school, [c]during breaks or recess.

B = 0.63 (CI: 0.06–1.21), perceived accessibility at home B = 1.47 (CI: 1.02–1.92), perceived parental rules B = −1.58 (CI: −2.01 to −1.15), purchase of food/drink at the school canteen (high vs. low) B = 2.10 (CI: 0.74–3.45), and purchase of food/drinks on the way to and from school (high vs. low) B = 2.87 (CI: 1.31–4.43). The factors found to be associated with snack consumption in the final adjusted models were perceived parental modeling B = 0.43 (95% CI: 0.01–0.85), perceived accessibility at home B = 1.0 (95% CI: 0.66–1.35), perceived parental rules B = −0.22 (95% CI: −0.43 to −0.01), self-efficacy related to healthy eating B = −0.90 (95% CI: −1.29 to −0.51), purchase of food/drink in the school canteen (high vs. low) B = 0.92 (95% CI: 0.13–1.71), and food/drink purchase around school during recessand breaks (high vs. low) B = 1.57 (95% CI: 0.73–2.41). Table 3 shows the results of the multivariable regression analyses exploring correlates of soft drink and snack consumption.

The factors found to be associated with fruit intake in the final adjusted models were perceived parental modeling B = 0.54 (95% CI: 0.02–1.06), perceived accessibility at home B = 1.38 (95% CI: 0.76–1.99), and self-efficacy regarding healthy eating B = 2.69 (95% CI: 2.01–3.38). The factors found to be associated with vegetable intake were perceived parental modeling B = 0.58 (95% CI: 0.09–1.07), perceived accessibility at home B = 2.98 (95% CI: 2.28–3.68), and self-efficacy regarding healthy eating B = 2.20 (95% CI: 1.46–2.94). Table 4 shows the results of the multivariable regression analyses exploring correlates of fruit and vegetable consumption.

Discussion

The aim of this study was to explore individual, home environmental, and school/neighborhood environmental correlates of fruit, vegetable, soft drink, and unhealthy snack consumption among adolescents. The adolescents'

Table 3. Correlates of soft drink and snack consumption among adolescents, $n = 742$

	B and CI	p
Soft drink consumption (dl/week)		
Gender (males)	1.33 (0.48–2.17)	0.002
Parental education	−0.21 (−1.08–0.66)	0.64
Perceived parental modeling	0.63 (0.06–1.21)	0.03
Perceived accessibility at home	1.47 (1.02–1.92)	<0.001
Perceived parental rules	−1.58 (−2.01 to −1.15)	<0.001
Self-efficacy regarding healthy eating	−0.58 (−1.24–0.08)	0.08
Perceived FV availability in neighborhood shops	−0.40 (−0.80–0.02)	0.06
Food/drink purchase in school canteen (high)	2.10 (0.74–3.45)	0.002
Food/drink purchase in school canteen (medium)	0.03 (−1.06–1.12)	0.96
Food/drink purchase in neighborhood shops[a] (high)	2.87 (1.31–4.43)	<0.001
Food/drink purchase in neighborhood shops[a] (medium)	−0.41 (−1.44–0.62)	0.44
Food/drink purchase in shops around school[b] (high)	−0.92 (−2.36–0.52)	0.21
Food/drink purchase in shops around school[b] (medium)	−0.85 (−2.0–0.30)	0.15
Intake of snacks (times/week)		
Perceived parental modeling	0.43 (0.01–0.85)	0.046
Perceived accessibility at home	1.0 (0.66–1.35)	<0.001
Perceived parental rules	−0.22 (−0.43 to −0.01)	0.04
Self-efficacy regarding healthy eating	−0.90 (−1.29 to −0.51)	<0.001
Perceived availability in neighborhood shops	0.14 (−0.08–0.35)	0.21
Perceived price compared to fruits and vegetables	0.20 (0.00–0.40)	0.05
Food/drink purchase in school canteen (high)	0.92 (0.13–1.71)	0.02
Food/drink purchase in school canteen (medium)	−0.27 (−0.9–0.37)	0.42
Food/drink purchase in neighborhood shops[a] (high)	0.29 (−0.64–1.21)	0.54
Food/drink purchase in neighborhood shops[a] (medium)	−0.28 (−0.89–0.32)	0.36
Food/drink purchase in shops around school[b] (high)	1.57 (0.73–2.41)	<0.001
Food/drink purchase in shops around school[b] (medium)	0.15 (−0.53–0.83)	0.67

FV, fruits and vegetables.
[a]On the way to and from school, [b]during recess or breaks.
Results were obtained using multiple linear regression analyses, and only factors significant at the 0.2 level on univariable regression were included in this model. Frequency of food purchase is defined as high when it occurs twice or more per week and as medium when it occurs once a week. The reference category includes those who report no purchase of food/drinks.

Table 4. Correlates of fruit and vegetable consumption among adolescents, $n = 741$

	B and CI	p
Fruit consumption (times/week)		
Ethnicity	1.28 (−0.23–2.79)	0.09
Perceived parental modeling	0.54 (0.02–1.06)	0.04
Perceived accessibility at home	1.38 (0.76–1.99)	<0.001
Perceived parental rules	−0.26 (−0.93–0.41)	0.45
Self-efficacy regarding healthy eating	2.69 (2.01–3.38)	<0.001
Perceived FV availability in neighborhood shops	0.07 (−0.36–0.50)	0.74
Perceived food rules at school	−0.23 (−0.54–0.08)	0.15
Vegetable consumption (times/week)		
Perceived parental modeling	0.58 (0.09–1.07)	0.02
Perceived accessibility at home	2.98 (2.29–3.68)	<0.001
Perceived parental rules	0.08 (−0.61–0.77)	0.82
Self-efficacy regarding healthy eating	2.20 (1.46–2.94)	<0.001
Perceived FV availability in neighborhood shops	−0.32 (−0.77–0.12)	0.15

FV, fruits and vegetables.
Results were obtained using multiple linear regression analyses, and only factors significant at the 0.2 level on univariable regression were included in this model.

food purchasing behavior at school and in the neighborhood was associated with soft drink and snack consumption. The other school and neighborhood environmental correlates were not associated with the dietary behaviors of the adolescents. Parental modeling and perceived accessibility at home were found to be positively associated with all the dietary behaviors. Parental rules were associated with soft drink and snack consumption; self-efficacy related to healthy eating was associated with fruit and vegetable consumption.

As hypothesized, home environmental variables were found to be the most important correlates of the dietary behaviors included. As previously documented in the literature, parental modeling (11–14) and perceived accessibility at home (13, 15) were found to be positively associated with all the dietary behaviors included. Self-efficacy related to healthy eating was also strongly positively related to the consumption of fruits and vegetables and inversely related to the consumption of unhealthy snacks. Self-efficacy has been found to be a strong correlate of healthy behaviors among adolescents including dietary behaviors (15). Parents can play a role in the enhancement of their adolescents' self-efficacy toward healthy eating that would result in favorable dietary behaviors, which might further enhance self-efficacy. There were also parental educational differences in soft drink consumption on univariable analysis. This association became insignificant in the final adjusted model, indicating that variables included in the model were potentially mediators of the socioeconomic differences in soft drink consumption. Indeed, separate analyses (results not shown) showed that there were socioeconomic differences in the correlates that were significantly associated with soft drink consumption. Factors such as parental modeling and accessibility at home have previously been found to mediate socioeconomic differences in soft drink consumption (33–35).

The frequency of food purchase in the school canteen was positively related to the intake of unhealthy snacks and soft drinks. The Norwegian recommendations for school food state that the offer of cakes and other sweet or fatty products be limited to special occasions. These recommendations also state that soft drinks should not be offered at school (36). However, in a qualitative component of the ESSENS study, which included observations of canteens in selected schools, it was found that some unhealthy foods and drinks were offered in some schools, in addition to healthier food alternatives (unpublished data). A previous study from the USA found that middle school students purchased unhealthy foods such as chips, soda, and soft drinks at school even when healthier alternatives were available (37). In another study, availability at school was related to the consumption of soft drinks and unhealthy snacks, but not with fruit and vegetable consumption (38). Limiting the availability of unhealthy foods and drinks from school canteens by ensuring that national guidelines for foods at school are properly implemented is therefore crucial.

The frequency of food purchase in neighborhood shops on the way to and from school was positively related to the consumption of soft drinks. The frequency of food purchase in shops around schools during breaks or recess was positively related to the consumption of unhealthy snacks. It is worth noting that there might be some overlap between these shops, as the shops around school might be the ones most accessible on the way to and from school for some, in particular those living in close proximity of their school. Food purchase away from home has been associated with unfavorable eating behaviors and weight outcomes in previous studies, although the type of food purchased and of food outlets explored varied between studies (39–41). In this regard, parents should encourage their children to purchase healthy foods and whenever possible limit their adolescents' food purchase by providing fewer financial resources for doing so. There was also a borderline statistically significant inverse association between the perceived price of snacks compared to fruits and vegetables and the consumption of snacks, that is, those who perceived the price of snacks to be lower consumed more snacks. Food prices have been shown to be key correlates of healthy and unhealthy food consumption (42–44) and can therefore serve as one of the entry points for interventions aimed at improving adolescents' dietary behaviors.

In this study, school and neighborhood environmental variables did not appear to have a significant influence on the dietary behaviors of the adolescents, in particular fruit and vegetable consumption. There might be several reasons for these findings. Existing data indicate that 95% of fifth to seventh graders in Norway bring their school lunch from home (24) which is likely similar among eighth graders. Therefore, most of the consumption of fruits and vegetables is likely to be either at home or from fruits and vegetables brought from home. It is also possible that there is homogeneity in the factors of interest between schools and neighborhoods although there was diversity in the perceptions reported. Consequently, actual school and neighborhood correlates might not have had enough variability that would allow for associations with dietary behaviors to be picked, for example, shops around schools might have similar availability/accessibility of foods across the included schools. Indeed, some ceiling effect was apparent for the measure of perceived fruit and vegetable availability in neighborhood shops. Future studies combining objective and subjective measures of the school and neighborhood environment in the same sample are needed in this regard. Such studies would allow for the assessment of similarities and differences in associations when subjective and objective measures are used. The latter might provide a more accurate assessment; however, how these environmental factors are perceived by the adolescents might be more relevant in influencing their behaviors.

The strengths of the study include the large number of correlates at multiple levels that were included. The sample size was also large; the response rate at the school level was very high and was moderate at the parental level. The weaknesses include the cross-sectional data that does not allow for any causal inference to be made. The use of self-report can lead to problems of validity and reliability, in particular among young children. Several of the correlates included, however, had displayed evidence of reliability and/or validity in previous studies among adolescents in a similar age group. There is, however, a scarcity of validity and reliability tested measures assessing the perceived school and neighborhood food environment including the measures used in this study. Finally, only carbonated sugar-sweetened soft drinks were included in this study; future studies should include other sugar-sweetened beverages such as cordials and energy drinks.

Conclusions

Food purchasing behavior at school and on the way to and from school was found to be related to the intake of soft drinks and snacks. Perceived accessibility and parental modeling were related to all dietary behaviors; parental rules were related to soft drink and snack intake. Other school and neighborhood environmental variables were unrelated to the dietary behaviors included. There is therefore a need to address the food purchasing behavior of the adolescents using different approaches such as limiting the availability of unhealthy foods and drinks from school canteens. The findings also highlight the important role of parents and the home environment for healthy and unhealthy dietary behaviors of adolescents.

Authors' contributions

MKG designed the study, planned the project, participated in the data collection, conducted the statistical analyses, and wrote the first draft of the manuscript. LET, LT, and SH participated in project planning and implementation. All authors have critically revised the manuscript, and read and approved the final version of the manuscript.

Acknowledgements

The ESSENS study is a collaborative project between the Oslo and Akershus University College of Applied Sciences and the public health project Folkehelseforum Øvre Romerike (FØR). The authors thank all the participants who took part in this study. They are particularly grateful to Elisabeth Hurum and Jorunn Utne for their work with recruitment and data collection.

Conflict of interest and funding

The authors declare that they have no competing interests. The ESSENS project was funded by internal funds from Oslo and Akershus University College of Applied Sciences.

References

1. Dietz WH. Health consequences of obesity in youth: childhood predictors of adult disease. Pediatrics 1998; 101: 518–25.
2. Daniels SR, Arnett DK, Eckel RH, Gidding SS, Hayman LL, Kumanyika S, et al. Overweight in children and adolescents: pathophysiology, consequences, prevention, and treatment. Circulation 2005; 111: 1999–2012.
3. Biro FM, Wien M. Childhood obesity and adult morbidities. Am J Clin Nutr 2010; 91: 1499S–505S.
4. Reilly JJ, Kelly J. Long-term impact of overweight and obesity in childhood and adolescence on morbidity and premature mortality in adulthood: systematic review. Int J Obes 2011; 35: 891–8.
5. Singh AS, Mulder C, Twisk JW, van Mechelen W, Chinapaw MJ. Tracking of childhood overweight into adulthood: a systematic review of the literature. Obes Rev 2008; 9: 474–88.
6. Swinburn BA, Sacks G, Hall KD, McPherson K, Finegood DT, Moodie ML, et al. The global obesity pandemic: shaped by global drivers and local environments. Lancet 2011; 378: 804–14.
7. Fismen AS, Smith OR, Torsheim T, Rasmussen M, Pedersen Pagh T, Augustine L, et al. Trends in food habits and their relation to socioeconomic status among Nordic adolescents 2001/2002–2009/20. PLoS One 2016; 11: e0148541.

8. Bjelland M, Lien N, Grydeland M, Bergh IH, Anderssen SA, Ommundsen Y, et al. Intakes and perceived home availability of sugar-sweetened beverages, fruit and vegetables as reported by mothers, fathers and adolescents in the HEIA (Health In Adolescents) study. Public Health Nutr 2011; 14: 2156–65.
9. Bere E, Glomnes ES, te Velde SJ, Klepp KI. Determinants of adolescents' soft drink consumption. Public Health Nutr 2008; 11: 49–56.
10. Sallis JF, Owen N, Fisher EB. Ecological models of health behaviour. In: Glanz Z, Rimer BK, Viswanath K, eds. Health behaviour and health education: theory, research and practice. 4th ed. San Francisco, CA: Jossey-Bass; 2008; 465–482.
11. Pearson N, Biddle SJH, Gorely T. Family correlates of fruit and vegetable consumption in children and adolescents: a systematic review. Public Health Nutr 2009; 12: 267–83.
12. De Vet E, De Ridder DT, De Wit JB. Environmental correlates of physical activity and dietary behaviours among young people: a systematic review of reviews. Obes Rev 2011; 12: e130–42.
13. Van der Horst K, Oenema A, Ferreira I, Wendel-Vos W, Giskes K, Van Lenthe F, et al. A systematic review of environmental correlates of obesity-related dietary behaviors in youth. Health Educ Res 2007; 22: 203–26.
14. McClain AD, Chappuis C, Nguyen-Rodriguez ST, Yaroch AL, Spruijt-Metz D. Psychosocial correlates of eating behavior in children and adolescents: a review. Int J Behav Nutr Phys Act 2009; 6: 54.
15. Rasmussen M, Krølner R, Klepp K-I, Lytle L, Brug J, Bere E, et al. Determinants of fruit and vegetable consumption among children and adolescents: a review of the literature. Part I: quantitative studies. Int J Behav Nutr Phys Act 2006; 3: 22.
16. Sleddens EF, Kroeze W, Kohl LF, Bolten LM, Velema E, Kaspers PJ, et al. Determinants of dietary behavior among youth: an umbrella review. Int J Behav Nutr Phys Act 2015; 12: 7.
17. Williams J, Scarborough P, Matthews A, Cowburn G, Foster C, Roberts N, et al. A systematic review of the influence of the retail food environment around schools on obesity-related outcomes. Obes Rev 2014; 15: 359–74.
18. Krølner R, Due P, Rasmussen M, Damsgaard MT, Holstein BE, Klepp KI, et al. Does school environment affect 11-year-olds' fruit and vegetable intake in Denmark? Soc Sci Med 2009; 68: 1416–24.
19. Vereecken CA, Bobelijn K, Maes L. School food policy at primary and secondary schools in Belgium-Flanders: does it influence young people's food habits? Eur J Clin Nutr 2005; 59: 271–7.
20. Van der Horst K, Timperio A, Crawford D, Roberts R, Brug J, Oenema A. The school food environment associations with adolescent soft drink and snack consumption. Am J Prev Med 2008; 35: 217–23.
21. Maes L, Lievens J. Can the school make a difference? A multilevel analysis of adolescent risk and health behaviour. Soc Sci Med 2003; 56: 517–29.
22. Johansen A, Rasmussen S, Madsen M. Health behavior among adolescents in Denmark: influence of school class and individual risk factors. Scand J Public Health 2006; 34: 32–40.
23. Gebremariam MK, Andersen LF, Bjelland M, Klepp KI, Totland TH, Bergh IH, et al. Does the school food environment influence the dietary behaviours of Norwegian 11-year-olds? The HEIA study. Scand J Public Health 2012; 40: 491–7.
24. Kunnskapsdepartementet. Skolemåltidet i grunnskolen. Kunnskapsgrunnlag, nytte og kostnadsvirkninger og vurdering av ulike skolemåltidsmodeller. Rapport fra arbeidsgruppe nedsatt av Kunnskapsdepartementet [The school meal in the primary school. Knowledge base, cost-benefit analysis and assessment of different models for school meals. Report from a working group appointed by the Ministry of Education and Research]. (In Norwegian). 2006; Available online at: https://www.regjeringen.no/globalassets/upload/kilde/kd/rap/2006/0008/ddd/pdfv/284882-skolemaltid_26.06.06.pdf
25. Lillegaard IT, Overby NC, Andersen LF. Evaluation of a short food frequency questionnaire used among Norwegian children. Food Nutr Res 2012; 56: 6399, doi: http://dx.doi.org/10.3402/fnr.v56i0.6399
26. Haraldsdóttir J, Thórsdóttir I, de Almeida MD, Maes L, Pérez Rodrigo C, Elmadfa I, et al. Validity and reproducibility of a precoded questionnaire to assess fruit and vegetable intake in European 11- to 12-year-old schoolchildren. Ann Nutr Metab 2005; 49: 221–7.
27. Lien N, Bjelland M, Bergh IH, Grydeland M, Anderssen SA, Ommundsen Y, et al. Design of a 20-month comprehensive, multicomponent school-based randomised trial to promote healthy weight development among 11-13 year olds: the health in adolescents study. Scand J Public Health 2010; 38(5 Suppl): 38–51.
28. Bjelland M, Hausken SE, Sleddens EF, Andersen LF, Lie HC, Finset A, et al. Development of family and dietary habits questionnaires: the assessment of family processes, dietary habits and adolescents' impulsiveness in Norwegian adolescents and their parents. Int J Behav Nutr Phys Act 2014; 11: 130.
29. De Bourdeaudhuij I, Klepp KI, Due P, Rodrigo CP, de Almeida M, Wind M, et al. Reliability and validity of a questionnaire to measure personal, social and environmental correlates of fruit and vegetable intake in 10-11-year-old children in five European countries. Public Health Nutr 2005; 8: 189–200.
30. Singh AS, Vik FN, Chinapaw MJ, Uijtdewilligen L, Verloigne M, Fernández-Alvira JM, et al. Test-retest reliability and construct validity of the ENERGY-child questionnaire on energy balance-related behaviours and their potential determinants: the ENERGY-project. Int J Behav Nutr Phys Act 2011; 8: 136.
31. Dewar DL, Lubans DR, Plotnikoff RC, Morgan PJ. Development and evaluation of social cognitive measures related to adolescent dietary behaviors. Int J Behav Nutr Phys Act 2012; 9: 36.
32. Lie B. Immigration and immigrants: statistisk sentralbyrå. Oslo, Norway: Statistics Norway; 2002.
33. De Coen V, Vansteelandt S, Maes L, Huybrechts I, De Bourdeaudhuij I, Vereecken C. Parental socioeconomic status and soft drink consumption of the child. The mediating proportion of parenting practices. Appetite 2012; 59: 76–80.
34. Totland TH, Lien N, Bergh IH, Bjelland M, Gebremariam MK, Klepp KI, et al. The relationship between parental education and adolescents' soft drink intake from the age of 11-13 years, and possible mediating effects of availability and accessibility. Br J Nutr 2013; 110: 926–33.
35. Hilsen M, te Velde SJ, Bere E, Brug J. Predictors and mediators of differences in soft drinks consumption according to gender and plans of further education among Norwegian secondary-school children. Public Health Nutr 2013; 16: 1250–6.
36. Helsedirektoratet. Mat og måltider i skolen. Nasjonal faglig retningslinje for mat og måltider i skolen. 2015 [The Directorate of Health. Food and meals in the school. National guidelines for school food and meals. 2015]. Available online at: https://helsedirektoratet.no/retningslinjer/mat-og-maltider-i-skolen
37. Park S, Sappenfield WM, Huang Y, Sherry B, Bensyl DM. The impact of the availability of school vending machines on eating behavior during lunch: the Youth Physical Activity and Nutrition Survey. J Am Diet Assoc 2010; 110: 1532–6.
38. Cisse-Egbuonye N, Liles S, Schmitz KE, Kassem N, Irvin VL, Hovell MF. Availability of vending machines and school stores in California schools. J Sch Health 2016; 86: 48–53.

39. Poti JM, Slining MM, Popkin BM. Where are kids getting their empty calories? Stores, schools, and fast-food restaurants each played an important role in empty calorie intake among US children during 2009–2010. J Acad Nutr Diet 2014; 114: 908–17.
40. French SA, Story M, Neumark-Sztainer D, Fulkerson JA, Hannan P. Fast food restaurant use among adolescents: associations with nutrient intake, food choices and behavioral and psychosocial variables. Int J Obes Relat Metab Disord 2001; 25: 1823–33.
41. Thompson OM, Ballew C, Resnicow K, Must A, Bandini LG, Cyr H, et al. Food purchased away from home as a predictor of change in BMI z-score among girls. Int J Obes Relat Metab Disord 2004; 28: 282–9.
42. Epstein LH, Dearing KK, Paluch RA, Roemmich JN, Cho D. Price and maternal obesity influence purchasing of low- and high-energy-dense foods. Am J Clin Nutr 2007; 86: 914–22.
43. Levy DT, Friend KB, Wang YC. A review of the literature on policies directed at the youth consumption of sugar sweetened beverages. Adv Nutr 2011; 2: 182S–200S.
44. French SA. Pricing effects on food choices. J Nutr 2003; 133: 841S–3S.

*Mekdes K. Gebremariam
Department of Nursing and Health Promotion
Faculty of Health Sciences
Oslo and Akershus University College of Applied Sciences
P.O. Box 4 Olavs Plass Street, NO-0130 Oslo
Norway
Email: mekdes.gebremariam@medisin.uio.no

7

Meals based on vegetable protein sources (beans and peas) are more satiating than meals based on animal protein sources (veal and pork) – a randomized cross-over meal test study

Marlene D. Kristensen[1,2], Nathalie T. Bendsen[1,3], Sheena M. Christensen[1], Arne Astrup[1] and Anne Raben[1]*

[1]Department of Nutrition, Exercise and Sports, Faculty of Science, University of Copenhagen, Copenhagen, Denmark; [2]Novo Nordisk A/S, Bagsværd, Denmark; [3]Ferring Farmaceuticals A/S, Copenhagen, Denmark

Abstract

Background: Recent nutrition recommendations advocate a reduction in protein from animal sources (pork, beef) because of environmental concerns. Instead, protein from vegetable sources (beans, peas) should be increased. However, little is known about the effect of these vegetable protein sources on appetite regulation.
Objective: To examine whether meals based on vegetable protein sources (beans/peas) are comparable to meals based on animal protein sources (veal/pork) regarding meal-induced appetite sensations.
Design: In total, 43 healthy, normal-weight, young men completed this randomized, double-blind, placebo-controlled, three-way, cross-over meal test. The meals (all 3.5 MJ, 28 energy-% (E%) fat) were either high protein based on veal and pork meat, HP-Meat (19 E% protein, 53 E% carbohydrate, 6 g fiber/100 g); high protein based on legumes (beans and peas), HP-Legume (19 E% protein, 53 E% carbohydrate, 25 g fiber/100 g); or low-protein based on legumes, LP-Legume (9 E% protein, 62 E% carbohydrate, 10 g fiber/100 g). Subjective appetite sensations were recorded at baseline and every half hour using visual analog scales until the *ad libitum* meal 3 h after the test meal. Repeated measurements analyses and summary analyses were performed using ANCOVA (SAS).
Results: HP-Legume induced lower composite appetite score, hunger, prospective food consumption, and higher fullness compared to HP-Meat and LP-Legume ($p < 0.05$). Furthermore, satiety was higher after HP-Legume than HP-Meat ($p < 0.05$). When adjusting for palatability, HP-Legume still resulted in lower composite appetite scores, hunger, prospective consumption, and higher fullness compared to HP-Meat ($p < 0.05$). Furthermore, HP-Legume induced higher fullness than LP-Legume ($p < 0.05$). A 12% and 13% lower energy intake, respectively, was seen after HP-Legume compared to HP-Meat or LP-Legume ($p < 0.01$).
Conclusion: Vegetable-based meals (beans/peas) influenced appetite sensations favorably compared to animal-based meals (pork/veal) with similar energy and protein content, but lower fiber content. Interestingly, a vegetable-based meal with low protein content was as satiating and palatable as an animal-based meal with high protein content.

Keywords: *legumes; appetite; fullness; hunger; dietary fiber; ad libitum*

Randomized controlled trials and some prospective cohort studies have demonstrated that a high protein intake can induce increased weight loss and improve weight maintenance after weight loss compared to a low protein intake (1–5). This effect appears to be associated with reduced feelings of hunger and increased satiety (6, 7), although increased energy expenditure may also be a contributing factor (8, 9).

In recent years, increasing attention has been put on the environmental impact of different foods, and it has become clear that meat products may contribute with more negative effects, for example, production of greenhouse gasses and CO_2 emission, than vegetable products (10–12). Therefore, a replacement of protein from animal sources such as beef and pork with protein from vegetable sources, such as legumes, would be an environmental-friendly approach. Such an approach would also lead to an increased intake of dietary fiber.

Recently, the Nordic Nutrition Recommendations were revised to reflect the issue on environmental impact of food production. Thus, a reduction in consumption of protein from animal sources such as beef and pork and an increase in vegetable sources such as legumes and pulses was recommended (13). Furthermore, focus should be on whole foods rather than single macronutrients.

When comparing CO_2 emission for legumes with meat, the CO_2 equivalent (in kg) is increased with a factor of 30 (12). Despite this, the consumption of protein-rich legumes is very low among Danes compared to the intake of, for example, red meat. Adults in Denmark consume on average 137 g of red meat and meat products per day (14), whereas the intake of legumes is approximately 7 g per day (15). The obstacles that could be accountable for the low intake could be palatability, gastrointestinal discomfort, but probably even more importantly, that legumes are not part of a typical Western dietary culture. A study investigated how chick pea supplementation in an Australian diet affected satiation and bowel health (16). They found that perceived satiation and perceived bowel function were improved. However, inconvenience and gastrointestinal upset were considered to discourage legume consumption.

Very little is still known about the effect of Nordic-grown vegetable sources of protein on appetite and body weight regulation. The aim of the present study was therefore to examine whether a meal based on vegetable sources (legumes: beans and peas) was comparable to a meal based on natural animal sources (pork and veal) regarding acute meal-induced appetite sensations and *ad libitum* energy intake.

Methods and materials

Study design

The study was designed as a randomized, double-blind, placebo-controlled, three-way cross-over intervention. Each meal test was separated by a washout period of at least 2 weeks. Subjects were instructed to refrain from alcohol consumption and intense physical activity for the 24 h proceeding each test day. In the evening before the test day, the subjects consumed a 4.0 MJ standardized evening meal (50.3 energy-% (E%) carbohydrate, 33 E% fat, 16.7 E% protein), consisting of pork and vegetable stew with rice (prepared by kitchen staff at the department) before 8:00 p.m. After this time subjects fasted (consumption of half a liter of water was allowed).

On each test day, the subjects met fasting in the morning at the department. After voiding, they were weighed to the nearest 0.05 kg on a decimal scale (Lindeltronic 8000, Copenhagen, Denmark). Before the test meal was served, subjects filled in the first visual analog scales (VASs). The test meal was served and consumed within 15 min. After the meal, subjects filled in VAS at time points 15, 30, 60, 90, 120, 150, and 180 min. VAS for palatability of the test meals were filled in immediately after finishing the meal. Three hours after the test meal, an *ad libitum* lunch meal was served, and subjects were instructed to eat until they felt comfortably satiated. The *ad libitum* lunch consisted of Pasta Bolognese and was served with 300 ml water. The meal had an energy content of 961 kJ/100 g and a macronutrient composition of 55 E% carbohydrates, 30 E% fat, and 15 E% protein. Food intake was registered and energy intake calculated. The subjects were not allowed to consume any other foods or drinks throughout the test day, but were allowed to read, listen to the radio, or use their computer.

Subjects

Healthy young men were recruited through university intranet systems and advertisements on websites. Subjects should be normal-weight to moderately overweight (body mass index (BMI) 22–28 kg/m^2), between 18 and 40 years of age, and free of any chronic health conditions. Subjects who smoked, were athletes (>10 h exercise/week), used regular medication, had food allergies, or used dietary supplements were excluded. In total, 60 subjects were screened; 7 subjects did not meet the inclusion/exclusion criteria, and 5 withdrew consent before starting the study. Thus, 48 subjects started the study. The subjects were given both verbal and written information, whereupon all gave written consent. Subjects meeting all the inclusion criteria were randomly allocated to the three meals. Meal sequences were generated by hand to make an even number of each sequence and a computer was used to generate a list of these sequences in random order. The list was kept by the investigator and not disclosed to the study coordinator who enrolled the subjects in the study.

The study was carried out at the Department of Nutrition, Exercise and Sports, Faculty of Science, University of Copenhagen, Frederiksberg, Denmark, April–July 2011. It was approved by the Municipal Ethical Committee of The Capital Region of Denmark to be in accordance with the Helsinki-II declaration. Subjects received $\sim$300 US$ as compensation on completion of all the test days. The trial was registered at clinicaltrials.gov as NCT01345487.

Test meals

The test meals were given as breakfast meals and each provided 3.5 MJ (Table 1). Three test meals were compared: one with a high protein content from meat, HP-Meat (19 E% protein, 53 E% carbohydrate, 28 E% fat, 6 g fiber/100 g); one with a high protein content from legumes, HP-Legume (19 E% protein, 53 E% carbohydrate, 28 E% fat, 25 g fiber/100 g); and one with a low protein content from legumes, LP-Legume (9 E% protein, 62 E% carbohydrate, 28 E% fat, 10 g fiber/100 g). The meals were all composed of oven-baked patties, made of veal and pork meat (HP-Meat) or of fava beans (HP-Legume and LP-Legume), and a mash of either potato

Table 1. Test meal ingredients and nutrient content (raw weight)

HP-Meat	g	HP-Legumes	g	LP-Legumes	g
Veal and pork patties		Fava bean patties		Fava bean patties	
Veal/pork, minced, 4% fat	135	Fava beans, dried	100	Fava beans, dried	29
Potato, raw, shredded	84			Potato, raw, shredded	124
Potato flour	6			Potato flour	39
Rapeseed oil	7	Rapeseed oil	10	Rapeseed oil	10
		Butter	5	Butter	4
Onions, fresh, diced	10	Onions, fresh, diced	10	Onions, fresh, diced	10
Breadcrumbs	20	Flour	5	Flour	8
Garlic, parsley, salt, cumin		Garlic, parsley, salt, cumin		Garlic, parsley, salt, cumin	
Mashed potatoes		Mash of split peas		Mash of split peas	
Potato	254	Split peas, dried	90	Split peas, dried	32
Potato flour	36			Potato	176
Butter	13	Butter	12	Butter	14
Rapeseed oil	2				
Salt		Salt and vinegar		Salt and vinegar	
Tomato ketchup	20	Tomato ketchup	20	Tomato ketchup	20
3,546 kJ		3,552 kJ		3,545 kJ	
19 E% protein		19 E% protein		9 E% protein	
39 g protein/100 g[a]		38 g protein/100 g[a]		18 g protein/100 g[a]	
28 E% fat		28 E% fat		28 E% fat	
53 E% carbohydrate		53 E% carbohydrate		62 E% carbohydrate	
6 g fiber/100 g[b]		25 g fiber/100 g[b]		10 g fiber/100 g[b]	
Serving weight: 591 g		Serving weight: 591 g		Serving weight: 591 g	

Water was added to the HP-Legume and LP-Legume recipes to achieve similar serving weight of all three meals. [a]Measured values. A 90% digestibility of protein from the vegetable sources was used in the calculations; [b]Analyzed values. Analyzed by a standard method (12). E%: Energy%. HP-Legume: high protein (19 E%) from legumes and HP-Meat: high protein (19 E%) from veal and pork meat. LP-Legume: low protein (9 E%) from legumes.

(HP-Meat), split peas (HP-Legume), or a combination of the two (LP-Legume) (Table 1). Water was added to the recipes of the HP-Legume and LP-Legume meals in order to achieve similar serving weight and energy density of all three meals. The final serving weight was 591 g for the three meals. The test meals were served with 300 ml of drinking water. The meals were prepared by the experienced kitchen staff at the department, but were blinded when served by the study responsible to the subjects. The energy content and nutrient composition of the test meals were calculated using Dankost 3000 dietary assessment software (Danish Catering Center, Herlev, Denmark). The software is based on the food database from the Danish Technical University. The energy factors used are 17 kJ/g for protein, 37 kJ/g for fat, 17 kJ/g for available carbohydrate, and 8 kJ/g for dietary fiber. Fiber content was analyzed by a standard method (17) and protein content was measured using the Kjeldahl method (18).

Measurements of subjective appetite

VASs were used to assess subjective perception of palatability of the test meals as well as appetite sensations before and for 180 min after consumption of the test meals. VAS, 100 mm in length with words anchored at each end, expressing the most positive and the most negative rating, were used to answer questions regarding the meal (palatability, taste, aroma, physical appearance, and off- taste) and appetite sensations (satiety, hunger, fullness, prospective food consumption, thirst, well-being, and desire to eat something fatty, sweet, salty, or meaty). The four standardized questions in relation to satiety feelings were: How satisfied do you feel? ('completely empty' to 'cannot eat another bite'); How hungry do you feel? ('not hungry at all' to 'as hungry as I have ever felt'); How full do you feel? ('not full at all' to 'totally full'); and How much do you think you can eat? ('nothing at all' to 'a large amount'). The four questions related to desire were: Do you feel like eating something sweet? ('yes, very much' to 'no, not at all'); Do you feel like eating something salty? ('yes, very much' to 'no, not at all'); Do you feel like eating something fatty? ('yes, very much' to 'no, not at all'); Do you feel like eating something meaty/fishy? ('yes, very much' to 'no, not at all'). The questionnaires were made as small booklets showing only one question at a time.

Subjects were not allowed to discuss or compare their ratings with each other and could not refer to their previous ratings when filling in the VAS booklets. The use, reproducibility, and validity of the VAS have been described before by Flint et al. (19).

In order to integrate the different feelings of appetite, a composite appetite score was calculated for each time point. The score has been described before (20) and is calculated with this formula:

[Satiety + hunger + (100-fullness) + (100-prospective food consumption)]/4.

Sample size calculation

Power calculation was done based on the primary endpoint, composite appetite score (area under the curve [AUC]) as well as on *ad libitum* energy intake. From unpublished data we estimated that a minimum of 42 subjects was required to detect an absolute difference of 275 mm*60 min in composite appetite score and 385 kJ in *ad libitum* energy intake between diets with a statistical power of 80%, and a two-sided significance level of 5%. To allow for an estimated ~10% drop out rate, 48 participants were recruited.

Statistical analyses

The statistical analyses were performed on participants who completed the intervention ($n = 43$) using SAS 9.3 (SAS Institute, Cary, NC, USA). The statistical significance level was defined as $p < 0.05$. Data are presented as estimated means ± SEM, unless otherwise stated. The appetite scores were analyzed using repeated measurements and AUC, calculated by the trapezoidal rule. Repeated measurements analyses were done using ANCOVA-type linear mixed models including a time-treatment interaction and adjusting for age, BMI, order of treatments, baseline appetite score, and with and without adjustment for assessed overall palatability of test meal. Additionally, differences between subjects were accounted for by means of random effects. AUCs were analyzed using ANCOVA models including treatment and adjusting for age, BMI, order of treatments, baseline appetite score, and with and without adjustment for assessed overall palatability of test meal. *Ad libitum* energy intake was analyzed using an ANCOVA model including treatment and adjusting for age, BMI, and order of treatments. For the repeated measurements we saw no significant time × treatment interactions. If a significant overall treatment effect was found, *post hoc* tests with Tukey-Kramer adjustment for multiplicity were carried out to identify significant differences between meals.

Table 2. Palatability assessments and AUCs of thirst and well-being of the three test meals (mm)

	HP-Meat	HP-Legume	LP-Legume
Palatability of test meal, mm	54 ± 3^a	29 ± 3^b	55 ± 4^a
Taste of test meal, mm	60 ± 3^a	31 ± 3^b	57 ± 4^a
Aroma of test meal, mm	61 ± 3^a	43 ± 3^b	57 ± 3^a
Physical appearance of test meal, mm	45 ± 4^a	29 ± 3^b	46 ± 3^a
Off-taste of test meal, mm	27 ± 4	37 ± 4	30 ± 4
Thirst AUC, mm × min	$9{,}923 \pm 470^{ab}$	$10{,}892 \pm 424^b$	$9{,}968 \pm 518^a$
Well-being AUC, mm × min	$11{,}325 \pm 313^a$	$10{,}528 \pm 331^b$	$11{,}106 \pm 328^a$

Numbers with different letters are significantly different ($p < 0.05$). AUC: Area under the curve. HP-Meat: high protein (19 E%) from veal and pork meat ($n = 43$). HP-Legume: high protein (19 E%) from legumes. LP-Legume: low protein (9 E%) from legumes.

Results

Of the 48 included subjects, 43 completed all three meal sessions and were included in the analyses (Age: 24.4 ± 4.8 years; height: 182.6 ± 7.2 cm; body weight: 76.8 ± 7.3 kg; BMI: 23.0 ± 2.1 kg/m^2). Two subjects withdrew after the first test meal because of gastrointestinal discomfort and three withdrew after the second test meal because of lack of time.

Ratings of palatability of test meals

The test meals were assessed in terms of physical appearance, aroma, taste, off-taste, and overall palatability (Table 2). The palatability of the HP-Legume meal was rated significantly poorer than that of the other two meals ($p < 0.0001$). No difference between the HP-Meat and the LP-Legume meal was observed for any of these parameters. The palatability of the *ad libitum* meal was rated similarly after the three test meals (data not shown).

Ratings of subjective appetite sensations

Postprandial responses in appetite ratings are illustrated by the scores for composite appetite and fullness sensations (Fig. 1). A significant effect of time was seen for all appetite parameters ($p < 0.0001$). Furthermore, an effect of meal was seen for all appetite parameters ($p < 0.05$). After adjusting for overall palatability, an effect of meal was still seen for composite appetite score ($p < 0.01$), prospective food consumption ($p < 0.05$), hunger ($p < 0.01$), and fullness ($p < 0.05$).

Pairwise comparisons (without adjusting for overall palatability) showed that the HP-Legume meal resulted in lower ratings for composite appetite scores, hunger, and prospective food intake compared to the HP-Meat and LP-Legume meal ($p < 0.05$ for all). Furthermore, the HP-Legume meal was significantly more satiating than the HP-Meat meal ($p < 0.05$), but not than the LP-Legume

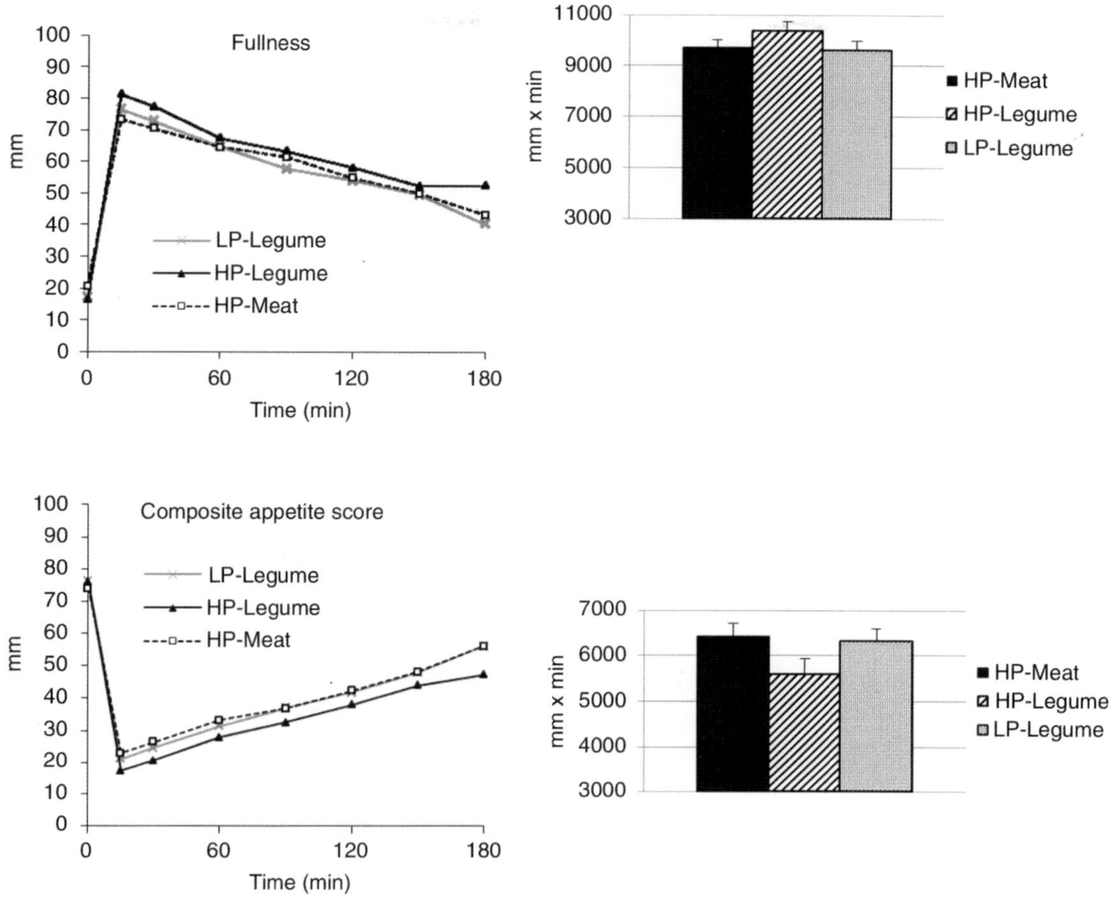

Fig. 1. Left panel: Line chart of unadjusted mean ratings. Right panel: Bar chart of mean (±SEM) area under the curves (AUC) for fullness and composite appetite score during 3 h after 3 iso-caloric test meals ($n = 43$). *Fullness*: Repeated measures (with and without adjustment for palatability): Meal $p < 0.05$, Time $p < 0.0001$. Fullness higher after HP-Legume compared with HP-Meat and LP-Legume ($p < 0.05$). AUC: HP-Legumes > LP–Legumes ($p < 0.05$). No differences in AUC after adjusting for palatability. *Composite appetite score* (CAS): Repeated measures (with and without adjustment for palatability): Meal $p < 0.05$, Time $p < 0.0001$. HP-Legume lower CAS than HP-Meat and LP-Legume, $p < 0.05$. After adjustment for palatability: HP-Legume lower than HP-Meat, $p < 0.05$ (but not than LP-Legume). AUC: HP-Legumes lower than LP-Legumes, $p < 0.05$. No differences in AUC after adjustment for palatability. HP-Meat: high protein (19 E%) from veal and pork meat. HP-Legume: high protein (19 E%) from legumes. LP-Legume: low protein (9 E%) from legumes.

meal ($p > 0.05$). When adjusting for overall palatability of the test meals, the HP-Legume meal still resulted in lower ratings of composite appetite, hunger, and prospective food intake compared to the HP-Meat meal ($p < 0.05$), but not the LP-Legume meal. Fullness after the HP-Legume meal was significantly higher than after the HP-Meat and LP-Legume meal, both with and without adjustment for overall palatability ($p < 0.05$ for both).

The AUCs showed lower composite appetite score, hunger, and prospective food intake and higher satiety after the HP-Legume meal compared to the HP-Meat meal ($p < 0.05$ for all). Additionally, the HP-Legume meal caused lower composite appetite fullness ratings compared to the LP-Legume meal ($p < 0.05$ for both). When adjusting for overall palatability of the test meal no significant differences in AUCs were seen any more.

Ad libitum energy intake

A significant meal effect was seen for *ad libitum* energy intake 3 h after the test meal ($p < 0.001$). Thus, energy intake was reduced by 400 kJ and 440 kJ (12 and 13%), ($p < 0.001$) after the HP-Legume meal compared to the HP-Meat and LP-Legume meals, respectively (Fig. 2).

Ratings of subjective sensory-specific desires

The overall well-being of the subjects was rated lower after consumption of the HP-Legume meal compared with the two other meals ($p < 0.01$ for pairwise comparisons) and the HP-Legume meal induced greater feelings of thirst than the LP-Legume meal ($p < 0.05$) (Table 2). The specific desires to eat something fatty, sweet, salty, or meaty were not different between meals ($p > 0.05$, data not shown).

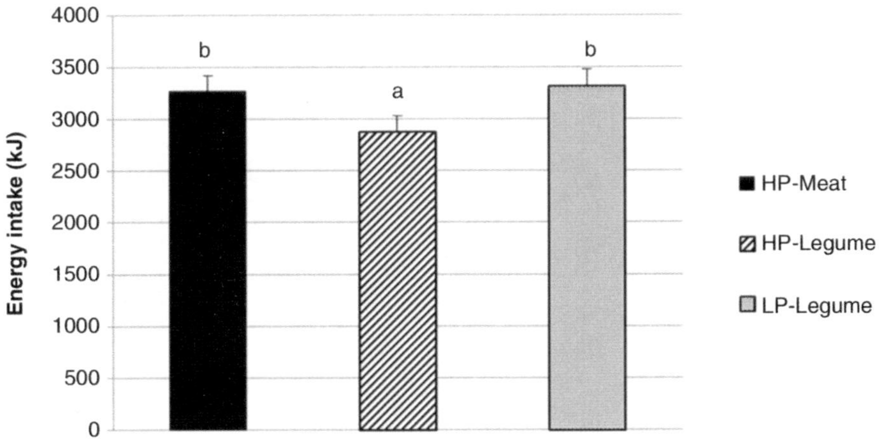

Fig. 2. *Ad libitum* energy intake (mean ± SEM) 3 h after the test meals. *Ad libitum* energy intake was reduced by 12% and 13%, respectively, after consumption of the HP-Legume meal, compared to HP-Meat and LP-Legume ($p < 0.01$ for both). HP-Meat: high protein (19 E%) from veal and pork meat. HP-Legume: high protein (19 E%) from legumes. LP-Legume: low protein (9 E%) from legumes.

Discussion

The current study showed that a high-protein meal based on vegetable sources (legumes: beans and peas), induced higher post-meal satiety ratings and lower energy intake compared with a high-protein meal based on animal sources (veal and pork). Even more interestingly, a low-protein meal based on legumes was both as satiating and as palatable as a high-protein meal based on veal and pork.

Although the vegetable meal was more favorable with regard to appetite regulation, this does not document that vegetable protein *per se* is more satiating than animal protein. Because of the choice of natural food sources, the HP vegetable meal had a higher fiber content than the HP animal meal, and this may have induced a higher satiety feeling. Also palatability of the HP legume meal was rated lower than the other two meals and this partly affected the results. Still, if choosing such vegetable protein sources, our results indicate that it is possible to obtain similar satiety, but for less protein, than with animal sources such as those chosen here.

To our knowledge, this is the first study to compare the effect on appetite regulation of vegetable meals based on beans and peas with animal meals based on pork and veal. There are several previous studies in this field. However, they have mainly examined soy vs dairy (whey, casein, milk) and used supplements and not real foods as test meals (e.g. soy or whey dissolved in water) (21). A few studies have compared pea vs dairy, but also as supplements (22, 23). Only a handful of studies have used real foods (solid) foods or meals and can therefore more readily be compared with the current study (24–28).

Douglas et al. (24) evaluated the effect of meals with beef or soy protein (34 E%) on appetite and hormonal signals in 21 young, normal-weight adults. Meals were macronutrient and fiber-matched or serving-size-matched. There were no significant differences in postprandial hunger, fullness, peptide YY (PYY), glucagon-like peptide-1 responses, or *ad libitum* energy intake after the beef or soy lunches, whether matched for macronutrients and fiber or for serving size. Another short-term cross-over study investigated iso-energetic, high-protein breakfasts and lunches (30 E% protein) based on meat (lean beef and ham) or soy (soy protein powder mixed in a shake) in 12 normal- or overweight men and women (25). No differences were seen in satiety during an 8 h postprandial period, however, lack of power could perhaps explain the lack of differences here (19).

Similar results were found in a more long-term cross-over study, which compared vegetarian (soy protein or soy-textured vegetable protein) and meat-based (chicken and beef) high-protein diets (30 E% protein) (23). Twenty overweight or obese men were included and each diet period lasted for 14 days with three meals per day. No differences in daily rated subjective appetite sensations or motivation to eat were found between the two diets (26). Still, differences in rated pleasantness of the diets might have biased the results.

Bayham et al. (27) compared egg vs cereal in energy- and macronutrient-matched breakfast meals (20 E% protein) using a 7-day cross-over design and 21 overweight men and women. They found that fullness and PYY was higher after egg vs cereal on the first study day, but there were no differences after 7 days' exposure.

The last meal test study using foods compared protein (17 E%) from mycoprotein (plant), tofu (plant), or chicken (meat) served as a pasta dish 4 h after breakfast to 42 overweight women in a cross-over design (28). The meals were isocaloric and macronutrient-matched, but the mycoprotein meal contained twice as much fiber (6 g) as the other two meals (3 g). Subjective appetite sensations did not differ, but *ad libitum* energy intake was significantly higher after intake of the chicken meal vs either of the two plant meals. This finding partly corresponds to our present findings.

As mentioned above, soy is in general the most studied vegetable protein source, whereas no or few studies have looked at brown beans or green peas, more commonly eaten in the Nordic countries. Furthermore, soy was most often given as a protein powder mixture. It can be assumed that the different vegetable sources matter when comparing studies, as the amino acid composition is not identical. Thus, in contrast to other vegetable protein sources, soy contains all essential amino acids, although in relatively small amounts. One previous study comparing soy with pea (supplements) did not see any differences, though (29). Because only 12 subjects were included here, lack of power could, however, also explain this finding (19).

One prospective cohort study which investigated the intake of animal and plant protein and subsequent weight changes is worth mentioning. The result was based on 89,432 European men and women who filled in country-specific food frequency questionnaires and were followed for a mean of 6.5 years. A positive association between animal protein and subsequent weight gain was found, but this was not the case with vegetable protein (30). This indicates less satiety from eating animal protein than plant protein. However, it is not possible to exclude whether other macronutrients or dietary factors in the food items (i.e. dietary fiber) influenced the results (30, 31).

A recent meta-analysis supports that dietary pulses can be a beneficial weight-loss strategy (32). Thus, analyses of data from 21 studies showed an overall significant weight reduction of -0.34 kg when diets included dietary pulses compared with when diets did not. The analyses also suggested that dietary pulses may reduce body fat mass.

The relatively large difference in fiber content between our test meals most likely plays an important role with regard to the satiating effects (33, 34). The fact that there was no difference between the LP-Legume meal and the HP-Meat meal indicates that a low-protein meal with fiber-rich beans/peas is as satiating as a high-protein meal with pork/veal and suggests that vegetable protein sources can be efficient alternatives for weight regulation with less use of protein than with animal protein sources. Thus, in respect to satiety, a high content of dietary fibers may be as effective as a high content of protein, when using real foods.

The strengths and weaknesses of the present study should be considered. We consider it a strength that we used real foods in realistic meals. Thus, such meals could be expected to be consumed outside the clinical setting. This is in contrast to many of the previous studies, where more unnatural meals and supplements were used. It could be argued, though, that a weakness in our design was that dietary fiber content was then not matched in the two HP meals. However, this is a consequence of using real foods. If a 2×2 factorial design had been used, we might have been able to obtain a clearer picture of the factor of interest (protein) without changing other factors that could influence the primary outcome.

The current study also highlights that a high protein level is difficult to obtain solely from vegetable sources without compromising palatability. Statistical analyses were therefore done with and without adjustment for palatability of the test meals. This resulted in similar, although less significant results for the appetite parameters. Such a finding is in line with the notion that food not considered palatable is perceived as more satiating than palatable food (35). It may be that our study subjects were not familiar with vegetable-based foods and meals and that this influenced their palatability ratings. Energy density and weight or volume are also factors important for energy intake and appetite sensations. We strived to compose meals with similar weight and hence energy density. Therefore, these factors were not likely to be of importance in the present study.

Conclusion

In conclusion, a vegetable-based meal (beans/peas) influenced appetite sensations and energy intake favorably compared to an animal-based meal (pork/veal) with similar energy and protein content. Interestingly, a vegetable-based meal with low protein content was as satiating and palatable as an animal-based meal with high protein content. Differences in dietary fiber and palatability are likely important contributing factors.

Authors' contributions

NTB and AA designed the study. NTB and SMC were responsible for collection of data. NTB and MDK performed the data analysis. NTB, MDK, and ARA drafted the manuscript. ARA was responsible for the final content. All authors participated in the discussion of the results and read and approved the final manuscript.

Acknowledgements

The study is part of the OPUS project 'Optimal well-being, development and health for Danish children through a healthy New Nordic Diet'. It is supported by a grant from the Nordea Foundation and from The Danish Agriculture & Food Council, Copenhagen, Denmark. We are grateful to the kitchen staff at the Department Nutrition, Exercise and Sports for their assistance and to the volunteers who participated in this study.

Conflict of interest and funding

AA is currently a consultant or member of advisory boards for Global Dairy Platform, USA; McCain Foods Ltd, USA; McDonald's, USA; and Weight Watchers,

USA. Furthermore, he is a member of extramural academic advisory committees: Data and safety monitoring board of the PREDIMED-PLUS multicenter trial led by University of Barcelona, Spain; International Carbohydrate Quality Consortium (ICQC) group, University of Toronto, Canada; and Global Energy Balance Network (GEBN), University of Colorado, USA. None of the other authors declared a conflict of interest.

References

1. Astrup A. The satiating power of protein – a key to obesity prevention? Am J Clin Nutr 2005; 82(1): 1–2.
2. Shai I, Schwarzfuchs D, Henkin Y, Shahar DR, Witkow S, Greenberg I, et al. Weight loss with a low-carbohydrate, Mediterranean, or low-fat diet. N Engl J Med 2008; 359(3): 229–41.
3. Skov A, Toubro S, Rønn B, Holm L, Astrup A. Randomized trial on protein vs carbohydrate in ad libitum fat reduced diet for the treatment of obesity. Int J Obes 1999; 23(5): 528–36.
4. Larsen TM, Dalskov S, van Baak M, Jebb SA, Papadaki A, Pfeiffer AF, et al. Diets with high or low protein content and glycemic index for weight-loss maintenance. N Engl J Med 2010; 363(22): 2102–13.
5. Maaslova E, Halldorsson TI, Astrup A, Olsen SF. Dietary protein-to-carbohydrate ratio and added sugar as determinants of excessive gestational weight gain: A prospective cohort study. BMJ Open 2015; 5: e005839, doi: http://dx.doi.org/10.1136/bmjopen-2014-005839
6. Paddon-Jones D, Westman E, Mattes RD, Wolfe RR, Astrup A, Westerterp-Plantenga M. Protein, weight management, and satiety. Am J Clin Nutr 2008; 87(5): 1558S–61S.
7. Belza A, Ritz C, Sorensen MQ, Holst JJ, Rehfeld JF, Astrup A. Contribution of gastroenteropancreatic appetite hormones to protein-induced satiety. Am J Clin Nutr 2013; 97(5): 980–9.
8. Raben A, Agerholm-Larsen L, Flint A, Holst JJ, Astrup A. Meals with similar energy densities but rich in protein, fat, carbohydrate, or alcohol have different effects on energy expenditure and substrate metabolism but not on appetite and energy intake. Am J Clin Nutr 2003; 77: 91–100.
9. Westerterp-Plantenga MS, Lemmens SG, Westerterp KR. Dietary protein–its role in satiety, energetics, weight loss and health. Br J Nutr 2012; 108(Suppl 2): S105–12.
10. Reijnders L, Soret S. Quantification of the environmental impact of different dietary protein choices. Am J Clin Nutr 2003; 78(Suppl 3): 664S–8S.
11. Temme EH, Toxopeus IB, Kramer GF, Brosens MC, Drijvers JM, Tyszler M, et al. Greenhouse gas emission of diets in the Netherlands and associations with food, energy and macronutrient intakes. Public Health Nutr 2015; 18: 2433–45.
12. Carlsson-Kanyama A, Gonzalez AD. Potential contributions of food consumption patterns to climate change. Am J Clin Nutr 2009; 89(5): 1704S–9S.
13. Nordic Council of Ministers. Nordic Nutrition Recommendations 2012: integrating nutrition and physical activity. Copenhagen, Denmark: Nordic Council of Ministers; 2014. doi: http://dx.doi.org/10.6027/Nord2014-002
14. Pedersen AN, Christensen T, Matthiessen J, Knudsen VK, Rosenlund-Sørensen M, Biltoft-Jensen A, et al. Danskernes Kostvaner 2011–2013. Søborg, Denmark: DTU Fødevareinstituttet; 2015.
15. Meyer C, Mithril C, Blauert E, Holt MK. Grundlag for Ny Nordisk Hverdagsmad, OPUS – WP1. Copenhagen, Denmark: Institut for Human Ernæring, Københavns Universitet; 2010.
16. Murty CM, Pittaway JK, Ball MJ. Chickpea supplementation in an Australian diet affects food choice, satiety and bowel health. Appetite 2010; 54(2): 282–8.
17. Prosky L, Asp NG, Schweizer TF, DeVries JW, Furda I. Determination of insoluble, soluble, and total dietary fiber in foods and food products: interlaboratory study. J Assoc Off Anal Chem 1988; 71(5): 1017–23.
18. Barkholt V, Jensen AL. Amino acid analysis: determination of cysteine plus half-cystine in proteins after hydrochloric acid hydrolysis with a disulfide compound as additive. Anal Biochem 1989; 177(2): 318–22.
19. Flint A, Raben A, Blundell JE, Astrup A. Reproducibility, power and validity of visual analogue scales in assessment of appetite sensations in single test meal studies. Int J Obes Relat Metab Disord 2000; 24(1): 38–48.
20. Gilbert JA, Gasteyger C, Raben A, Meier DH, Astrup A, Sjödin A. The effect of tesofensine on appetite sensations. Obesity 2012; 20: 553–61.
21. Gilbert J, Bendsen N, Tremblay A, Astrup A. Effect of proteins from different sources on body composition. Nutr Metab Cardiovasc Dis 2011; 21: B16–31.
22. Abou-Samra R, Keersmaekers L, Brienza D, Mukherjee R, Macé K. Effect of different protein sources on satiation and short-term satiety when consumed as a starter. Nutr J 2011; 10: 139. doi: http://dx.doi.org/10.1186/1475-2891-10-139
23. Overduin J, Guérin-Deremaux L, Wils D, Lambers TT. NUTRALYS(®) pea protein: characterization of in vitro gastric digestion and in vivo gastrointestinal peptide responses relevant to satiety. Food Nutr Res 2015; 59: 25622, http://dx.doi.org/10.3402/fnr.v59.25622
24. Douglas SM, Lasley TR, Leidy HL. Consuming beef vs soy protein has little effect on appetite, satiety, and food intake in healthy adults. J Nutr 2015; 145: 1010–16.
25. Tan SY, Batterham M, Tapsell LC. Energy expenditure does not differ, but protein oxidation rates appear lower in meals containing predominantly meat versus soy sources of protein. Obes Facts 2010; 3(2): 101–4. doi: http://dx.doi.org/10.1159/000290061
26. Neacsu M, Fyfe C, Horgan G, Johnstone AM. Appetite control and biomarkers of satiety with vegetarian (soy) and meat-based high-protein diets for weight loss in obese men: a randomized crossover trial. Am J Clin Nutr 2014; 100(2): 548–58.
27. Bayham BE, Greenway FL, Johnson WD, Durandhar NV. A randomized trial to manipulate the quality instead of quantity of dietary proteins to influence the markers of satiety. J Diabetes Complications 2014; 28: 547–52.
28. Williamson DA, Geiselman PJ, Lovejoy J, Greenway F, Volaufova J, Martin CK, et al. Effects of consuming mycoprotein, tofu or chicken upon subsequent eating behaviour, hunger and safety. Appetite 2006; 46: 41–8.
29. Lang V, Bellisle F, Oppert JM, Craplet C, Bornet FR, Slama G, et al. Satiating effect of proteins in healthy subjects: a comparison of egg albumin, casein, gelatin, soy protein, pea protein, and wheat gluten. Am J Clin Nutr 1998; 67(6): 1197–204.
30. Halkjær J, Olsen A, Overvad K, Jakobsen M, Boeing H, Buijsse B, et al. Intake of total, animal and plant protein and subsequent changes in weight or waist circumference in European men and women: the Diogenes project. Int J Obes 2011; 35(8): 1104–13.
31. Smith JD, Hou T, Ludwig DS, Rimm EB, Willett W, Hu FB, et al. Changes in intake of protein foods, carbohydrate amount and quality, and long-term weight change: results from 3 prospective cohorts. Am J Clin Nutr 2015; 101: 1216–24. doi: http://dx.doi.org/10.3945/ajcn.114.100867
32. Kim SJ, de Souza RJ, Choo VL, Ha V, Cozma AI, Chiavaroli L, et al. Effects of dietary pulse consumption on body weight: a systematic review and meta-analysis of randomized controlled trials. Am J Clin Nutr 2016; 103: 1213–23.

33. Burton-Freeman B. Dietary fiber and energy regulation. J Nutr 2000; 130(Suppl 2S): 272S–5S.
34. Slavin JL. Dietary fiber and body weight. Nutrition 2005; 21(3): 411–18.
35. Drewnowski A. Energy density, palatability, and satiety: implications for weight control. Nutr Rev 1998; 56(12): 347–53.

*Anne Raben
Department of Nutrition, Exercise and Sports
Faculty of Science
University of Copenhagen
DK-1958 Frederiksberg, Denmark
Email: ara@nexs.ku.dk

8

Enhanced polyunsaturated fatty acids production in *Mortierella alpina* by SSF and the enrichment in chicken breasts

Shengli Yang[1]* and Hui Zhang[2]*

[1]The College of Pharmaceutical Science, Zhejiang University of Technology, Hangzhou, People's Republic of China;
[2]Physical and Chemical Test Center, Zhejiang Institute of Quality Inspection Science, Hangzhou, China

Abstract

Background: Distiller's dried grains with solubles (DDGS) and soybean meal were used as the substrates for the production of polyunsaturated fatty acids (PUFA) in solid-state fermentation (SSF) by *Mortierella alpine*. These fermented products were fed to laying hens. PUFA enrichment from chicken breasts was studied.

Methods: The maximum productivity of PUFA was achieved under optimized process condition, including 1% w/w yeast extract as additive, an incubation period of 5 days at 12°C, 10% v/w inoculum level, 75% moisture content, and pH 6.0. The hens were then fed with ration containing soybean DDGS, rapeseed oil, soybean oil, and peanut oil. The control group was fed with basal ration.

Results: Under the optimal condition, *M. alpine* produced total fatty acids (TFA) of 182.34 mg/g dry substrate. It has better mycelial growth when soybean meal was added to DDGS (SDDGS). PUFA in fermentation product increased with higher soybean meal content. The addition of 70% soybean meal to DDGS substrate yielded 175.16 mg of TFA, including 2.49 mg eicosapentaenoic acid (EPA) and 5.26 mg docosahexaenoic acid (DHA). The ratios of ω-6/ω-3 found in chicken breasts fat were all lower than that found in control by 36.98, 31.51, 18.15, and 12.63% for SDDGS, rapeseed oil, soybean oil, and peanut oil, respectively.

Conclusions: This study identified an optimized SSF process to maximize PUFA productivity by *M. alpine* as the strain. This PUFA-enriched feed increased the PUFA contents as well as the proportions of ω-6 and ω-3 in chicken breasts and liver.

Keywords: *PUFA*; *DDGS*; Mortierella alpina; *soybean meal*; *solid-state fermentation*; *chicken breasts*; *enrichment*

Fatty acids are the major energy source and reservoir for animals to grow and survive (1–3). However, not all the fatty acids are equal. Dietary saturated fat intake has been associated with increased risk of cardiovascular disease. As substitutes of saturated fatty acids, polyunsaturated fatty acids (PUFA) provide many health benefits (4, 5), for example, a reduction in low-density lipoprotein or bad cholesterol and an increase in high-density lipoproteins or good cholesterol (6). Moreover, PUFA contain essential fatty acids like omega-3 and omega-6, which the body need but are not able to synthesize. Eicosapentaenoic acid (EPA), found in fatty cold-water fish and fish oil supplements along with docosahexaenoic acid (DHA) (7), is one of the several omega-3 fatty acids used by the body. Omega-3 fatty acids help lower the risk of heart disease. Increased intake of EPA has beneficial effects on coronary heart disease, high blood pressure, and inflammatory disorders, such as rheumatoid arthritis (8). Most people in the Western countries do not get enough omega-3 fatty acids in their diet, which is one of the reasons that PUFA production has become a prominent research focus.

Microorganisms have been used in PUFA production in recent years (9–15). Several *Mortierella* strains are reported (16–18). The most common *Mortierella* species are *M. alpine* (19, 20) and *M. isabellina* (21, 22). Among the large amounts of published information on microbial PUFA production, EPA (23–28), arachidonic acid (AA) (29–32), and γ-linolenic acid (GLA) (33, 34) are the most popular targets.

Agricultural coproducts such as soybean meal, distiller's dried grains with solubles (DDGS), rice bran, and wheat bran are abundantly produced. Both soybean meal and DDGS are good substrates for enzymes to produce oil. Being economically competitive, soybean meal and DDGS were used as the base substrate in the present study to produce PUFA using *M. alpina* by solid-state fermentation (SSF).

Adding lipids in feed has been in place for more than 50 years, since 1953. Lipids improve the energy density of the diet and provide essential fatty acids for poultry. Lipids also improve the palatability and processing properties of feed. Essential fatty acids can inhibit the inflammation, promote brain development, inhibit tumor growth, as well as can reduce the plasma triglyceride and cholesterol levels to inhibit thrombosis and atherosclerosis (35).

Fermentation using agricultural coproducts as a substrate can produce a variety of unsaturated fatty acids. PUFA, especially EPA and DHA deposition in poultry, are very important as we essentially need them for our health. The objectives of this study were to determine the parameters for the growth of the fungi selected and to examine the PUFA changes after fermentation. This study at the current stage is a proof of concept in nature. This PUFA-enriched feed increased the PUFA contents as well as the proportions of ω-6 and ω-3 in chicken breasts and liver.

Materials and methods

Microorganisms

Mortierella alpina was maintained on potato dextrose (PD) agar slants at 4°C and transferred every 3 months.

Seed culture and inoculum preparation

The fungi were cultivated on PD agar containing 2.0% agar and incubated at 20°C for 7 days until complete sporulation. The spores from the agar were suspended in 15% glycerol. The suspension was used as inoculums (10^7 spores/mL).

Solid-state fermentation

Two miniliter spore suspensions of *M. alpina* were transferred to shake flasks (250 mL) containing 50-mL PD medium. Flasks were shaken at 20°C and 150 rpm for 24 h. Inoculum (10% v/w) was transferred to 40 g (as is) substrate in a 250-mL Erlenmeyer flask. The moisture contents of soybean meal and DDGS were adjusted to 75% and the pH to 6.0 before inoculation. Samples were incubated for 10 days. A water reservoir was placed in the incubator to maintain constant moisture content. All treatments were performed in triplicate.

Optimization of process parameters

SSF was conducted to optimize various process parameters influencing PUFA production, including incubation temperature (10, 12, 15, 20, and 25°C), incubation time, initial moisture content of the substrate (60, 65, 70, 75, and 80%), inoculation volume (5, 8, 10, 12, 15, and 20%), and initial pH (5, 5.5, 6, 6.5, 7, 7.5, and 8). All treatments were performed in triplicate.

Effect of carbon source on DDGS SSF

DDGS was supplemented with different carbon sources (1% w/w) such as glucose, maltose, fructose, sucrose, and starch to study their effects on PUFA production. The substrate moisture content was 75% and pH was 6.0. All samples were incubated for 5 days at 20°C and then at 12°C for an additional 5 days. All treatments were performed in triplicate.

Effect of nitrogen source on DDGS SSF

Given the poor growth of the fungi on DDGS, nitrogen sources (1% w/w), such as ammonium sulfate, urea, peptone, casein, and yeast extract, were added into DDGS to examine their effect on PUFA production. All treatments were performed in triplicate.

Effect of soybean meal addition on DDGS SSF

The moisture contents of soybean meal and DDGS were adjusted to 75%. Soybean meal was added at various concentrations (0, 30, 40, 50, 60, and 70%, as is) to the DDGS substrate to enhance the PUFA production. The substrate pH was adjusted to 6.0, and fermentation was conducted for 5 days at 20°C and then at 12°C for an additional 5 days. All treatments were performed in triplicate.

Test animals and feeds

Sixty healthy 52-week-old laying hens were selected and divided into four treatment groups based on weights. Each treatment was repeated five times, with four laying hens for each repetition. Single-factor completely randomized design was adopted in the test. Test Groups 1, 2, 3, and 4 were fed with a recipe containing soybean DDGS (SDDGS), 3% rapeseed oil, 3% soybean oil, and 3% peanut oil, respectively. The control group was fed with base recipe. The test period was 45 days.

Sample collection and analytical methods

During the study period, eggs were collected and counted; the weight of the eggs and the ration consumption were determined. This study was approved by the Animal Ethics Committee in Zhejiang University (*Institutional Animal Welfare and Ethics Committee* in Zhejiang University, China). At the end of the test period, the laying hens were sacrificed by cervical dislocation, and their liver and breast were obtained for later use.

PUFA analysis

Fermented flour (1 g) was soaked in 30 mL of chloroform/methanol (2:1, v/v) supplemented with 1.5 mL sulfuric acid. Mixture was refluxed for 1 h and reaction was stopped by adding 5 mL deionized water. The lipid phase was then dried. Fatty acid methyl esters were extracted using hexanes and analyzed using capillary gas chromatography (GC; Hewlett-Packard model 5890 series II) equipped with flame ionization detector. The conditions used for GC were as follows: injection temperature, 230°C; detector temperature, 230°C, oven temperature was programmed from 130 to 220°C with a heating rate of 10°C/min. The column used was a supelco sp-2330

(Bellefonte, PA) capillary column, 15 m (length) × 0.25 nm (i.d.) × 0.2 μm (film thickness).

Statistical analyses

All treatments were repeated as described under each experiment. ANOVA was performed using SAS and the least significant difference mean comparison was used to compare treatment mean differences at $p = 5\%$.

Results

PUFA accumulation by SSF with M. alpina using DDGS and soybean meal as substrates

As shown in Table 1, each gram of soybean meal substrate yielded 58.75 mg of total fatty acids (TFA), including 0.91 mg EPA, 2.10 mg DHA, 23.65 mg linoleic acid (LA), and 2.29 mg α-linolenic acid (ALA) after a 10-day incubation. As shown in Table 2, each gram of DDGS yielded only 0.42 mg EPA and 0.95 mg DHA, in comparison. This also indicates that soybean meal may be a better nitrogen source for *M. alpina* than DDGS. Therefore, the addition of soybean meal to DDGS may help improve SSF performance.

Effect of incubation temperature and time on PUFA content of DDGS SSF

The maximum PUFA yield was obtained at 12°C; however, the microbial growth was better at 20°C. The strains hardly synthesized EPA and DHA when the temperature exceeded 20°C. The detailed results are presented in Table 3. A decrease in the PUFA yield was observed when the incubation temperature was higher or lower than 12°C, indicating that 12°C is more advantageous for PUFA production by *M. alpina*. Although a higher temperature was beneficial to mycelial growth, some adverse effects on the metabolic activities were nevertheless observed. Therefore, we designed a two-phase incubation process with programmed temperatures, that is, 5-day preincubation at 20°C and an additional incubation period (2, 3, 4, 5, 6, and 7 days) at 12°C. The maximum PUFA yield was obtained after 5-day preincubation at 20°C followed by another 5-day incubation at 12°C (Table 4).

Table 1. Polyunsaturated fatty acids accumulation from *M. alpina* for SSF on soybean meal after 10-day incubation

PUFA name	PUFA formation (original), mg/g dry substrate	PUFA formation (fermented), mg/g dry substrate
16:0	1.33 ± 0.17	9.96 ± 0.82*
18:0	0.50 ± 0.04	2.63 ± 0.23*
18:1	1.63 ± 0.24	12.91 ± 1.18*
18:2	2.01 ± 0.21	23.65 ± 2.84*
18:3	0.27 ± 0.02	2.29 ± 0.331*
20:5	0.00	0.91 ± 0.04*
22:6	0.00	2.10 ± 0.22*
Total	6.08	58.75

PUFA, polyunsaturated fatty acids; SSF, solid-state fermentation.
*$p < 00.05$ compared with unfermented group.

Table 2. Polyunsaturated fatty acids accumulation from *M. alpina* for SSF on DDGS after 10-day incubation

PUFA name	PUFA formation (original), mg/g dry substrate	PUFA formation (fermented), mg/g dry substrate
16:0	14.81 ± 1.08	15.48 ± 1.40
18:0	2.00 ± 0.19	2.32 ± 0.18*
18:1	25.70 ± 2.32	25.50 ± 2.06
18:2	57.46 ± 4.88	56.42 ± 5.71
18:3	2.11 ± 0.24	2.43 ± 0.28
20:5	0.00	0.42 ± 0.03*
22:6	0.00	0.95 ± 0.08*
Total	105.16	108.32

DDGS, distiller's dried grains with solubles; PUFA, polyunsaturated fatty acids; SSF, solid-state fermentation.
*$p < 00.05$ compared with unfermented group.

Effect of initial substrate moisture content on PUFA content

A high PUFA yield was attained with an initial moisture level of 75% (Fig. 1a). The moisture content of the SSF substrate affects dissolved oxygen and, consequently, the biosynthesis and secretion of products (36). Low moisture content decreases the solubility of nutrients in the substrate. Also, low degree of swelling and low water activity limit the growth of microorganisms (37). This explains low PUFA content at low moisture content (Fig. 1a). An increase in moisture level is believed to reduce substrate porosity, thus limiting oxygen transfer (38). Therefore, the moisture content of the medium should be controlled within a suitable range. The most suitable moisture content of the medium for PUFA production of *M. alpina* was 75%.

Effect of inoculation volume on DDGS SSF and PUFA content

The inoculation volume significantly affected fermentation, considering the maximum PUFA production was obtained at 10% (v/w) inoculum compared with other higher inoculation volumes. The results are presented in Fig. 1b. A lower inoculum level may give insufficient biomass, causing reduced product formation, whereas a higher inoculum level may produce too much biomass, leading to poor product formation.

Effect of initial pH on DDGS SSF and PUFA content

The pH level is another important factor affecting the growth and product yield during SSF. Each microorganism has an optimal pH and pH range for its growth and activity. The initial pH values were adjusted with the addition of HCl or NaOH to 5.0, 5.5, 6.0, 6.5, 7.0, or 7.5 to

Table 3. Effect of incubation temperature on PUFA from *M. alpina* for SSF on DDGS

	PUFA (mg/g dry substrate)							
Temp. (°C)	16:0	18:0	18:1	18:2	18:3	20:5	22:6	Total
10	15.35 ± 1.32^{b}	2.17 ± 0.28^{c}	24.16 ± 2.59^{c}	57.43 ± 4.66^{b}	2.39 ± 0.24^{b,c}	0.32 ± 0.03^{b}	0.74 ± 0.05^{b}	109.26^{b}
12	15.89 ± 1.44^{a}	2.51 ± 0.17^{a}	24.33 ± 2.31^{a,b}	58.04 ± 5.27^{a}	2.58 ± 0.26^{a}	0.41 ± 0.04^{a}	0.93 ± 0.08^{a}	111.69^{a}
15	14.78 ± 1.39^{c}	2.22 ± 0.21^{b,c}	24.03 ± 2.48^{d}	57.49 ± 5.06^{b}	2.58 ± 0.24^{a}	0.28 ± 0.03^{b}	0.66 ± 0.07^{b}	109.14^{b}
20	15.37 ± 1.52^{b}	2.32 ± 0.22^{b}	24.58 ± 2.34^{a}	56.42 ± 4.77^{c}	2.43 ± 0.21^{b}	0.02 ± 0.01^{c}	0.15 ± 0.01^{c}	107.56^{c}
25	15.28 ± 1.48^{b}	2.03 ± 0.19^{d}	24.22 ± 2.26^{b,c}	57.63 ± 5.13^{b}	2.34 ± 0.16^{c}	0.00	0.06 ± 0.01^{c}	107.21^{c}

DDGS, distiller's dried grains with solubles; PUFA, polyunsaturated fatty acids.
Mean SD, $n = 3$. Means in the same column that do not share alphabetic superscript show significant difference at 0.05 level according to Duncan's multiple range test.
[a–d]Means in the same column per parameter with different letters are significantly different at $P < 0.05$ by Tukey's range test.

evaluate the effects of the initial pH value of the solid substrate on PUFA synthesis. Microbial growth achieved a high rate in the pH range of 5–7.5 and decreased dramatically when the pH falls out of this range. Maximum PUFA production was obtained at pH 6.0 (Fig. 1c).

Effect of additional carbon source on DDGS SSF and PUFA content

The substrate moisture content was maintained at 75%, the pH at 6.0, and the inoculation volume at 10% (v/w). All samples were initially incubated for 5 days at 20°C and then at 12°C for an additional 5 days. PUFA production was assayed for the control with DDGS alone as the substrate. Very low PUFA were obtained. The TFA obtained were about 103.52 mg/g dry substrate, composing of 0.42 mg EPA and 0.95 mg DHA, during the 10-day incubation. The addition of different sugars (1% w/w) into DDGS resulted in better PUFA production, the highest was obtained with starch (Fig. 2a), followed by glucose, maltose, fructose, and sucrose. With starch, TFA obtained were about 164.25 mg/g dry substrate, composing of 2.34 mg EPA, 72.38 mg LA, 7.48 mg ALA, and 4.66 mg DHA, during the 10-day incubation.

Effect of additional nitrogen source on DDGS SSF and PUFA content

The nitrogen source or nitrogen availability is an important factor in microbial growth and enzyme production. Since DDGS led to poor fungal growth, different nitrogen sources were added into DDGS to further optimize SSF efficiency. Figure 2b shows the differences in PUFA contents produced with various nitrogen sources. The results showed that PUFA production in nitrogen-supplemented DDGS increased remarkably in comparison with the control. Among these nitrogen sources, the addition of yeast extract yielded the highest PUFA, about 182.34 mg/g dry substrate including 2.84 mg EPA, 79.03 mg LA, 7.78 mg ALA, and 6.05 mg DHA, after the 10-day incubation. Peptone yielded the second highest PUFA yield, followed by casein. Furthermore, organic nitrogen sources were significantly better than inorganic nitrogen sources, indicating that organic nitrogen sources may be more suitable for the growth of *M. alpina* and PUFA formation.

Effect of soybean meal addition in DDGS on PUFA content

PUFA production was relatively low in DDGS with poor growth. The strains grew better when soybean meal was

Table 4. Effect of incubation time on PUFA from *M. alpina* for SSF on DDGS at 12°C

	PUFA (mg/g dry substrate)							
Time (days)	16:0	18:0	18:1	18:2	18:3	20:5	22:6	Total
2	14.87 ± 1.25^{d}	2.04 ± 0.22^{c}	25.67 ± 2.47^{a,b}	56.88 ± 5.28^{b}	2.16 ± 0.19^{b}	0.09 ± 0.01^{c}	0.32 ± 0.03^{d}	107.42^{c}
3	14.99 ± 1.39^{d}	2.26 ± 0.23^{a,b}	25.59 ± 2.27^{b}	57.19 ± 5.09^{a}	2.13 ± 0.24^{b}	0.14 ± 0.01^{c}	0.51 ± 0.03^{c}	108.29^{c}
4	15.72 ± 1.51^{b}	2.01 ± 0.25^{c}	25.48 ± 2.26^{b}	56.07 ± 4.97^{c}	1.96 ± 0.16^{c}	0.27 ± 0.01	0.76 ± 0.04^{b}	110.58^{b}
5	16.02 ± 1.47^{a}	2.28 ± 0.26^{a,b}	25.74 ± 2.31^{a}	56.18 ± 5.17^{c}	2.49 ± 0.22^{a}	0.45 ± 0.02^{a}	0.92 ± 0.05^{a}	111.68^{a}
6	15.87 ± 1.45^{b}	2.31 ± 0.18^{a}	24.93 ± 2.29^{c}	57.04 ± 4.83^{a,b}	2.36 ± 0.20^{a,b}	0.41 ± 0.02^{a,b}	0.87 ± 0.06^{a,b}	110.86^{b}
7	15.26 ± 1.43^{c}	2.26 ± 0.21^{a,b}	24.27 ± 2.34^{d}	56.13 ± 5.28^{c}	2.05 ± 0.17^{c}	0.31 ± 0.02^{b}	0.65 ± 0.05^{b,c}	108.43^{c}

DDGS, distiller's dried grains with solubles; PUFA, polyunsaturated fatty acids.
Mean SD, $n = 3$. Means in the same column that do not share alphabetic superscript show significant difference at 0.05 level according to Duncan's multiple range test.
[a–d]Means in the same column per parameter with different letters are significantly different at $P < 0.05$ by Tukey's range test.

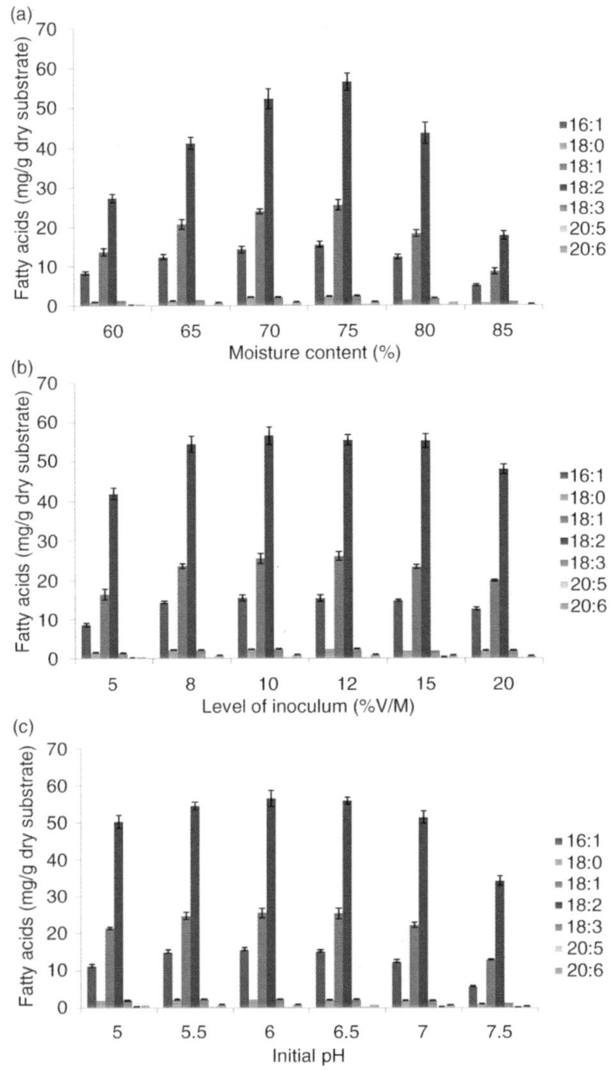

Fig. 1. Effects of initial moisture content, inoculums concentration, and initial pH on PUFA production from *Mortierella alpina* by SSF using DDGS as the substrate after 10-day incubation.

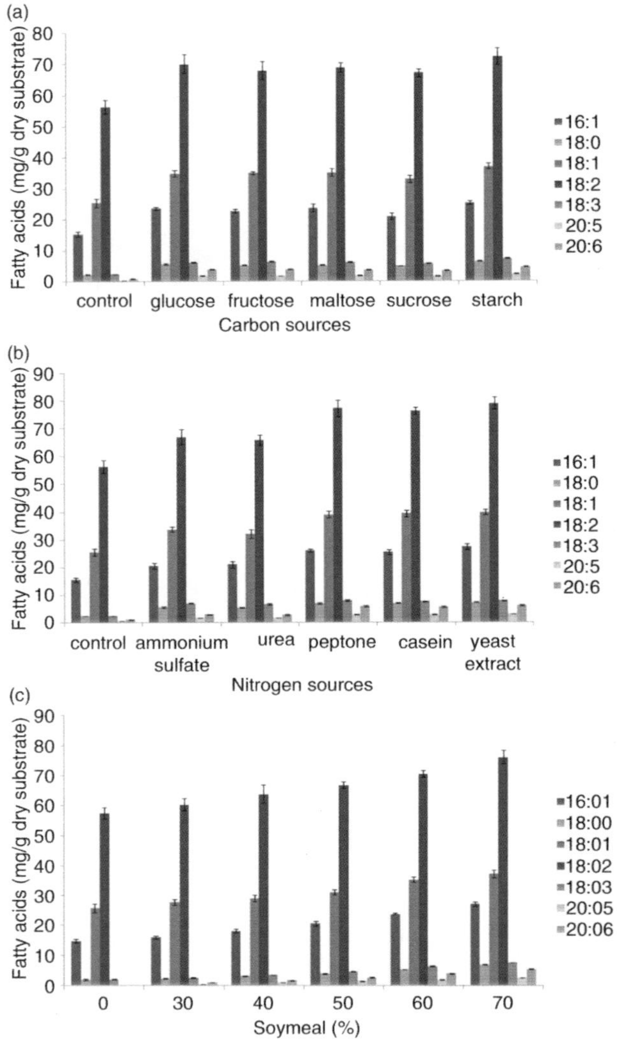

Fig. 2. Effects of carbon sources addition, nitrogen sources addition, and soybean meal addition in DDGS on PUFA production from *Mortierella alpina* by SSF after 10-day incubation.

added to DDGS, as mentioned early. PUFA production also increased with increasing soybean meal content. PUFA production from fermented DDGS with different soybean meal concentrations is presented in Fig. 2c. A positive relation between PUFA and soybean meal percentage in DDGS was observed. The addition of 70% soybean meal to the DDGS substrate yielded 175.16 mg of TFA, including 2.49 mg EPA, 75.94 mg LA, 7.52 mg ALA, and 5.26 mg DHA for 10-day incubation.

PUFA enrichment and proportion in chicken breasts and liver

The changes in the enrichment and proportion of PUFA in chicken breasts and liver are shown in Table 5. In the test groups fed with SDDGS and vegetable oil-added ration, the PUFA contents in the chicken breasts and liver were higher than those in the control group ($p < 0.05$). Table 5 shows that the proportions of ω-6 and ω-3 in chicken breasts in Test Groups 1, 2, 3, and 4 were 36.98, 31.51, 18.15, and 12.63% lower than that of the control group, respectively. The content of ω-6 in Test Group 3 was significantly different from that of the control group ($p < 0.01$). In addition, the proportions of both in liver and in the test groups were slightly higher than that of the control group, with the values for Test Groups 1, 2, and 3 higher by 0.76, 0.50, and 0.31%, respectively. A significant difference in the ω-6 content in the liver was observed among the test groups ($p < 0.05$). No difference was found in the ω-6 content in chicken breasts among Test Groups 1, 2, and 4. The ω-3 content in the liver of Test Group 1 was significantly different from that of the control group ($p < 0.01$). Furthermore, the ω-3 content was significantly different among the test groups ($p < 0.05$).

Table 5. PUFA enrichment and proportion in chicken breasts and liver

Group	Liver			Chicken breasts		
	ω-6 (g/100g TFA)	ω-3 (g/100g TFA)	Proportion	ω-6 (g/100g TFA)	ω-3 (g/100g TFA)	Proportion
1 (SDDGS)	24.50 ± 2.62^{a}	4.01 ± 0.64^{a}	$6.11{:}1^{a}$	23.70 ± 3.14^{a}	0.94 ± 0.33^{a}	$25.21{:}1^{a}$
2 (3% rapeseed oil)	22.70 ± 2.87^{b}	$3.88 \pm 0.71^{b,c}$	$5.85{:}1^{b}$	22.40 ± 2.72^{c}	0.63 ± 0.45^{b}	$30.68{:}1^{b}$
3 (% soybean oil)	22.30 ± 1.93^{b}	3.94 ± 0.43^{b}	$5.66{:}1^{c}$	22.90 ± 2.44^{b}	0.52 ± 0.17^{c}	$44.04{:}1^{c}$
4 (3% peanut oil)	21.20 ± 2.46^{c}	$3.98 \pm 0.35^{a,b}$	5.33:1	$22.80 \pm 2.91^{b,c}$	0.46 ± 0.25^{c}	$49.56{:}1^{d}$
Control group	17.40 ± 2.22	3.25 ± 0.62	5.35:1	19.90 ± 2.78	0.32 ± 0.28	62.19:1

PUFA, polyunsaturated fatty acids; SDDGS, soybean distiller's dried grains with solubles; TFA, total fatty acids.
Mean SD, $n = 3$. Means in the same column that do not share alphabetic superscript show significant difference at 0.05 level according to Duncan's multiple range test.
[a–d]Means in the same column per parameter with different letters are significantly different at $P < 0.05$ by Tukey's range test.

Discussion

Nitrogen source supplement could provide additional nutrients for microbial growth and consequently increase PUFA production. Ben-Amotz (39) indicated that high concentrations of nitrogen source could stimulate EPA production. Nitrogen content of the solid substrate could stimulate ω-3 PUFA production, especially EPA. The organic nitrogen sources and inorganic nitrogen sources were used to improve PUFA production by SSF using DDGS as the substrate. Some researchers have suggested that different strains have different preferences for either inorganic or organic nitrogen for growth and PUFA production, although organic nitrogen sources are usually used for PUFA production (40). In our studies, PUFA production was higher when organic nitrogen sources were used (Fig. 2b and c). Furthermore, organic nitrogen sources were proven more effective than inorganic nitrogen sources in enhancing cell growth and PUFA production. Thus, the soybean meal and DDGS mixture showed good potential as base substrate for PUFA production with *M. alpina*. Sajbidor et al. (41) and Jang et al. (42) reported that carbon/nitrogen ratio of solid substrate was very important in PUFA production.

PUFA production of the fungi was significantly influenced by the moisture content of substrate in SSF. The moisture content in SSF substrate affects dissolved oxygen and thus the biosynthesis and secretion of PUFA. Low moisture content causes a reduction in the solubility of nutrients in the substrate and a low degree of swelling (37), and low water activity limits the growth of microorganisms (43). Lekha and Lonsane (44) also indicated that high moisture contents decreased the porosity and the gas exchange, induced the loss of particle structure and the production of stickiness, reduced the gas volume, and enhanced the aerial mycelium formation. Jang et al. (45) reported that the initial moisture content of solid substrate ranging from 60 to 65% was good for PUFAs production. Moisture content at 70–75% favored the production of ω-6 series PUFAs; while moisture content at 60–65% was good for the production of ω-3 series PUFA. Therefore, we determined that the moisture content of 75% is most suitable for PUFA production in our system (Fig. 1).

The suitable range of ratios between ω-6 and ω-3 recommended by WHO are 1:1–8:1 (46), that by USA are 4:1–15:1 (47), respectively. However, with more demand for ω-3 due to health concerns, this ratio needs to be further reduced (48, 49). This study shows that the proportion of both in the liver was within the suitable range. The proportion of these two fatty acids in chicken breasts was obviously beyond the suitable range. The result indicates that, after adding either of the three vegetable oils and SDDGS, the increment in ω-6 content was higher than that of ω-3. This observation may be related to the different LA contents in the three vegetable oils and SDDGS. These fatty acids, after being absorbed through the intestines of domestic birds, are transported to the liver, and go into the tissue. During this period, palmitic acid, saturated fatty acids can be converted into linoleic and linolenic acids through desaturase and chain extension, while stearic acid can be converted into oleic and LAs. Therefore, after adding vegetable oil and SDDGS into the feed, the proportions of ω-6 and ω-3 in the liver tended to stabilize. Furthermore, the proportions of ω-6 and ω-3 in chicken breasts fed by SDDGS were more close to the suitable range, indicating that SDDGS as a feed for chicken breasts is more helpful in balancing ω-6 and ω-3 in chicken breasts than vegetable oil.

The balance between ω-6 and ω-3, which is very important for stable internal environment and normal growth, can reduce the incidence of cardiovascular diseases and other chronic diseases, and is conducive to mental health (50–54). Both of them cannot be converted in but can interact with the body (55–57). Therefore, the focus should be given on their proportion while their adequate supply is ensured. Many experiments have verified that regulated feed was feasible to produce poultry products with high ω-3 and controlled ratio of ω-6 and ω-3 (58). These studies provided a reliable basis for further investigation and production of poultry products rich in ω-3.

Conclusions

In this study, soybean meal and DDGS were successfully utilized as SSF substrates for PUFA production by *M. alpina*. Higher biomass and PUFA yield were achieved using DDGS supplemented with soybean meal compared with DDGS alone. PUFA production can also be optimized by added carbon and nitrogen sources, especially organic nitrogen, for the growth of *M. alpina* and PUFA production. SSF enrichment of PUFA is feasible using *M. alpina* as the starting strain. The product from this SSF process improved the laying rate, increased the PUFA contents in chicken breasts and liver, and enhanced the proportions of ω-6 and ω-3. The optimized SSF process we verified is a unique process to maximize PUFA yield by *M. alpina.*

Acknowledgements

Great appreciation is given to all members of our laboratory for their enthusiastic participation in the research, as well as Wang Guang and Michael Pu for their editorial help.

Conflict of interest and funding

The authors have not received any funding or benefits from industry or elsewhere to conduct this study.

References

1. Jain JL, Jain S, Jain N. Fundamentals of biochemistry. India: Chand (S.) & Co Ltd; 2005, pp. 565.
2. Yngvar O. Resources for fish feed in future mariculture. Aquacult Environ Interact 2011; 1: 187–200.
3. Annison EF, Bryden WL. Perspectives on ruminant nutrition and metabolism. II. Metabolism in ruminant tissues. Nutr Res Rev 1999; 12: 147–77.
4. Ciftci O, Cetin A, Aydin M, Kaya K, Oguz F. Fish oil contained in eicosapentaenoic acid and docosahexaenoic acid, attenuates testicular and spermatological damage induced by cisplatin in rats. Andrologia 2014; 46: 1161–8.
5. Yoshida H, Ito K, Sato R. Clinical relevance of decreased ratios of serum eicosapentaenoic acid/arachidonic acid (AA) and docosahexaenoic acid/AA to impaired arterial stiffness. Int J Cardiol 2014; 177: 517–9.
6. Siri-Tarino PW, Krauss RM, Sun Q, Hu FB. Saturated fatty acids and risk of coronary heart disease: modulation by replacement nutrients. Curr Atheroscler Rep 2010; 12: 384–90.
7. James GM, Jerry K, Bradley R, James CL, Paul R, Ross Z. Biochemical characterization of polyunsaturated fatty acid synthesis in Schizochytrium: release of the products as free fatty acids. Plant Physiol Bioch 2009; 47: 472–8.
8. Jeffery LE, Calder P, Raza K. Plasma levels of polyunsaturated omega-3-eicosapentaenoic acid are associated with anti-TNF response in rheumatoid arthritis and inhibit the etanercept driven rise in Th17 cell differentiation in vitro. Immun 2014; 143: 143.
9. Ashwini T, Ramin A, Ajay KD, Uday SA, Janusz AK. Extraction and fractionation of polyunsaturated fatty acids from *Mortierella sp.* using supercritical fluid: experimental and kinetic studies. Asia Pac J Chem Eng 2014; 9: 507–18.
10. Eiji S, Akinori A, Sakayu S, Jun O. Metabolic engineering for the production of polyunsaturated fatty acids by oleaginous fungus *Mortierella alpina* 1S–4. J Bioscie Bioeng 2013; 116: 417–22.
11. Hao G, Chen H, Wang L, Gu Z, Song Y, Zhang H, et al. Role of malic enzyme during fatty acid synthesis in the oleaginous fungus *Mortierella alpina*. Appl Environ Microbiol 2014; 80: 2672–8.
12. Jung IS, Lovitt RW. Integrated production of long chain polyunsaturated fatty acids (PUFA)-rich Schizochytrium biomass using a nutrient supplemented marine aquaculture wastewater. Aquacult Eng 2010; 43: 51–61.
13. Nisha A, Venkateswaran G. Effect of culture variables on mycelial arachidonic acid production by *Mortierella alpine.* Food Bioproc Tech 2011; 4: 232–40.
14. Spencer DS, Roberto EA, Kevin TB, Andrew WN. Use of raw glycerol to produce oil rich in polyunsaturated fatty acids by a thraustochytrid. Enzyme Microb Technol 2011; 48: 267–72.
15. Sun Q, Liu J, Zhang Q, Qing X, Gary D, Li X. Characterization of three novel desaturases involved in the delta-6 desaturation pathways for polyunsaturated fatty acid biosynthesis from *Phytophthora infestans.* Appl Microbiol Biotechnol 2013; 97: 7689–97.
16. Jin MJ, Huang H, Xiao AH, Gao Z, Liu X, Peng C. Enhancing arachidonic acid production by *Mortierella alpine* ME-1 using improved mycelium aging technology. Bioprocess Biosyst Eng 2009; 32: 117–22.
17. Worapol J, Tsunehiro A, Rieko T, Kazuhiro I, Seiji K, Kazuhisa O. Purification and characterization of intracellular lipase from the polyunsaturated fatty acid-producing fungus *Mortierella alliacea*. N Biotechnol 2011; 28: 158–64.
18. Yu AQ, Zhu JC, Zhang B, Xing LJ, Li MC. Effects of different carbon sources on the growth, fatty acids production, and expression of three desaturase genes of *Mortierella alpina* ATCC 16266. Curr Microbiol 2011; 62: 1617–22.
19. Ganesan V, Govindarajulu V. Production and enhancement of omega-3 fatty acid from *Mortierella alpina* CFR-GV15: its food and therapeutic application. BioMed Res Int 2014; 2014: 9–17.
20. Hiroshi K, Eiji S, Shigenobu K, Si-Bum P, Akinori A, Jun S, et al. Characterization of a trifunctional fatty acid desaturase from oleaginous filamentous fungus *Mortierella alpine* 1S–4 using a yeast expression system. J Biosci Bioeng 2013; 116: 672–6.
21. Gao D, Zeng J, Yu X, Dong T, Chen S. Improved lipid accumulation by morphology engineering of oleaginous fungus *Mortierella isabellina*. Biotechnol Bioeng 2014; 111: 1758–66.
22. Zhang J, Hu B. Microbial lipid production from corn stover via *Mortierella isabellina*. Appl Biochem Biotechnol 2014; 174: 574–86.
23. Annali J, Alf B, Willem HVZ. The production of eicosapentaenoic acid by representatives of the genus *Mortierella* grown on brewers' spent grain. Biologia 2009; 64: 871–6.
24. Fu Y, Fan X, Li X, Wang H, Chen H. The Desaturase OPIN17 from *Phytophthora infestans* converts arachidonic acid to eicosapentaenoic acid in CHO cells. Appl Biochem Biotechnol 2013; 171: 975–88.
25. Sakuradani E, Akinori A, Jun O, Sakayu S. Improved production of various polyunsaturated fatty acids through filamentous fungus *Mortierella alpine* breeding. Appl Microbiol Biotechnol 2009; 84: 1–10.
26. Snehak KA, Rafael AG, When ZY. Use of biodiesel-derived crude glycerol for producing eicosapentaenoic acid (EPA) by the fungus *Pythium irregulare.* J Agric Food Chem 2009; 57: 2739–44.
27. Wu L, Charles LR, Wen Z. The safety assessment of *Pythium irregulare* as a producer of biomass and eicosapentaenoic acid for use in dietary supplements and food ingredients. Appl Microbiol Biotechnol 2013; 97: 7579–85.

28. Zhang R, Zhu Y, Ren L, Zhou P, Hu J, Yu L. Identification of a fatty acid Δ6-desaturase gene from the eicosapentaenoic acid-producing fungus *Pythium splendens* RBB-5. Biotechnol Lett 2013; 35: 431–8.
29. Alpettiyil N, Navin KR, Govindarjulu V. Optimization of media components for enhanced arachidonic acid production by *Mortierella alpine* under submerged cultivation. Biotechnol Bioproc Eng 2011; 16: 229–37.
30. Jin MJ, Huang H, Xiao AH, Zhang K, Liu X, Li S, et al. A novel two-step fermentation process for improved arachidonic acid production by *Mortierella alpine*. Biotechnol Lett 2008; 30: 1087–91.
31. Lio JY, Wang T. Pythium irregulare fermentation to produce arachidonic acid (ARA) and eicosapentaenoic acid (EPA) using soybean processing co-products as substrates. Appl Biochem Biotechnol 2013; 169: 595–611.
32. Lu JM, Peng C, Ji XJ, You JY, Cong LL, Ouyang PK, et al. Fermentation characteristics of *Mortierella alpine* in response to different nitrogen sources. Appl Biochem Biotechnol 2011; 164: 979–90.
33. Hou CT. Production of arachidonic acid and dihomo-γ-linolenic acid from glycerol by oil-producing Wlamentous fungi, *Mortierella* in the ARS culture collection. J Ind Microbiol Biotechnol 2008; 35: 501–6.
34. Xian M, Kang YJ, Yan JC. Production of linolenic acid by *Mortierella isabellina* grown on octadecanol. Curr Microbiol 2002; 44: 141–4.
35. Das UN. Essential fatty acids: biochemistry, physiology and pathology. Biotechnol J 2006; 1(4): 420–39.
36. Laukevics JJ, Apsite AF, Viesturs US, Tengerdy RP. Steric hindrance of growth of filamentous fungi in solid substrate fermentation of wheat straw. Biotechnol Bioeng 1985; 27: 1687–91.
37. Feniksova RV, Tikhomirova AS, Rakhleeva EE. Conditions for forming amylase and proteinase in surface cultures of Bacillus subtilis. Microbiologia 1960; 29: 745–8.
38. Babu KR, Satyanarayana T. α-Amylase production by thermophilic *Bacillus coagulance* in solid-state fermentation. Process Biochem 1995; 30: 305–9.
39. Ben-Amotz A, Tornabene TG, Thomas WH. Chemical profile of selected species of microalgae with emphasis on lipids. J Phycol 1985; 21: 72–81.
40. Devyani S, Rupali M, Ramchandra G, Sanjay N, Harsulkar AM. Production of polyunsaturated fatty acids in recombinant *Lipomyces starkeyi* through submerged fermentation. Bioprocess Biosyst Eng 2015; 38: 1407–14.
41. Sajbidor J, Dobronova S, Certik M. Arachidonic acid production by *Mortierella sp.* S-17: influence of C/N ratio. Biotechnol Lett 1990; 12: 455–6.
42. Jang HD, Lin YY, Yang SS. Effect of culture media and conditions on polyunsaturated fatty acids production by *Mortierella alpina*. Bioresour Technol 2005; 96: 1633–44.
43. Zandrazil F, Brunert H. Investigation of physical parameters important for solid-state fermentation of straw by white rot fungi. Eur J Appl Microbiol Biotechnol 1981; 11: 183–8.
44. Lekha PK, Lonsane BK. Comparative titres, location and properties of tannin acyl hydrolase produced by *Aspergillus niger* PKL104 in solid state, liquid surface and submerged fermentation. Process Biochem 1994; 29: 497–503.
45. Jang HD, Lin YY, Yang SS. Polyunsaturated fatty acid production with Mortierella alpina by solid substrate fermentation. Bot Bull Acad Sin 2000; 41: 41–8.
46. Joint WHO/FAO expert consultation. In: World Health Organization, ed. Diet, nutrition and the prevention of chronic diseases. Geneva, Switzerland: World Health Organization; 2003, p. 89.
47. Institute of Medicine. In: Institute of Medicine, ed. Food and Nutrition Board. Dietary reference intakes for energy, carbohydrate, fiber, fat, fatty acids, cholesterol, protein and amino acids. Washington, DC: National Academies Press; 2002, pp. 769–70.
48. Lands WEM, Libelt B, Morris A, Kramer NC, Prewitt TE, Bowen P, et al. Maintenance of lower proportions of n-6 eicosanoid precursors in phospholipids of human plasma in response to added dietary n-3 fatty acids. Biochim Biophys Acta 1992; 1180: 147–62.
49. Lands B. Historical perspectives on the impact of n-3 and n-6 nutrients on health. Prog Lipid Res 2014; 55: 17–29.
50. Lands B. Measuring blood fatty acids as a surrogate indicator for coronary heart disease risk in population studies. In: Simopoulos AP, De Meester F, eds. A balanced omega-6/omega-3 fatty acid ratio, cholesterol and coronary heart disease. Vol. 100. Basel: Karger; 2009, pp. 22–34.
51. Ramsden CE, Faurot KR, Zamora D, Suchindran CM, Macintosh BA, Gaylord S, et al. Targeted alteration of dietary n-3 and n-6 fatty acids for the treatment of chronic headaches: a randomized trial. Pain 2013; 154: 2441–51.
52. Gomez Candela C, Bermejo Lopez LM, Loria Kohen V. Importance of a balanced omega 6/omega 3 ratio for the maintenance of health: nutritional recommendations. Nutr Hosp 2011; 26: 323–9.
53. Zhang B, Wang P, Zhou Q, Chen CG. The relationships between erythrocyte membrane n-6 to n-3 polyunsaturated fatty acids ratio and blood lipids and C-reactive protein in Chinese adults: an observational study. Biomed Environ Sci 2011; 24: 234–42.
54. Yamashita T, Oda E, Sano T, Yamashita T, Ijiru Y, Giddings JC, et al. Varying the ratio of dietary n-6/n-3 polyunsaturated fatty acid alters the tendency to thrombosis and progress of atherosclerosis in apo$E^{-/-}$ $LDLR^{-/-}$ double knockout mouse. Thromb Res 2005; 116: 393–401.
55. Lucas M, Mirzaei F, O'Reilly EJ, Pan A, Willett WC, Kawachi I, et al. Dietary intake of n-3 and n-6 fatty acids and the risk of clinical depression in women: a10-y prospective follow-up study. Am J Clin Nutr 2011; 93: 1337–43.
56. Lands B, Lamoreaux E. Describing essential fatty acid balance as 3–6 differences rather than 3/6 ratios. Nutr Metab 2012; 9: 46–54.
57. Hibbeln JR, Nieminen LR, Blasbalg TL, Riggs JA, Lands WE. Healthy intakes of n-3 and n-6 fatty acids: estimations considering world wide diversity Internet. Am J Clin Nutr 2006; 83(6 Suppl): 1483S–93.
58. Kartikasari LR, Hughes RJ, Geier MS, Makrides M, Gibson RA. Dietary alpha-linolenic acid enhances omega-3 long chain polyunsaturated fatty acid levels in chicken tissues. Prostaglandins, Leukot Essent Fatty Acids 2012; 87: 103–9.

***Shengli Yang**
The College of Pharmaceutical Science
Zhejiang University of Technology
Hangzhou City, Chaowang Road 18#, 310014
China
Email: yangshengli01@zjut.edu.cn

***Hui Zhang**
Physical and Chemical Test Center
Zhejiang Institute of Quality Inspection Science
Hangzhou, Xiasha Road 300#, 310018
China
Email: zhanghui0461@sina.com.cn

9

Metabolic effects of quail eggs in diabetes-induced rats: comparison with chicken eggs

Eric Lontchi-Yimagou[1]*, Agatha Tanya[2], Carine Tchankou[3], Judith Ngondi[3] and Julius Oben[3]

[1]Laboratory for Molecular Medicine and Metabolism, Biotechnology Center, University of Yaoundé I, Yaoundé, Cameroon; [2]Department of Public Health, Faculty of Medicine and Biomedical Sciences, University of Yaoundé I, Yaoundé, Cameroon; [3]Laboratory of Nutrition and Nutritional Biochemistry, Faculty of Sciences, University of Yaoundé I, Yaoundé, Cameroon

Abstract

Background: Quail eggs as a food item have recently been introduced into the diet of some Cameroonians. These eggs are being sold in local markets, but with many unfounded health claims. One claim is that quail eggs can reduce blood glucose levels in diabetics. It was therefore necessary to evaluate the effect of consuming quail eggs on blood glucose levels, lipid profiles, and oxidative stress parameters in diabetes-induced rats.
Methods: Twenty Wistar rats weighing, on average, 250 g were divided into four groups of five rats each. Group 1 consisted of rats with normal blood glucose, and the other three groups (2, 3, and 4) consisted of diabetes-induced rats achieved by intravenous injection of streptozotocin. During 16 days, rats in groups 1 and 2 received distilled water; and rats in groups 3 and 4 received quail and chicken eggs, respectively, with gastroesophageal probe at a dose of 1 mL/200 g body weight. Fasting blood glucose levels were determined in all the groups on the 1st, 7th, 14th, and 17th days after induction of diabetes. On the 17th day, the fasting rats were sacrificed, and blood and liver samples were collected for biochemical analyses.
Results: In 17 days, the consumption of quail and chicken eggs had no effect on blood glucose levels of diabetic rats. Total cholesterol levels were higher in groups 3 (75.59 mg/dL) and 4 (59.41 mg/dL) compared to group 2 (55.67 mg/dl), although these differences were not significant (all $p > 0.05$). Triglyceride levels were significantly higher ($p < 0.05$) in groups 3 (106.52 mg/dL) and 4 (109.65 mg/dL) compared to group 2 (65.82 mg/dL). Quail eggs had no effect on oxidative stress parameters (malondialdehyde, hydroperoxides, and catalase).
Conclusions: The consumption of quail eggs by diabetic rats at the tested dose had no effect on blood glucose level and oxidative stress parameters and may have a negative effect on lipid profile.

Keywords: *diabetes; hyperlipidemia; oxidative stress; quail eggs; chicken eggs*

Responsible Editor: Per Ole Iversen, University of Oslo, Norway.

The prevalence of type 2 diabetes mellitus (T2DM) has increased worldwide (1, 2), including in Africa, where the greatest proportional increase (90%) in the number of diabetic cases is projected to occur by 2030 (3, 4). Sedentary lifestyles, obesity, and unhealthy dietary behaviors are the most common risk factors of T2DM (5). T2DM leads to serious complications such as nervous system disorders, kidney diseases, and eye pathologies; thus, its prevention and treatment should be considered a priority (6). Diet has been used in the prevention and management of T2DM. Strategies used to manage obesity include the use of high-fiber, low-carbohydrate, and low-fat diets (7, 8). Conventional dietary and behavioral treatments have failed in long-term management.

The Japanese quail (Galliformes: Phasianidae) has existed since ancient times. Consumption of Japanese quail eggs has been claimed to improve metabolism; prevent stress; and help in the treatment of obesity, asthma, and various allergies (9). These eggs are rich sources of antioxidants, minerals, vitamins, and other nutrients (10). Reportedly, quail eggs strengthen the immune system, promote memory health, increase brain activity, and stabilize the nervous system (11). They apparently help relieve anemia by increasing the level of hemoglobin in the body while removing toxins and heavy metals. After the consumption of quail eggs, Anca et al. (12) stated that 'in Brasil, people claim to be relieved of many physiological disorders such as anemia, tuberculosis, ulcers, hypertension, diabetes, arteriosclerosis, asthma and many others'.

Aba and Onah (13) showed that alloxanized rats that were administered a quail egg solution demonstrated hypolipidemia and ameliorated lesions in the pancreas. Quail eggs have recently been introduced in Cameroon. They are sold in local markets and some supermarkets at exorbitant prices and with many nutritional claims. They are appreciated for their nutritional value and functional properties. However, without any real justification, people believe that consuming these eggs can relieve diabetes, hypertension, asthma, sinusitis, cardiovascular diseases, and many other conditions. The public health consequences of such allegations may be serious; therefore, this work was undertaken to address this information gap by evaluating of the effects of quail egg consumption on the blood glucose level, lipid profile, and oxidative stress parameters in diabetes-induced rats.

Methods

Animal management and ethical considerations

Adult male Wistar albino rats 12 weeks of age and weighing, on average, 250 g were used in this study. Rats ($n = 20$) were purchased from the animal house of the Faculty of Medicine and Biomedical Sciences, University of Yaoundé I, Cameroon. The animals were maintained at 25°C in a room with a 12/12-h light/dark cycle and had free access to water and food. The study was approved by the institutional animal ethical committee.

Quail and chicken eggs

To enable a comparative study on different groups of rats, we used both quail and chicken eggs. Both types of eggs were purchased from the same breeder in the Biyem-Assi neighborhood (Yaoundé-Cameroon) to avoid variations related to food quality that could modify the composition of eggs (14).

Egg administration

Every morning, quail and chicken eggs were administered to each rat with a gastroesophageal probe at a dose of 1 mL/200 g body weight. This dose reflected the dose used by most Cameroonians for their treatment. The egg was broken, introduced into a beaker, and then homogenized using a glass rod. The volume of eggs that was given to the rats was drawn with a graduated syringe into the gastroesophageal probe for administration to the rats.

Evaluation of nutritional effects of quail and chicken eggs on blood glucose *of diabetes-induced rats*

Induction of diabetes in rats

A single intraperitoneal dose of 55 mg/kg streptozotocin (STZ; Sigma-Aldrich, Germany) was administered to induce diabetes (15). After 72 h, rats with marked hyperglycemia (fasting blood glucose of 250 mg/dL) were considered diabetics. The animals were divided into four groups of five rats each. The four groups were treated as follows:

Group	Description
1	Normal/untreated rats (negative control) receiving distilled water at the dose of 1 mL/200 g BW.
2	Diabetics/untreated rats (positive control) receiving distilled water at the dose of 1 mL/200 g BW.
3	Diabetics/treated rats receiving quail eggs at the dose of 1 mL/200 g BW.
4	Diabetics/treated rats receiving chicken eggs at the dose of 1 mL/200 g BW.

Blood collection

The effects of quail and chicken eggs on blood glucose, lipid profile, and oxidative stress parameters of the four groups of rats were determined. Group 1 consisted of rats with normal blood glucose and the other three groups (2–4) consisted of diabetes-induced rats by intravenous injection of STZ. For 16 days, groups 1 and 2 received distilled water; groups 3 and 4 received quail and chicken eggs, respectively, from a gastroesophageal probe at a dose of 1 mL/200 g BW. The rats were on these specific treatments for 16 days and had free access to water and were on the same diet. Fasting blood glucose levels were determined in all the groups on the 1st, 7th, 14th, and 17th days after induction of diabetes. On the 17th day, the fasting rats were sacrificed by jugular venesection after light chloroform anesthesia.

For each rat, blood was collected into ethylenediaminetetraacetic acid tubes and allowed to clot at room temperature. Thereafter, plasma was separated from the clot by centrifuging at 1,126*g* for 15 min. The plasma was collected in clean bottles and stored at −20°C until required. After the animals were dissected, organs were put on ice and processed as rapidly as possible.

- *Preparation of liver homogenates*: Approximately 10% (w/v) tissue homogenates were prepared in 10% phosphate-buffered saline (pH 6.4) by using a microhomogenizer (Physcotron, Niti-on Inc., Chiba, Japan). The supernatant was obtained from the homogenate after centrifugation at 3,000 rpm for 15 min. The sample was then stored at −20°C until used for the determination of malondialdehyde (MDA) concentration, hydroperoxides concentration, and the activities of catalase.
- *Preparation of hemolysates of erythrocytes*: After centrifuging total blood, 100 μL of pellets was pipetted into another tube and then washed twice with 2 mL of 0.9% NaCl and centrifuged at 1,126*g*

for 10 min at room temperature. Hemolysates were obtained by adding 2 mL of distilled water and was stored at $-20°C$. This hemolysate was used for protein assays and determination of catalase activity.

Biochemical analyses

Plasma was prepared from blood samples collected from rats on day 17 in the morning after an overnight fast of 12 h. Plasma glucose was determined using a GlucoPlus™ glucometer. Total cholesterol and triglycerides were measured enzymatically using standard enzymatic kits (Sigma Diagnostics). Oxidative stress markers such as MDA level, hydroxyl (OH) radical level, and activity of catalase were also measured.

Evaluation of effect of quail and chicken eggs on lipid profile of diabetes-induced rats

Plasma total cholesterol and triglycerides were estimated enzymatically according to Watson (16) and Fossati and Prencipe (17), respectively, by using commercial kits from Ran-dox, Ltd., Co. (UK).

Evaluation of antioxidant properties of quail eggs on diabetes-induced rats

- Total protein content was evaluated in all collected samples (hemolysate of erythrocytes, plasma and homogenates of liver) using the 'total protein colorimetric test Biuret' kit commercialized by Cypress Diagnostics.
- MDA level was estimated spectrophotometrically by thiobarbituric acid according to methods described by Wilbur et al. (18). Thiobarbituric acid reacts with plasma MDA that is produced by hydrolysis of lipid hydroperoxides to form a pink-red colored complex with high absorbance at 532 nm. The results are expressed as micromoles per liter. This complex is usually quantified against MDA standards that are generated from 1,1,3,3-tetraethoxypropane under the same reaction conditions.
- OH radical level was measured in blood plasma and homogenates of liver according to the protocol described by Jiang et al. (19). This method is based on the principle that in acid medium, the peroxide ion oxidizes Fe^{2+} into Fe^{3+} that then reacts with xylenol orange to form a complex that absorbs at 560 nm.
- Catalase activity in hemolysates and liver homogenates was assayed as previously described by Sinha (20). An aliquot of hydrogen peroxide (0.8 mL) was dispensed into an Eppendorf tube. Phosphate buffer (1.0 mL) and (0.002%, v/v) diluted homogenate/hemolysate (125 μL) were added. The reaction mixture (0.5 mL) was dispensed into 5% dichromate reagent (1.0 mL) and vigorously shaken. The mixture was heated in a Clifton water bath for 10 min and allowed to cool. The absorbance at 570 nm was taken using a spectrophotometer (BioMate 3S UV-Visible, Thermo Scientific, Wohlen, Switzerland). The absorbance obtained was extrapolated from the following standard curve: $y = 0.0028x + 0.0132$. The catalase activity was thereafter expressed as units per minute per milligram of protein: catalase (unit/mg protein) = (Abs/min × 30,000 units)/(40 cm/M × mg protein) × df, where df is dilution factor and Abs is absorbance.

Statistical analysis

Statistical analysis of the results was performed using SPSS 10.1 for Windows (SPSS, Chicago, IL, USA). The results are presented as mean ± standard deviation. The comparison was done using one-way analysis of variance followed by Duncan's multiple range post hoc test. A value of $p < 0.05$ was considered as significant.

Results

Evaluation of nutritional effects of quail and chicken eggs on blood glucose of diabetes-induced rats

The results of nutritional effect of quail and chicken eggs on blood glucose in diabetic rats are presented in Fig. 1. The administration of quail and chicken eggs for 16 days in diabetic rats had no effect on blood glucose. After 7, 14, and 16 days of treatment, there was no significant differences in blood glucose between the positive control diabetic rats receiving distillated water and diabetic rats treated with quail and chicken eggs ($p > 0.05$).

Evaluation of effect of quail and chicken eggs on lipid profile of diabetes-induced rats

Plasma total cholesterol was significantly elevated in untreated diabetic rats compared to normal untreated rats. Total cholesterol level was higher in diabetic rats receiving quail eggs (75.59 mg/dL) and those receiving chicken eggs (59.41 mg/dL) compared to non-treated diabetic rats (55.67 mg/dL), although this difference was not significant ($p > 0.05$) (Fig. 2). Also, triglyceride levels were significantly higher ($p < 0.05$) in diabetic rats receiving quail eggs (106.52 mg/dL) and chicken eggs (109.65 mg/dL) compared to diabetic untreated rats receiving distilled water (65.82 mg/dL) (Fig. 3).

Evaluation of effect of quail eggs on OH radical and MDA levels in diabetes-induced rats

Plasma and liver homogenates OH radical and MDA levels were significantly elevated in untreated diabetic rats compared to normal untreated rats ($p < 0.05$). During the 16 days, no difference was observed in these parameters in untreated diabetic rats compared to

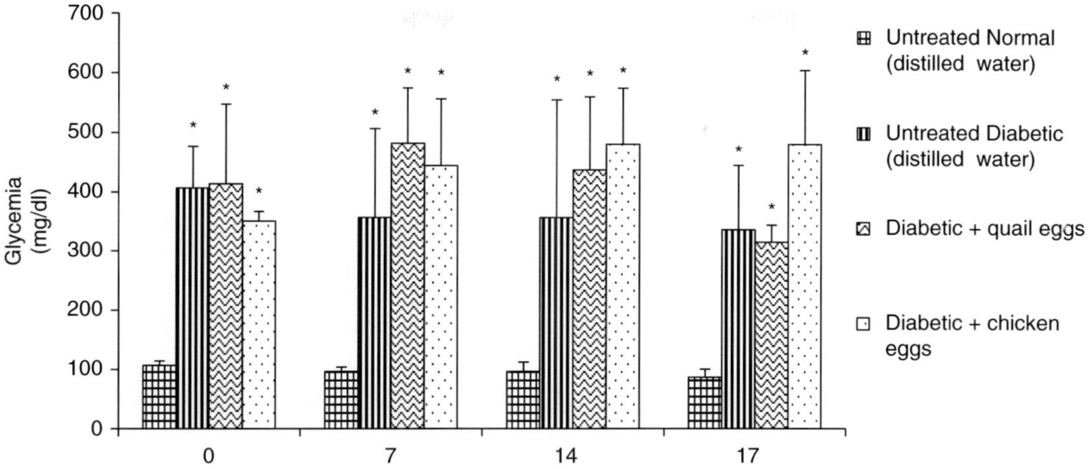

Fig. 1. Nutritional effect of quail and chicken eggs at dose of 1 mL/200 g BW for 16 days on blood glucose in diabetes-induced rats. Data are means + standard deviation. *$p < 0.05$, significantly different from untreated normal control (distilled water 1 mL/200 g BW).

diabetic rats treated with quail and chicken eggs ($p > 0.05$) (Tables 1 and 2).

Evaluation of effect of quail eggs on catalase activity in diabetes-induced rats

The effect of the consumption of quail eggs on the activity of catalase on hemolysates and liver homogenates in diabetes-induced rats is shown in Figs. 4 and 5, respectively. The catalase activity in hemolysates and liver homogenates was significantly elevated in untreated diabetic rats compared to normal untreated rats ($p < 0.05$). Higher catalase activity was observed in hemolysates and liver homogenates in the untreated diabetic rats compared to the treated diabetic rats, although the difference was not significant ($p > 0.05$).

Discussion

Diabetes induced with STZ lead to a significant elevation of blood glucose. This result is consistent with that of Bibak et al. (15). We observed an increase of total cholesterol and triglyceride levels and markers of lipid peroxidation (MDA and hydroperoxides) and catalase in STZ-induced diabetic rats. Diabetes induced with STZ in rats is a good disease model that can be used to test substances that are supposed to have hypoglycemic, hypolipidemic, and antioxidant activity *in vivo*. STZ is an antibiotic that produces pancreatic islet β-cell destruction and is widely used experimentally to produce a model of type 1 diabetes mellitus. These animals are used for assessing the pathological consequences of diabetes and for screening potential therapies for the treatment of this condition (21, 22).

The consumption of quail eggs had no significant effect on blood glucose levels in treated rats compared to untreated diabetic rats. This could be an indication that quail eggs had no substance that can affect blood glucose. These results are contrary to those reported by Anca et al. (12)

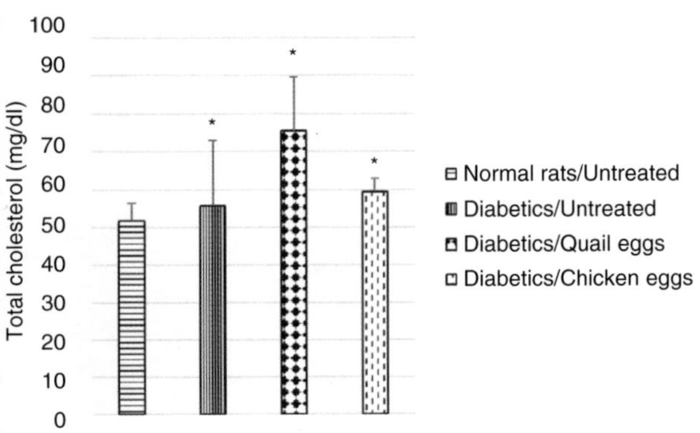

Fig. 2. Nutritional effect of quail and chicken eggs at dose of 1 mL/200 g BW for 16 days on total cholesterol in diabetes-induced rats. Data are means + standard deviation. *$p < 0.05$, significantly different from untreated normal control (distilled water 1 mL/200 g BW).

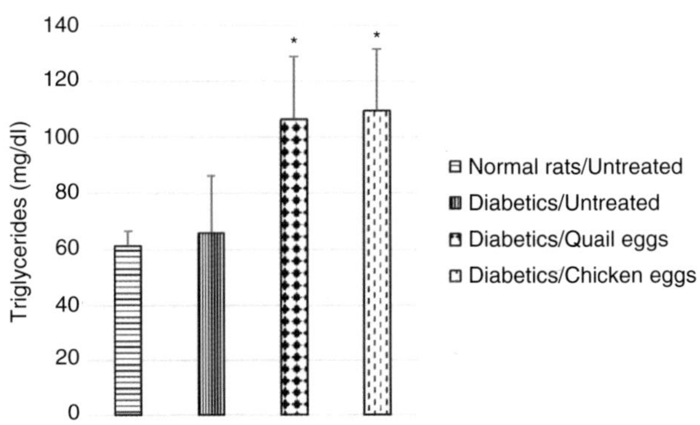

Fig. 3. Nutritional effect of quail and chicken eggs at dose of 1 mL/200 g BW for 16 days on triglycerides in diabetes-induced rats. Data are means + standard deviation. *$p < 0.05$, significantly different from untreated normal control (distilled water 1 mL/200 g BW) and untreated diabetic (distilled water 1 mL/200 g BW) rats.

Table 1. Effect of quail and chicken eggs on hydroperoxides in diabetes-induced rats

Group of rats	Oxidative stress parameter (hydroperoxides)	
	Plasma	Liver homogenate
Untreated normal (distilled water 1 mL/200 g BW)	0.3 ± 0.01	0.5 ± 0.1
Untreated diabetic (distilled water 1 mL/200 g BW)	0.6 ± 0.1*	0.8 ± 0.1*
Diabetic + quail eggs (1 mL/200 g BW)	0.7 ± 0.1*	0.9 ± 0.3*
Diabetic + chicken eggs (1 mL/200 g BW)	0.5 ± 0.04*	0.9 ± 0.1*

Data are means ± standard deviation. BW = body weight. *$p < 0.05$, significantly different from untreated normal control (distilled water 1 mL/200 g BW).

and the beliefs of Cameroonians who use quail eggs for the treatment of diabetes. It is possible that for some people with diabetes who consume quail eggs and are also taking oral hypoglycemic agents or insulin, the components of quail eggs could have a synergistic effect with the bioactive compounds contained in drug formulations. For those who consume quail eggs without any medication, the improvement in their disease may simply be a psychological effect. Therefore, it will be interesting to also carry out this study directly in humans. However, at this stage of the research, one should be wary of the exclusive use of quail eggs in the management of diabetes.

An increase was observed in the levels of lipid profile parameters in rats rendered diabetic with STZ. In 16 days, treatment of diabetic rats with quail and chicken eggs resulted in an increase of the concentration of total cholesterol and triglyceride levels compared to those of untreated diabetic rats, although this difference was not significant regarding the level of total cholesterol. This trend of increased total cholesterol levels in rats treated with quail and chicken eggs compared to the untreated diabetic rats could be due to the high level of cholesterol in the eggs. Bragagnolo and Rodriguez-Amaya (23) showed that the concentration of cholesterol in quail eggs is similar to that found in chicken eggs: 12.1 mg of cholesterol per gram of yolk in quail eggs compared to 12.0 mg in chicken eggs. These results are contrary to the results of Aba et al. (13) who observed a reduction in the serum levels of total cholesterol, low-density lipoprotein cholesterol, and very-low-density lipoprotein cholesterol and an increase in high-density lipoprotein cholesterol in a concentration-dependent manner compared to the untreated diabetic group. The American Heart Association recommends a daily cholesterol intake of <300 mg for healthy individuals and <200 mg for at-risk individuals. Eggs are one of the main sources of dietary cholesterol, with a large egg containing about 200 mg of cholesterol (24). Cameroonians consume for their treatment, on average, 12–14 quail eggs per day. It would be advisable for them to reduce their daily consumption of quail eggs.

Diabetes induced with STZ is a good disease model that can be used to test substances that are supposed to contain antioxidant activity *in vivo*. Increased oxidative stress is widely accepted as a major factor in the development and progression of diabetes mellitus (25). The obtained experimental diabetes in laboratory animals such as rats is a good model to study oxidative stress due to chronic hyperglycemia, which thereby depresses the activity of the antioxidant defense system and induces the generation of free radicals *de novo*. The free radicals thus formed react with all biological substances. The reactions with these constituents of the cell membrane lead to lipid peroxidation (26). The liver contains a high content of antioxidant enzymes such as catalase and superoxide dismutase that can trap these free radicals. Compounds with antioxidant properties should be able to reduce the concentration of free radicals. The lipid peroxidation in diabetes leads to increased plasma and hepatic levels of MDA and hydroperoxides. This study did show an effect

Table 2. Effect of quail and chicken eggs on the malondialdehydes in diabetes induced rats

Group of rats	MDA (μmol/L)	
	Plasma	Liver homogenate
Untreated normal (distilled water 1 mL/200 g BW)	5.9 ± 0.6	3.5 ± 0.2
Untreated diabetic (distilled water 1 mL/200 g BW)	10.8 ± 1.3*	10.8 ± 0.3*
Diabetic + quail eggs (1 mL/200 g BW)	9.3 ± 1.4*	8.3 ± 1.3*
Diabetic + chicken eggs (1 mL/200 g BW)	7.1 ± 1.2*	7.4 ± 1.7*

Data are means ± standard deviation. BW = body weight; MDA = malondialdehyde. *$p < 0.05$, significantly different from untreated normal control (distilled water 1 mL/200 g BW).

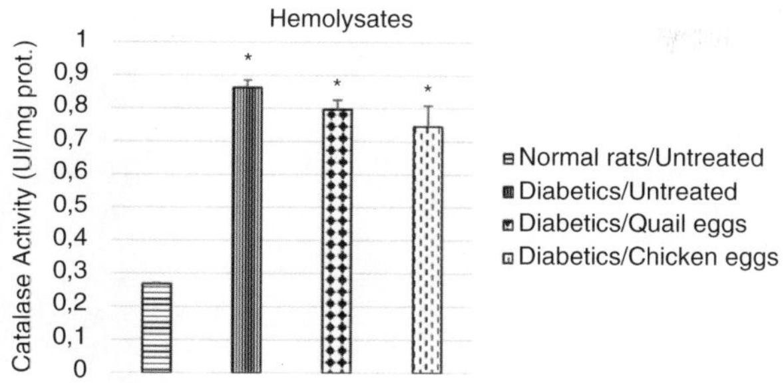

Fig. 4. Effect of quail and chicken eggs on the catalase activity (hemolysates) in diabetes-induced rats. Data are means + standard deviation. $*p < 0.05$, significantly different from untreated normal control (distilled water 1 mL/200 g BW).

of the consumption of quail and chicken eggs on markers of oxidative stress. Notably, the levels of MDA and hydroperoxides in the plasma and liver homogenates increased in untreated diabetic rats, showing an increased generation of free radicals compared to those of normal rats. The increase in MDA and hydroperoxide levels in untreated diabetic rats might have resulted from the decreased activity of antioxidant enzymes. A decrease in the activity of catalase was also observed. There was no significant difference in oxidative stress markers between the groups treated with quail and chicken eggs with respect to untreated groups. These results suggest that quail eggs might not contain any substance with antioxidant properties.

Conclusions

The present investigation has revealed that the consumption of quail eggs by diabetic rats has no direct effect on blood glucose, but oxidative stress parameters may have a negative effect on the lipid profile. Depending on the parameters that have been studied in diabetic rats, quail eggs may be considered to have the same properties as chicken eggs. Quail eggs are richer in cholesterol compared to chicken eggs and require caution in their consumption.

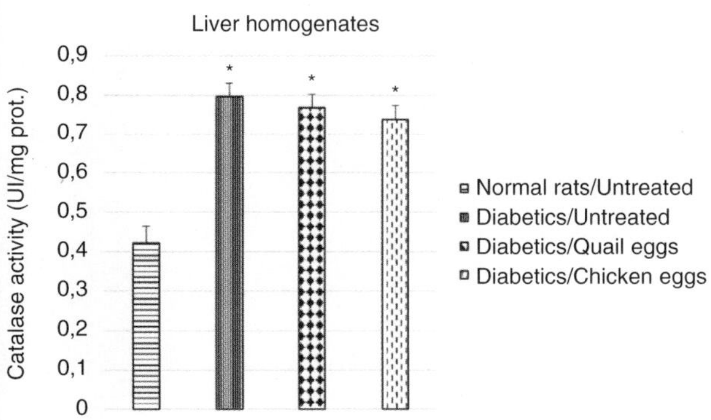

Fig. 5. Effect of quail and chicken eggs on the catalase activity (liver homogenates) in diabetes-induced rats. Data are means + standard deviation. $*p < 0.05$, significantly different from untreated normal control (distilled water 1 mL/200 g BW).

Authors' contributions

ELY, AT, CT, JN, and JO: study design and conception, data collection and analysis, and drafting of the manuscript. ELY, AT: data interpretation, editing and review of the manuscript. All authors read and approved of the final manuscript.

Acknowledgements

We acknowledge the Laboratory of Nutrition and Nutritional Biochemistry, Faculty of Sciences, University of Yaoundé I, Yaoundé, Cameroon, for support to obtain materials and reagents.

Conflict of interest and funding

The authors declare that they have no conflict of interests.

References

1. Wiréhn AB, Andersson A, Ostgren CJ, Carstensen J. Age-specific direct healthcare costs attributable to diabetes in a Swedish population: a register-based analysis. Diabet Med 2008; 25(6): 732–7.
2. King H, Aubert RE, Herman WH. Global burden of diabetes: prevalence, numerical estimates, and projections, 1995–2025. Diabetes Care 1998; 21(9): 1414–31.
3. Kengne AP, Echouffo-Tcheugui JB, Sobngwi E, Mbanya JC. New insights on diabetes mellitus and obesity in Africa-part 1: prevalence, pathogenesis and comorbidities. Heart 2013; 99(14): 979–83.
4. Peer N, Kengne AP, Motala AA, Mbanya JC. Diabetes in the Africa region: an update. Diabetes Res Clin Pract 2014; 103(2): 197–205.
5. Kiencke S, Handschin R, VonDahlen R, Muser J, Brunner-Larocca HP, Schumann J, et al. Pre-clinical diabetic cardiomyopathy: prevalence, screening, and outcome. Eur J Heart Fail 2010; 12(9): 951–7.
6. Lutale JK, Thordarson H, Sanyiwa A, Mafwiri M, Vetvik K, Krohn J. Diabetic retinopathy prevalence and its association with microalbuminuria and other risk factors in patients with type 1 and type 2 diabetes in Dar es Salaam, Tanzania. JOECSA 2013; 15(1): 263–7.
7. Bray GA. Complications of obesity. Ann Intern Med 1985; 103(6 (Pt 2)): 1052–62.
8. Harris MI. Epidemiological correlates of NIDDM in Hispanics, whites, and blacks in the U.S. population. Diabetes Care 1991; 14(7): 639–48.
9. Truffier JC. Approach to treatment of allergy by consumption of quail egg. La Clinique 1978; 22: 2–4.
10. Lalwani P. Quail egg nutrition. 2011. Available from: http://www.buzzle.com/articles/quail-egg nutrition.html [cited 15 April 2012].
11. Tunsaringkarn T, Tungjaroenchai W, Siriwong W. Nutrient's benefit of quail eggs (*Coturnix coturnix japonica*). Int J Sci Res Publ 2013; 3: 1–7.

12. Anca T, Vacaru-opris I, Teusan V. Aspects regarding some morphological values of the domestic quail eggs (*Coturnix coturnix japonica*). Lucr Ştiinţ Zooteh Biotech 2008; 41(2): 709–16.
13. Aba PE, Onah JA. Evaluation of the possible hypolipidemic properties of quail egg on alloxan-induced diabetic rats. J. Worlds Poult Res 2015; 5(4): 84–9.
14. Silva WA da, Elias AHN, Aricetti JA, Sakamoto MI, Murakami AE, Gomes STM, et al. Quail egg yolk (*Coturnix coturnix japonica*) enriched with omega-3 fatty acids. LWT Food Sci Technol 2009; 42(2): 660–3.
15. Bibak B, Khalili M, Rajaei Z, Soukhtanloo M, Hadjzadeh MA, Hayatdavoudi P. Effects of melatonin on biochemical factors and food and water consumption in diabetic rats. Adv Biomed Res 2014; 3: 173.
16. Watson D. Calorimetric test for cholesterol lipid clearing factor. Clin Chem Acta 1960; 5: 637.
17. Fossati P, Prencipe L. Serum triglycerides determined colorimetrically with an enzyme that produces hydrogen peroxide. Clin Chem 1982; 28(10): 2077–80.
18. Wilbur KM, Bernheim F, Shapiro OW. The thiobarbituric acid reagent as a test for the oxidation of unsaturated fatty acids by various agents. Arch Biochem 1949; 24(2): 305–13.
19. Jiang ZY, Hunt JV, Wolff SP. Ferrous ion oxidation in the presence of xylenol orange for detection of lipid hydroperoxide in low density lipoprotein. Anal Biochem 1992; 202(2): 384–9.
20. Sinha AK. Colorimetric assay of catalase. Anal Biochem 1972; 47(2): 389–94.
21. Furman BL. Streptozotocin-induced diabetic models in mice and rats. Curr Protoc Pharmacol 2015; 70: 5.47.1–20.
22. Akbarzadeh A, Norouzian D, Mehrabi MR, Jamshidi Sh, Farhangi A, Verdi AA, et al. Induction of diabetes by Streptozotocin in rats. Indian J Clin Biochem 2007; 22(2): 60–4.
23. Bragagnolo N, Rodriguez-Amaya DB. Comparison of the cholesterol content of Brazilian chicken and quail eggs. J Food Compos Anal 2002; 16(2): 147–53.
24. Song WO, Kerver JM. Nutritional contribution of eggs to American diets. J Am Coll Nutr 2000; 19(Suppl 5): 556S–62.
25. Ceriello A. Oxidative stress and glycemic regulation. Metabolism 2000; 49(2 Suppl 1): 27–9.
26. Memisogullari R, Bakan E. Levels of ceruloplasmin, transferrin, and lipid peroxidation in the serum of patients with type 2 diabetes mellitus. J Diabetes Complications 2004; 18(4): 193–7.

*Eric Lontchi-Yimagou
Laboratory for Molecular Medicine and Metabolism
Biotechnology Center,
University of Yaoundé I
Yaoundé, Cameroon
Email: lontchifrenzy@yahoo.fr

10

Effects of royal jelly supplementation on regulatory T cells in children with SLE

Asmaa M. Zahran[1], Khalid I. Elsayh[2], Khaled Saad[2]*, Esraa M.A. Eloseily[2], Naglaa S. Osman[2], Mohamd A. Alblihed[3], Gamal Badr[4] and Mohamed H. Mahmoud[5,6]

[1]Clinical Pathology Department, South Egypt Cancer Institute, Assiut University, Assiut, Egypt; [2]Pediatric Department, Faculty of Medicine, Assiut University, Assiut, Egypt; [3]Medical Biochemistry Department, College of Medicine, Taif University, Taif, Kingdom of Saudi Arabia; [4]Zoology Department, Laboratory of Immunology & Molecular Physiology, Faculty of Science, Assiut University, Assiut, Egypt; [5]Deanship of Scientific Research, King Saud University, Riyadh, Kingdom of Saudi Arabia; [6]Food Science and Nutrition Department, National Research Center, Dokki, Cairo, Egypt

Abstract

Background and objective: To our knowledge, no previous studies have focused on the immunomodulatory effects of fresh royal jelly (RJ) administration on systemic lupus erythematosus (SLE) in humans. Our aim was to study the effect of fresh RJ administration on the disease course in children with SLE with some immunological markers ($CD4^+$ and $CD8^+$ regulatory T cells and T lymphocytes apoptosis).
Methods: This was an open-label study in which 20 SLE children received 2 g of freshly prepared RJ daily, for 12 weeks.
Results: The percentages of $CD4^+CD25^{+\,high}$ $FOXP3^+$cells ($CD4^+$ regulatory T cells) and $CD8^+$ $CD25^{+\,high}$ $FOXP3^+$cells ($CD8^+$ regulatory T cells) were significantly increased after RJ treatment when compared with baseline values. Apoptotic CD4 T lymphocytes were significantly decreased after RJ therapy when compared with baseline values and the control group.
Conclusion: This is the first human study on the effect of RJ supplementation in children with SLE. Our results showed improvements with 3-month RJ treatment with regard to the clinical severity score and laboratory markers for the disease. At this stage, it is a single study with a small number of patients, and a great deal of additional wide-scale randomized controlled studies are needed to critically validate the efficacy of RJ in SLE.

Keywords: *royal jelly*; *regulatory T cells*; *children*; *systemic lupus erythematosus*

Systemic lupus erythematosus (SLE) is a common autoimmune disease characterized by abnormal T- and B-cell activation, cytokines disorders, and considerable production of autoantibodies (1). Despite central mechanisms of tolerance, some T cells recognizing self-antigens are released into the periphery. One of the mechanisms employed to eliminate or control these potentially damaging cells is regulatory T cells (Tregs). A number of immune Tregs have been described (2). $CD4^+$ Tregs play an important role in the maintenance of peripheral tolerance and are characterized by the expression of the CD25 surface marker and the transcription factor forkhead box protein 3 (FOXP3), making up to 5–10% of the normal $CD4^+$ T-cell population. Abrogation of CD4 Tregs development and/or peripheral function may cause autoimmune diseases (3).

$CD8^+CD25^+FOXP3^+$ T cells with regulatory function in maintaining self-tolerance have been identified and can be generated by continuous antigen stimulation. Human $CD8^+$ Tregs are implicated in autoimmune disorders: multiple sclerosis and inflammatory bowel disease (2, 4). Suppressive CD8 Tregs appear after T-cell receptor stimulation, suppressing cellular proliferation of $CD4^+$ naïve and effector T cells via cell–cell contact lysis or soluble factors like interleukin (IL) 10 and transforming growth factor beta (TGF-β). CD8 Tregs have suppressive ability typically associated with $CD4^+$ Tregs. Interaction between subsets of Tregs that protect against autoimmune diseases remains unclear (4, 5). FOXP3-expressing $CD8^+$ T cells proved vital for $CD4^+CD25^+$ Tregs induced by a tolerogenic peptide to suppress murine lupus (5).

Apoptosis is a programmed cell death and, normally, the resulted apoptotic cells are removed by phagocytes. Failure to remove apoptotic bodies leads to the release of autoantigens which may induce autoimmunity. Increased lymphocyte apoptosis is found to be part of the pathogenesis of SLE. Studies in human SLE have revealed increased lymphocyte apoptosis and defects in macrophage removal of apoptotic cells (6–8).

Royal jelly (RJ) is a creamy product secreted by young nurse worker bees (*Apis mellifera*), and it is synthesized in the hypopharyngeal and mandibular glands. RJ comprises 60–70% water, 10–12% carbohydrates, 12–15% proteins and 3–7% lipids. Based on unique composition of RJ, recently *in vivo* and *in vitro* studies focused on its health-promoting characteristics such as hypotensive, anti-hypercholesterolemia, anti-inflammatory, antitumor, antioxidant and weight management effects and immunomodulatory properties (9, 10). The immunomodulatory properties were approved in animal studies of SLE, as RJ administration to mice caused a significant decrease in the serum level of IL-10 and in the autoantibodies against single-stranded deoxyribonucleic acid (ssDNA), double-stranded deoxyribonucleic acid (dsDNA), and erythrocytes, as well as a reduction in the number of splenic autoreactive B cells (9). We hypothesized that RJ has a role in controlling the disease activity of SLE through its immunomodulatory effect on Tregs. To our knowledge, no previous studies have focused on the immunomodulatory effect of RJ administration on SLE patients in humans. Our aim was to study the effect of RJ supplementation on the disease course of pediatric SLE with some immunological markers (the CD4 and CD8 Tregs) and lymphocytes apoptosis.

Patients and methods

The Ethical Committee of Assiut University, Assiut, Egypt, approved the study. Participants were given a complete description of the study, and a written informed consent in accordance with Assiut University Ethical Committee guidelines was taken from parents of all the participants. The participants can leave the study at any time. The work has been carried out in accordance with the code of ethics of the World Medical Association (Declaration of Helsinki) for experiments involving humans.

Study setting

The study was conducted in the Pediatric Immunology and Rheumatology Unit, Assiut University Children Hospital, Assiut, Upper Egypt, from June 2015 to January 2016.

Study subjects

A total of 20 SLE children, with 18 girls and 2 boys, who regularly followed up at Assiut University Children Hospital were included in this study. The inclusion criteria included children <18 years old, who are fulfilling at least four of the American College of Rheumatology Revised Criteria for SLE (11), and 20 sex- and age-matched healthy controls were enrolled in this study.

Exclusion criteria were children who were known to have hypersensitivity to honey, and children with congenital abnormalities of respiratory and GI systems. In addition, children younger than 1 year who had severe malnutrition and who had taken any recent vaccination were excluded.

Study design

This was an open-label study in which SLE children received 2 g of freshly prepared RJ daily, for 12 weeks. RJ was advised to be taken on an empty stomach at least 30 min before meals. All children in the study were assessed by taking medical history, performing clinical examinations. Serologic records were collected at the time of enrollment, and after 3 months of the RJ therapy. Anti-dsDNA antibodies, antinuclear antibodies (ANA), C3, C4, complete blood count, serum albumin, serum creatinine, serum urea, erythrocyte sedimentation rate (ESR), C-reactive protein (CRP), protein in urine, and urine red blood cells (RBCs) were done for all SLE patients before and after RJ therapy. Immunological markers (the CD4 and CD8 Tregs) and lymphocytes apoptosis were done for healthy controls and SLE children at baseline and at the end of the study.

Flow cytometric detection of apoptosis of lymphocytes

Apoptosis was measured by the annexin V–fluoroisothiocyanate (FITC) binding assay according to the manufacturer's instructions (BD Biosciences, San Jose, CA, USA). Fifty microliters of whole blood was stained with 5 μl of peridinium-chlorophyll-protein (Per-CP)-conjugated anti-CD8 and phycoerythrin (PE)-conjugated anti-CD4, washed twice with 2 ml of phosphate-buffered saline (PBS), and RBCs were lysed. The cells were washed and resuspended in 100 μl of the annexin V-conjugate binding buffer to which 5 μl of FITC-conjugated annexin V was added. The mixture was incubated in dark at room temperature for 15 min, after which 400 μl of the binding buffer was added and 10,000 cells were acquired and analyzed by FACSCalibur flow cytometry. Anti-human immunoglobulin G (IgG) was used as an isotype-matched negative control for each sample. Forward and side scatter histogram was used for lymphocytes populations. Then, the percentages of $CD4^+$ (T-helper lymphocytes) and $CD8^+$ (T cytotoxic lymphocytes) were assessed in the lymphocyte populations. Then, the expression of annexin V in $CD4^+$ and $CD8^+$ lymphocytes was detected (Fig. 1).

Flow cytometric detection of regulatory T lymphocytes

Tregs in whole blood samples were enumerated using FITC-conjugated anti-FOXP3 (eBioscience, San Diego, CA, USA), PE-conjugated anti CD25 (IQ Product, Groningen, the Netherlands), Per-CP-conjugated anti-CD4, and allophycocyanin (APC)-conjugated anti-CD8 (Becton Dickinson,

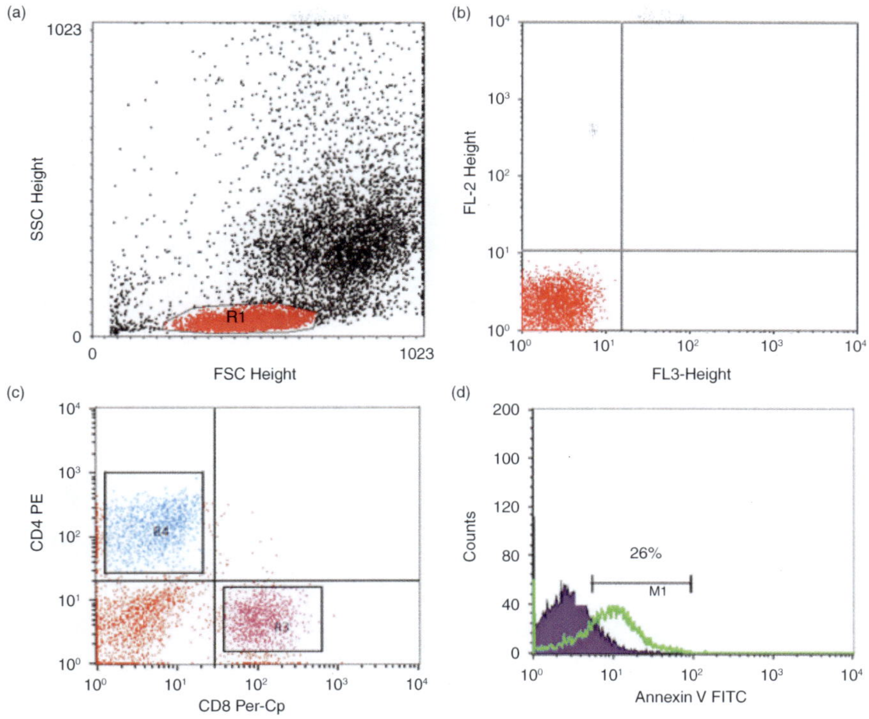

Fig. 1. Flow cytometric analysis of T lymphocytes apoptosis. (a) Forward and side scatter histogram was used to define the lymphocytes. (b, c) The expression of CD8 and CD4 was assessed in lymphocytes population compared with the negative isotype control. The T-helper cells ($CD4^+$) and T cytotoxic cells ($CD8^+$) were gated for further analysis of annexin V expression. (d) Example of annexin V expression on T cells ($CD4^+$ or CD8). The positivity was defined as fluorescence (green histogram) higher than that of the isotype control (blue histogram).

Bioscience, USA). Fifty microliters of blood sample was incubated with 5 µl of CD4, CD8, and CD25 for 15 min at room temperature in the dark. Following incubation, RBC lysis, washing with PBS, addition of fixed solution to fix the cells, and incubation for 10 min were done. After incubation, cells were washed with PBS, and then permeabilized solution and 5 µl of FOXP3 were added and incubated for 30 min at room temperature. After one wash, the cells were resuspended in PBS. Flow cytometric analysis was done by FACSCalibur flow cytometry with CellQuest software (BD Biosciences). Anti-human IgG was used as an isotype-matched negative control for each sample. Forward and side scatter histogram was used to define the lymphocytes population (R1). Then, the percentages of $CD4^+$ (T-helper cells) and $CD8^+$ (T cytotoxic cells) were assessed in lymphocytes population. Total $CD4^+CD25^+$, $CD4^+CD25^{+low}$ and $CD4^+CD25^{+High}$ (defined as the population of CD4-positive T cells whose CD25 expression exceeded the level of CD25 positivity seen in the CD4-negative T cells), and $CD4^+CD25^{+High}$ $FOXP3^+$Tregs were evaluated as a percentage of $CD4^+$. Also, total $CD8^+CD25^+$, $CD8^+CD25^{+intermediate\ (low)}$ and $CD8^+CD25^{+High}$, and $CD8^+CD25^{+High}$ $FOXP3^+$Tregs were evaluated as a percentage of $CD8^+$. The expression of $FOXP3^+$ in $CD4^+CD25^{+high}$ and in $CD8^+CD25^{+high}$ cells was expressed as a geometric mean of fluorescence intensity (MFI) as shown in Fig. 2.

Outcome assessment

SLE children in our study were followed up for 3 months. Disease activity was assessed by SLE Disease Activity Index (SLEDAI). Active disease was defined as SLEDAI >4 (12). Regarding the clinical assessment, each patient served as his or her own control, and differences after 12 weeks of RJ therapy were calculated and compared with each patient's baseline values (at Week 0). Caregivers of participating children received a weekly telephone call from the research team reminding them to administer the therapy. They were not allowed to change the provided dose or to add any supplements throughout the study period. At follow-up visits, the parents were asked to report any difficulties or adverse effects during the study period. Side effects were recorded throughout the study and were assessed using a checklist every month. With regard to serologic, laboratory, and flow cytometric records, the patients were compared before and after RJ with healthy controls.

Statistical analysis

Data analysis was performed with the Statistical Package for Social Sciences (SPSS version 17). Data are expressed as mean ± standard deviation (SD) for all parameters. Because of the small sample size and a propensity for outliers in some of the variables, statistical differences between the groups

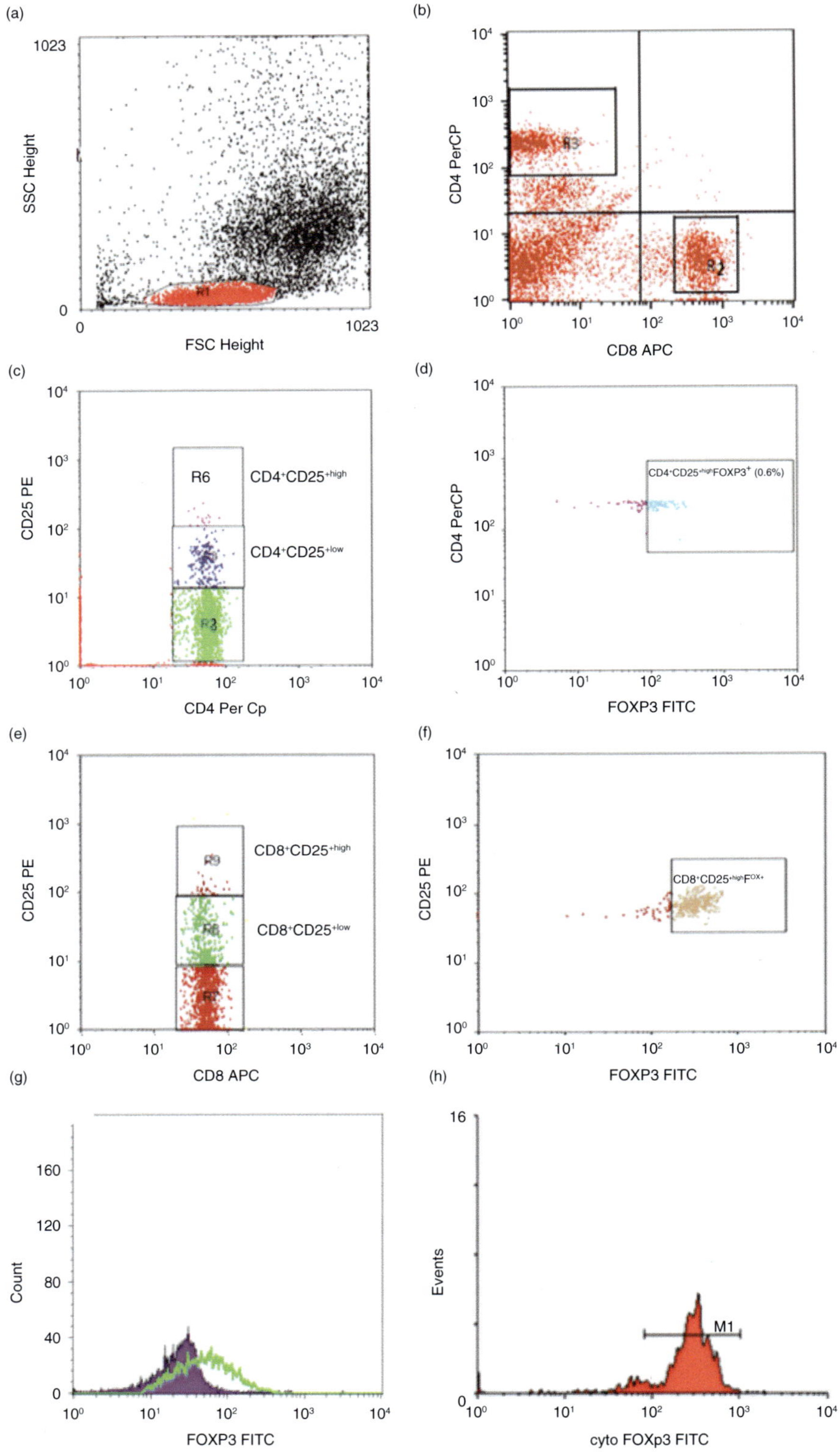

Fig. 2. Flow cytometric detection of regulatory T cells. (a) Forward and side scatter histogram was used to define the lymphocytes population (R1). (b) The expression of $CD8^+$ (R2) and $CD4^+$ (R3) was assessed in lymphocytes population. (c) The expression of CD25 in $CD4^+$ was detected and compared with the negative isotype control (not shown), and different gates were drowned to define $CD4^+CD25^{+low}$ cells (R5) and $CD4^+CD25^{+High}$ cells (R6). (d) The percentage of $CD4^+CD25^{+high}$ $FOXP3^+$cells ($CD4^+$ regulatory T cells) was determined. (e, f) The detection of $CD8^+$ regulatory T cells in $CD8^+$ cells. The expression of CD25 in $CD8^+$ was detected. Then, $CD8^+CD25^{+low}$ cells (R8), and $CD8^+CD25^{+High}$ (R9) cells and $CD8^+CD25^{+high}$ $FOXP3^+$cells ($CD8^+$ regulatory T cells) were determined. (g, h) The expression of $FOXP3^+$ in $CD4^+CD25^{+High}$ cells $CD8^+CD25^{+high}$ cells.

were examined using the Mann-Whitney test and Wilcoxon test. Spearman's correlation was used to determine the correlation between studied parameters. A value of $p \leq 0.05$ denoted a statistically significant difference.

Results

Table 1 shows some demographic characteristics of SLE children. The mean age of the patients was 9.4±3.7 years (range 7–16 years) with a mean disease duration of 3.5±2.8 years (range 1–8 years). The mean SLEDAI score was 11.3±7.6 (range 2–31). Fifty percent of the patients were positive for anti-dsDNA and ANA antibodies. All clinical characteristics of SLE patients were summarized in Table 1.

Table 2 shows laboratory data of SLE children and SLEDAI before and after RJ supplementation and the controls. SLEDAI score was significantly improved after 3 months of RJ therapy (mean±SD, 11.3±7.6 vs. 8.3±6.1; $p = 0.01$). Complement C3 ($p = 0.009$) and C4 ($p = 0.014$) levels were significantly increased after RJ therapy.

Table 1. Baseline clinical data of all studied SLE children and controls

Parameter	SLE patients (20)	Control (20)	*p*
Age (years)			
Range	7–16	7–16	NS
Mean±SD	9.4±3.7	9.0±4.5	NS
Disease duration (years)	4.5±2.8	–	–
Male/female	2/18	2/18	NS
SLEDAI			
Range	2–31	–	–
Mean±SD	11.3±7.6	–	–
ACR criteria of SLE: no. (%)			
Malar rash	7 (35%)	–	–
Discoid rash	2 (10%)	–	–
Photosensitivity	2 (10%)	–	–
Oral ulcers	1 (5%)	–	–
Arthritis	11 (55%)	–	–
Serositis	5 (25%)	–	–
Renal disorders	8 (40%)	–	–
Neuropsychiatric disorders	9 (45%)	–	–
Hematological disease	13 (65%)	–	–
Positive antinuclear antibodies	10 (50%)	–	–
Positive anti-dsDNA antibodies	10 (50%)	–	–
Other clinical data			
Fatigue	16 (80%)	–	–
Pulmonary disorders	3 (15%)	–	–

ACR, American College of Rheumatology; NS, not significant; SD, standard deviation; SLE, systemic lupus erythematosus; SLEDAI, Systemic Lupus Erythematosus Disease Activity Index.

Regarding the hematological parameters, there were no statistically significant differences in platelet counts in the peripheral blood among patients and the controls. The mean hemoglobin level was significantly improved after 3 months of RJ therapy (mean±SD, 9.71±0.51 vs. 11.57±0.26; $p = 0.025$).

White blood cell counts, serum albumin, serum creatinine, serum urea, ESR, CRP, and protein in urine were significantly improved after 3 months of RJ therapy; however, no significant changes were observed in urine RBCs and anti-dsDNA antibodies at the end of the therapy (Table 2).

The percentages of $CD4^+CD25^{+high}$ and $CD4^+CD25^{+high}$ $FOXP3^+$ cells ($CD4^+$ regulatory T cells) were significantly increased after RJ treatment versus baseline value, however, the values prior and after RJ therapy were statistically significantly lower than control group (Table 3).

The frequencies of $CD8^+CD25^{+high}$ and $CD8^+CD25^{+high}$ $FOXP3^+$cells ($CD8^+$ regulatory T cells) were significantly increased after RJ treatment versus baseline value. The percentages of $CD8^+CD25^{+high}$ and $CD8^+$ regulatory T cells at baseline were significantly lower than control group. After RJ supplementation, there were no significant difference between patients and controls (Table 3).

Table 4 shows that patients with SLE (both before and after RJ treatment) had significantly lower counts of CD4 lymphocytes versus the normal control group. There was also significantly lower $CD4^+/CD8^+$ cell ratio in patients than the controls. The percentage of $CD4^+$ T lymphocytes was significantly increased after RJ treatment versus baseline value (mean%±SD%, 31.06%±1.23% vs. 37.48%±1.54%; $p = 0.008$). This was not true for $CD8^+$ T lymphocytes as it did not show any significant changes with RJ treatment or any difference between the SLE children and normal control group.

With regard to the apoptosis data, at baseline, SLE patients exhibited a significant increase in the percentage of apoptotic $CD4^+$ T lymphocytes (mean%±SD%, 32.35%±3.75% vs. 8.09%±0.26%; $p = 0.001$) and an insignificant increase in the percentage of apoptotic CD8 T lymphocytes (mean%±SD%, 9.53%±0.47% vs. 8.29%±0.40%; $p = 0.07$) when compared with healthy children (Table 4). Apoptotic $CD4^+$ T lymphocytes were significantly decreased after RJ therapy (mean%±SD%, 32.35%±3.75% vs. 8.45±0.23%; $p = 0.018$) when compared with baseline values (Table 4). The frequency of apoptotic $CD8^+$ T lymphocytes was decreased after RJ therapy; however, this was statistically insignificant (mean%±SD%, 9.53%±0.47% vs. 9.31%±0.41%; $p = 0.678$). The frequencies of both apoptotic CD4 and CD8 T cells were comparable between SLE patients after RJ therapy and controls (Table 4).

Table 2. Some laboratory data and SLEDAI in SLE patients before and after Royal Jelly supplementation and the controls

	SLE patients before RJ supplementation (20)	SLE patients after RJ supplementation (20)	Controls (20)	p^a	p^b	p^c
SLEDAI	8.3±4.1	3.3±2.9	ND	–	0.01	–
C3 (mg/dl)	0.44±0.09	1.1±0.13	ND	–	0.009	–
C4 (mg/dl)	0.17±0.030	0.82±0.17	ND	–	0.014	–
Hemoglobin (g/dl)	9.71±0.51	11.57±0.26	12.3±0.28	0.001	0.025	NS
Platelets (10^3/μl)	252.06±47.69	270.89±28.7	290±24.5	NS	NS	NS
WBC (10^3/μl)	5.32±0.54	7.01±0.83	7.29±0.41	0.004	0.018	NS
Albumin (g/dl)	2.93±0.21	4.02±0.13	4.03±0.09	<0.001	0.001	NS
Creatinine (mg/dl)	2.99±0.38	1.32±0.22	0.73±0.06	<0.001	0.002	0.004
Urea (mg/dl)	151.86±29.6	55.15±4.75	19.51±2.37	<0.001	0.003	0.001
ESR (mm/h)	77.68±10.12	20.22±2.4	9.2±0.75	<0.001	0.004	0.001
Protein in urine (mg/dl)	369.6±123.17	23.11±4.8	Negative	–	0.041	–
Anti-dsDNA	0.78±0.14	0.71±0.09	Negative	–	NS	–
CRP	3.68±0.2	1.88±0.18	Negative	–	<0.001	–
Urine RBCs	3.43±0.35	2.87±0.12	Negative	–	NS	–

Data are represented as means±SD. $P \leq 0.05$ is significant.

CRP, C-reactive protein; ESR, erythrocyte sedimentation rate; ND, not determined; NS, not significant; RBC, red blood cells; RJ, royal jelly; SLE, systemic lupus erythematosus; SLEDAI, Systemic Lupus Erythematosus Disease Activity Index; WBC, white blood cells; [a]SLE patients before RJ supplementation versus controls (Mann–Whitney *U*-test); [b]SLE patients before RJ supplementation versus SLE patients after RJ supplementation (Wilcoxon test); [c]SLE patients after RJ supplementation versus controls (Mann–Whitney *U*-test).

Adverse events

RJ supplementation was generally well tolerated. We reported temporally associated side effects in four patients (20%) during the study period: skin rash (one patient), itching (one patient), and stomach pain (two patients). All side effects were mild and transient, and all patients continued the 3-month RJ treatment.

Discussion

SLE is a common autoimmune disease characterized by abnormal immune regulation and the production of autoantibodies to self-nuclear, cytoplasmic, and cell surface molecules with the resulting generalized multisystem chronic autoimmune inflammatory disease (1, 2, 13). RJ is known to have multipotent health beneficial actions; the immunomodulatory effects in particular are being increasingly proven in the literature (9). RJ was found to stimulate antibody production and immunocompetent cell proliferation in mice (14). Furthermore, RJ was found to have anti-inflammatory effects through different mechanisms, one was due to the inhibition of proinflammatory cytokine production by macrophages (15). In addition, RJ was suggested to modulate the immune responses in rats through affecting their dendritic cells by its fatty acid contents (16). RJ was found to suppress type-I allergic reactions and

Table 3. Regulatory T cells in patients with systemic lupus erythematosus before and after royal jelly supplementation and the controls

	SLE patients before RJ supplementation (20)	SLE patients after RJ supplementation (20)	Controls (20)	p^a	p^b	p^c
$CD4^+$ regulatory T cells	1.32±0.25	1.74±0.28	2.24±0.52	<0.001	0.001	0.001
$CD8^+$ regulatory T cells	0.93±0.37	1.58±0.84	2.01±0.98	<0.001	0.003	NS
MFI of $FOXP3^+$ expression in $CD4^+$ $CD25^{+High}$	102.98±6.94	118.16±29.96	149.72±19.3	<0.001	0.032	0.001
MFI of $FOXP3^+$ expression in $CD8^+$ $CD25^{+High}$	96.85±12.51	113.09±14.49	116.98±33.54	0.016	0.01	NS

Data are represented as means±SD. $P \leq 0.05$ is significant.

FOXP3, forkhead box protein 3; MFI, mean of fluorescence intensity; NS, not significant; RJ, royal jelly; SLE, systemic lupus erythematosus; [a]SLE patients before RJ supplementation versus controls (Mann–Whitney *U*-test); [b]SLE patients before RJ supplementation versus SLE patients after RJ supplementation (Wilcoxon test); [c]SLE patients after RJ supplementation versus controls (Mann–Whitney *U*-test).

Table 4. T lymphocytes and their apoptosis in children with SLE before and after royal jelly supplementation and the controls

	SLE patients before RJ supplementation (20)	SLE patients after RJ supplementation (20)	Controls (20)	p^a	p^b	p^c
CD4 T lymphocytes	31.06±1.23	37.48±1.54	46.47±2.85	0.002	0.008	0.023
CD8 T lymphocytes	29.11±1.42	28.54±0.92	31.12±1.12	NS	NS	NS
CD4/CD8 ratio	1.25±0.06	1.53±0.09	1.69±0.107	0.001	0.02	NS
Apoptotic CD4 T lymphocytes	32.35±3.75	8.45±0.23	8.09±0.26	0.001	0.018	NS
Apoptotic CD8 T lymphocytes	9.53±0.47	9.31±0.41	8.29±0.40	NS	NS	NS

Data are represented as means±SD. $P \leq 0.05$ is significant.
NS, not significant; RJ, royal jelly; SLE, systemic lupus erythematosus; [a]SLE patients before RJ supplementation versus controls (Mann–Whitney *U*-test); [b]SLE patients before RJ supplementation versus SLE patients after RJ supplementation (Wilcoxon test); [c]SLE patients after RJ supplementation versus controls (Mann–Whitney *U*-test).

was associated with the restoration of macrophage function and Th1/Th2 cytokine responses (17). RJ was also found to inhibit the development of atopic dermatitis-like lesions in mice (18).

Based on these immunomodulatory properties, RJ was challenged in some *in vivo* and animal studies of autoimmune diseases, and the results were promising. With regard to SLE, there is only one animal study that explored this effect. In an animal model of SLE in New Zealand Black × New Zealand White F1 mice that genetically exhibit many manifestations similar to human SLE, RJ oral administration showed a significant delay in the onset of the disease and its active progression. Mice that received RJ showed decreased proteinuria and a prolongation of lifespan. RJ caused a significant decrease in the serum level of IL-10, and in the autoantibodies against ssDNA, dsDNA, and erythrocytes, as well as a reduction in the number of splenic autoreactive B cells (9).

In our cohort of children with SLE, before treatment there was an observed imbalance between $CD4^+$ and $CD8^+$ lymphocytes; this may be explained by the immune dysregulation in cases of SLE. Our results showed that patients with SLE (both before and after RJ treatment) had significantly lower percentages of $CD4^+$ lymphocytes versus the normal control group. There was also significantly lower $CD4^+/CD8^+$ cell ratio in patients than the controls. The frequency of $CD4^+$ T lymphocytes was significantly increased after RJ treatment versus baseline value. This was not true for $CD8^+$ T lymphocytes as it did not show any significant changes with RJ treatment or any difference between the SLE children and normal control group.

Our results are in accordance with what was found by McInerney et al. (19) who examined the levels and function of peripheral blood immunoregulatory T-cell subpopulations in SLE. They found normal percentages of $CD8^+$ T cells in peripheral blood in all SLE patients. Interestingly, about $CD4^+$, they found about half of the SLE patients had markedly depressed $CD4^+$ cell levels and in turn significantly lower $CD4^+/CD8^+$ cell ratio, whereas the remaining half of the patients had normal levels of $CD4^+$ cells (normal $CD4^+/CD8^+$ cell ratio) (19).

FOXP3 is a key transcription factor that is critically important in controlling Treg development and function. There are many evidence that FOXP3 is involved in the pathogenesis of autoimmune diseases. In our previous study, we found that $CD4^+CD25^{+High}$ and $CD4^+$ $CD25^{+High}$ $FOXP3^+$ were significantly decreased in total lymphocytes and in $CD4^+$ cells in the recently diagnosed diabetes type I pediatric patients (20). Moreover, in a mouse model (collagen induced) of rheumatoid arthritis, FOXP3 transduction led to inhibition of T-cell activation and attenuation of the cell proliferation. It decreased IL-2 and interferon (IFN)-gamma expression, and increased IL-10 expression in activated $CD4^+CD25^-$ T cells. FOXP3-transduced $CD4^+CD25^-$ T cells attenuated proliferation of activated $CD4^+CD25^-$ T cells. FOXP3 transduction delayed disease incidence remarkably and alleviated autoimmune symptoms of collagen-induced arthritis mice (21).

In this study, we found that the children with SLE (in both before and after RJ treatment) had significantly lower levels of CD4 regulatory T cells and FOXP3 expression in $CD4^+CD25^{+High}$ versus normal control group. Also, the levels of $CD4^+$ regulatory T cells and FOXP3 expression were negatively correlated with disease activity as detected by SLEDAI. This is in accordance with Hu et al. (1) and Lyssuk et al. (22) who showed that the $CD4^+$ regulatory T cells and FOXP3 levels in SLE patients were significantly lower than normal controls. Also, they found a significant negative correlation between Tregs level and the disease activity index (SLEDAI scores). $CD4^+$ regulatory T cells is suggested to play an important role in the pathogenesis of SLE (1, 22). On the contrary, there has been very contradicting results between studies of $CD4^+FOXP3^+$ cells in SLE. Barath et al. (23) found decreased $CD4^+CD25^+FOXP3^+$ cells in SLE without any correlation with disease activity. Other studies have reported normal values for $CD4^+CD25^+FOXP3^+$ cells (24, 25). Surprisingly, other researchers have reported increased percentages of $CD4^+$ $FOXP3^+$ in lupus and found that this result correlated with disease activity (26).

The significant increase in the level of $CD4^+$ regulatory T cells in our SLE patients after treatment with RJ may be explained by its immunomodulatory effects through its ability to increase proliferation of immune competent cells (14). It is also found to modulate the immune responses in rats through affecting their dendritic cells through affecting their fatty acid content (16). A recent study has shown a special active substance that exists only in RJ that is called 'hydroxyl-2-decenoic acid'. It was found to promote the growth of T lymphocyte subsets and IL-2 production (27). In an animal model of SLE, oral administration of RJ showed significant delay in the disease onset and its active progression. In our patients, there was a decrease in disease activity after administration of RJ as detected by SLEDAI. Our patients also showed a negative correlation between the disease activity and CD4 and FOXP3, which may suggest that the rate of increase of the regulatory T cells has an impact on decreasing the disease activity. La Cava et al. (28) demonstrated that the production of autoantibodies by B cells in SLE patients could be interrupted via induction of regulatory T cells, and the regulatory T cells could inhibit the production of dsDNA antibodies by B cells via cell contact inhibition induced by membrane-bound TGF-β and Glucocorticoid-induced tumour necrosis factor receptor (GITR) molecules.

The $CD8^+$ regulatory T cells interact with effector cells significantly, limiting immune response (1). The decreased level of $CD8^+$ regulatory T cells in our patients before treatment indicates a poor ability of these cells to suppress the autoreactive T cells in SLE patients. Also, $CD8^+$ regulatory T cells are essential for $CD4^+CD25^+$ regulatory T cell functions in the suppression of autoimmunity (29). This contributed to the ongoing immune dysregulation in our patients. After treatment with RJ, the level of $CD8^+$ regulatory T cells was significantly increased and became non-significantly different from that of the controls. This can be explained by the effect of hydroxy-2-decenoic acid in promoting IL-2. $CD8^+$ regulatory T cells expand in response to IL-2 treatment and can be characterized phenotypically and functionally, at steady state and under IL-2 stimulation. $CD8^+$ regulatory T cells are highly suppressive and responsive to IL-2 (30).

Apoptosis is a programmed cell death, and normally the resulted apoptotic cells are removed by phagocytes. Failure to remove apoptotic bodies leads to the release of autoantigens, which may induce autoimmunity (7, 8). Our study revealed a significantly higher frequency in $CD4^+$ T cells apoptosis, which could explain the reduction of $CD4^+$ T cells in our patients with SLE. Increased lymphocyte apoptosis is found to be part of the pathogenesis of SLE. Studies in human SLE have revealed increased lymphocyte apoptosis and defects in macrophage removal of apoptotic cells, although the mechanism by which the macrophages are defective in removal of apoptotic cells is not yet clear. Taylor et al. (31) found that complement deficiency may be involved in this process. Ren et al. (8) have shown that macrophages from SLE patients were less capable of ingesting apoptotic neutrophils and that this was secondary to the presence or lack of serum factors rather than an intrinsic defect of the macrophages. Jin et al. (32) found that the macrophages activity was actually increased in SLE in response to increased lymphocytes apoptosis. This was confirmed by the finding that serum levels of neopterin and IFN-γ was increased in SLE. Also, they found that neopterin correlated positively with the increased number of apoptotic lymphocytes and the overall SLE disease activity. Moreover, they found that lymphocyte apoptosis and increased macrophages activity were correlated with the disease activity.

With regard to the effect of RJ treatment on lymphocytes apoptosis in our study, we found that the apoptotic $CD4^+$ T lymphocytes showed significant reduction to about its quarter of the baseline values before treatment to values about normal as the healthy control group. Again in correlation with the previous $CD8^+$ T lymphocytes count, the changes in apoptotic $CD8^+$ T lymphocytes were insignificant between patients and controls.

Conclusion

To the best of our knowledge, this is the first human study on the effect of RJ supplementation in children with SLE. Our results showed improvements with 3-month RJ treatment in regard to the clinical severity score and laboratory markers for the disease. At this stage, it is a single study with a small number of patients, and a great deal of additional wide-scale randomized controlled studies are needed to critically validate the efficacy of RJ in SLE.

Limitations of the study and the impact on future research

There were some limitations of this study. First, this was an open, uncontrolled study. Second, we investigated a small group of children with SLE. Further randomized controlled longitudinal studies with a larger sample size are warranted to confirm our findings and to explore the mechanism of action of RJ in SLE. SLE patients have higher serum levels of IL-17 than healthy controls. Moreover, the frequency of IL-17-producing T cells is increased in peripheral blood of SLE patients (33). We recommend to analyze the regulation of IL-17 in context to RJ therapy in patients with SLE in the future studies.

Acknowledgment

The authors extend their appreciation to the Laboratory of Immunology and Molecular Physiology, Faculty of Science, Assiut University, for funding this work. The authors would also like to extend their sincere appreciation to the Deanship of Scientific Research at King Saud University for funding this research group (No. RG - 1435-019).

Conflict of interest and funding

All authors declare no potential conflicts of interest with respect to the research, authorship, and/or publication of this article.

References

1. Hu S, Xiao W, Kong F, Ke D, Qin R, Su M. Regulatory T cells and their molecular markers in peripheral blood of the patients with systemic lupus erythematosus. J Huazhong Univ Sci Technol Med Sci 2008; 28(5): 549–52.
2. Wing K, Sakaguchi S. Regulatory T cells exert checks and balances on self tolerance and autoimmunity. Nat Immunol 2010; 11(1): 7–13.
3. Sakaguchi S, Ono M, Setoguchi R, Yagi H, Hori S, Fehervari Z, et al. FoxP3+ CD25+ CD4+ natural regulatory T cells in dominant self-tolerance and autoimmune disease. Immunol Rev 2006; 212: 8–27.
4. Tsai YG, Yang KD, Niu DM, Chien JW, Lin CY. TLR2 agonists enhance CD8+FoxP3+ regulatory T cells and suppress Th2 immune responses during allergen immunotherapy. J Immunol 2010; 184(12): 7229–37.
5. Tsai YG, Lee CY, Lin TY, Lin CY. $CD8^+$ Treg cells associated with decreasing disease activity after intravenous methylprednisolone pulse therapy in lupus nephritis with heavy proteinuria. PLoS One 2014; 9(1): e81344.
6. Elsayh KI, Mohammed WS, Zahran AM, Saad K. Leukocytes apoptosis and adipocytokines in children with beta thalassemia major. Clin Exp Med 2016; 16(3): 345–50.
7. Shao WH, Cohen PL. Disturbances of apoptotic cell clearance in systemic lupus erythematosus. Arthritis Res Ther 2011; 28; 13(1): 202.
8. Ren Y, Tang J, Mok MY, Chan AW, Wu A, Lau CS. Increased apoptotic neutrophils and macrophages and impaired macrophage phagocytic clearance of apoptotic neutrophils in systemic lupus erythematosus. Arthritis Rheum 2003; 48: 2888–97.
9. Mannoor MK, Shimabukuro I, Tsukamotoa M, Watanabe H, Yamaguchi K, Sato Y. Honeybee royal jelly inhibits autoimmunity in SLE-prone NZB × NZW F1 mice. Lupus 2009; 18(1): 44–52.
10. Erem C, Deger O, Ovali E, Barlak Y. The effects of royal jelly on autoimmunity in Graves' disease. Endocrine 2006; 30(2): 175–83.
11. Hochberg MC. Updating the American College of Rheumatology revised criteria for the classification of systemic lupus erythematosus. Arthritis Rheum 1997; 40(9): 1725.
12. Bombardier C, Gladman DD, Urowitz MB, Caron D, Chang CH. Derivation of the SLEDAI. A disease activity index for lupus patients. The Committee on Prognosis Studies in SLE. Arthritis Rheum 1992; 35: 630–40.
13. Choi J, Kim S, Craft J. The pathogenesis of systemic lupus erythematosus – an update. Curr Opin Immunol 2012; 24: 651–7.
14. Okamoto I, Taniguchi Y, Kunikata T, Kohno K, Iwaki K, Ikeda M, et al. Major royal jelly protein 3 modulates immune responses *in vitro* and *in vivo*. Life Sci 2003; 73: 2029–45.
15. Kohno K, Okamoto I, Sano O, Arai N, Iwaki K, Ikeda M, et al. Royal jelly inhibits the production of proinflammatory cytokines by activated macrophages. Biosci Biotechnol Biochem 2004; 68: 138–45.
16. Vucevic D, Melliou E, Vasilijic S, Gasic S, Ivanovski P, Chinou I, et al. Fatty acids isolated from royal jelly modulate dendritic cell-mediated immune response *in vitro*. Int Immunopharmacol 2007; 7: 1211–20.
17. Oka H, Emori Y, Kobayashi N, Hayashi Y, Nomoto K. Suppression of allergic reactions by royal jelly in association with the restoration of macrophage function and the improvement of Th1/Th2 cell responses. Int Immunopharmacol 2001; 1: 521–32.
18. Taniguchi Y, Kohno K, Inoue S, Koya-Miyata S, Okamoto I, Arai N, et al. Oral administration of royal jelly inhibits the development of atopic dermatitis-like skin lesions in NC/Nga mice. Int Immunophamacol 2003; 3: 1313–24.
19. McInerney MF, Clough JD, Senitzer D, Cathcart MK. Two distinct subsets of patients with systemic lupus erythematosus. Clin Immunol Immunopathol 1988; 49(1): 116–32.
20. Zahran AM, Elsayh KI, Metwalley KA. Regulatory T cells in children with recently diagnosed type 1 diabetes. Indian J Endocrinol Metab 2012; 16(6): 952–7.
21. Liu X, Ji B, Sun M, Wu W, Huag L, Sun A, et al. Cell-penetrable mouse forkhead box protein 3 alleviates experimental arthritis in mice by up-regulating regulatory T cells. Clin Exp Immunol 2015; 181(1): 87–99.
22. Lyssuk EY, Torgashina AV, Soloviev SK, Nassonov EL, Bykovskaia SN. Reduced number and function of CD4+ CD25highFoxP3+ regulatory T cells in patients with systemic lupus erythematosus. Adv Exp Med Biol 2007; 601: 113–9.
23. Barath S, Aleksza M, Tarr T, Sipka S, Szegedi G, Kiss E. Measurement of natural (CD4+CD25high) and inducible (CD4+IL−10+) regulatory T cells in patients with systemic lupus erythematosus. Lupus 2007; 16: 489–96.
24. Venigalla RK, Tretter T, Krienke S, Max R, Eckstein V, Blank N, et al. Reduced CD4+,CD25− T cell sensitivity to the suppressive function of CD4+,CD25high,CD127−/low regulatory T cells in patients with active systemic lupus erythematosus. Arthritis Rheum 2008; 58: 2120–30.
25. Yates J, Whittington A, Mitchell P, Lechler RI, Lightstone L, Lombardi G. Natural regulatory T cells: number and function are normal in the majority of patients with lupus nephritis. Clin Exp Immunol 2008; 153: 44–55.
26. Zhang B, Zhang X, Tang FL, Zhu LP, Liu Y, Chen W, et al. Clinical significance of increased CD4+CD25−Foxp3+T cells in patients with new-onset systemic lupus erythematosus. Ann Rheum Dis 2008; 67: 1037–40.
27. Barnutio LI, Marghistas LA, Dizmireun DS, Mihai CM, Bobiso O. Chemical composition and antimicrobial activity of royal jelly – review. Anim Sci Biotechnol 2011; 44(2): 27–72.
28. La Cava A, Fang CJ, Singh RP, Ebling F, Hahn BH. Manipulation of immune regulation in systemic lupus erythematosus. Autoimmun Rev 2005; 4(8): 515–19.
29. Sharabi A, Mozes E. The suppression of murine lupus by a tolerogenic peptide involves foxp3-expressing CD8 cells that are required for the optimal induction and function of foxp3-expressing CD4 cells. J Immunol 2008; 181: 3243–51.
30. Churlaud G, Pitoiset F, Jebbawi F, Lorenzon R, Bellier B, Rosenzwajg M, et al. Human and mouse CD8(+)CD25(+) FOXP3(+) regulatory T cells at steady state and during interleukin-2 therapy. Front Immunol 2015; 6: 171.
31. Taylor PR, Carugati A, Fadok VA, Cook HT, Andrews M, Carroll MC, et al. A hierarchical role for classical pathway complement proteins in the clearance of apoptotic cells *in vivo*. J Exp Med 2000; 192(3): 359–66.

32. Jin O, Sun LY, Zhou KX, Zhang XS, Feng XB, Mok MY, et al. Lymphocyte apoptosis and macrophage function: correlation with disease activity in systemic lupus erythematosus. Clin Rheumatol 2005; 24(2): 107–10.
33. Nalbandian A, Crispín JC, Tsokos GC. Interleukin-17 and systemic lupus erythematosus: current concepts. Clin Exp Immunol 2009; 157(2): 209–15.

*Khaled Saad
Department of Pediatrics
Assiut University
Assiut 71516, Egypt
Emails: ksaad8@yahoo.com; khaled.ali@med.au.edu.eg

Chronic leucine supplementation improves lipid metabolism in C57BL/6J mice fed with a high-fat/cholesterol diet

Jun Jiao[1†], Shu-Fen Han[1†], Wei Zhang[1], Jia-Ying Xu[2,3], Xing Tong[1], Xue-Bin Yin[4], Lin-Xi Yuan[4] and Li-Qiang Qin[1,5*]

[1]Department of Nutrition and Food Hygiene, School of Public Health, Soochow University, Suzhou, China; [2]School of Radiation Medicine and Protection, Soochow University, Suzhou, China; [3]Collaborative Innovation Center of Radiation Medicine of Jiangsu Higher Education Institutions, Soochow University, Suzhou, China; [4]Jiangsu Bio-Engineering Research Centre of Selenium, Suzhou, China; [5]Jiangsu Key Laboratory of Preventive and Translational Medicine for Geriatric Disease, Soochow University, Suzhou, China

Abstract

Background: Leucine supplementation has been reported to improve lipid metabolism. However, lipid metabolism in adipose tissues and liver has not been extensively studied for leucine supplementation in mice fed with a high-fat/cholesterol diet (HFCD).
Design: C57BL/6J mice were fed a chow diet, HFCD, HFCD supplemented with 1.5% leucine (HFCD + 1.5% Leu group) or 3% leucine (HFCD + 3% Leu group) for 24 weeks. The body weight, peritoneal adipose weight, total cholesterol (TC), triglyceride in serum and liver, and serum adipokines were analyzed. In addition, expression levels of proteins associated with hepatic lipogenesis, adipocyte lipolysis, and white adipose tissue (WAT) browning were determined.
Results: Mice in the HFCD group developed obesity and deteriorated lipid metabolism. Compared with HFCD, leucine supplementation lowered weight gain and TC levels in circulation and the liver without changing energy intake. The decrease in body fat was supported by histological examination in the WAT and liver. Furthermore, serum levels of proinflammatory adipokines, such as leptin, IL-6, and tumor necrosis factor-alpha, were significantly decreased by supplemented leucine. At the protein level, leucine potently decreased the hepatic lipogenic enzymes (fatty acid synthase and acetyl-coenzyme A carboxylase) and corresponding upstream proteins. In epididymal WAT, the reduced expression levels of two major lipases by HFCD, namely phosphorylated hormone-sensitive lipase and adipose triglyceride lipase, were reversed when leucine was supplemented. Uncoupling protein 1, β3 adrenergic receptors, peroxisome proliferator-activated receptor g coactivator-1α, and fibroblast growth factor 21 were involved in the thermogenic program and WAT browning. Leucine additionally upregulated their protein expression in both WAT and interscapular brown adipose tissue.
Conclusion: This study demonstrated that chronic leucine supplementation reduced the body weight and improved the lipid profile of mice fed with a HFCD. This beneficial effect was ascribed to hepatic lipogenesis, adipocyte lipolysis, and WAT browning.

Keywords: *leucine*; *lipid metabolism*; *brown adipose tissue*; *white adipose tissue*; *WAT browning*

The prevalence of obesity is increasing at an alarming rate in many parts of the world. About 2 billion people are overweight, and one-third of them are obese (1). Obesity is a major health problem because it increases the risk of several clinical conditions, including diabetes and cardiovascular diseases (2, 3). From a public health perspective, the current obesity epidemic must be reduced. Besides regular physical activity, choosing healthy food is the main way to prevent obesity (4). In this case, manipulating the dietary composition of macronutrients merits careful investigation because macronutrients not only provide calories, but they also work as signaling molecules that can affect cellular metabolic processes (5–7). Leucine, which is an essential branched chain amino acid (BCAA), is one such example (8, 9). Our multi-ethnic population-based international study also

[†]These authors contributed equally to this work.

demonstrated that the intake of BCAA including leucine is inversely associated with the prevalence of overweight status and obesity (10).

In 2006, Cota found that the central administration of leucine decreases food intake and body weight in rats by stimulating the intracellular energy-sensing mammalian target of rapamycin (mTOR) pathway (7). Consequently, Zhang found that increasing leucine intake for 14 weeks results in reduced weight and adiposity in high-fat diet (HFD)-fed mice (11). Since then, several studies have observed the effects of leucine supplementation on HFD-induced obesity and metabolic profile through multiple mechanisms, but the results were inconsistent (12–19). Obesity results from the expansion of adipose tissue, which is categorically divided into white adipose tissue (WAT) and brown adipose tissue (BAT). WAT is characterized by lipid storage as triglyceride and endocrine functions. In this case, the promotion of lipolysis in WAT is beneficial for the prevention and treatment of obesity. Meanwhile, the main BAT function is energy dissipation, which is largely in the form of heat (20). Certain white depots have been found to develop brownish characteristics (21). Thus, inducible brown-like adipocytes from WAT (WAT browning) may be a promising strategy to combat obesity.

Despite the intricate mechanisms dictating obesity, lipid metabolism in adipose tissues itself and liver, other major site for lipid metabolism has not been extensively studied for the beneficial effect of leucine supplementation on obesity prevention. Therefore, we investigated whether or not chronic leucine supplementation with a high-fat/cholesterol diet (HFCD) in rats has a direct action on target tissues, focusing on the expression of proteins related to hepatic lipogenesis, adipocyte lipolysis, and WAT browning.

Materials and methods

Experimental animals and diets

Seven-week-old male C57BL/6J mice were purchased from SLAC Laboratory Animal Company (Shanghai, China). The mice were housed in standard cages (four to five mice per cage) with a constant temperature of 22°C ± 2°C, 60% relative humidity, and an artificial 12-h light–darkness cycle. All of the animal studies were pre-approved by the Soochow University Animal Welfare Committee. After 1 week of acclimatization to the laboratory conditions, the animals were weighed and randomly assigned to one of four dietary groups (14 mice per group), namely those fed with chow diet (CD group), HFCD group, HFCD supplemented with 1.5% leucine (HFCD + 1.5% Leu group) or 3.0% leucine (HFCD + 3% Leu group). The CD contained 3.90 kcal/g with 20.8, 67.7, and 11.5% calories from protein, carbohydrates, and fat, respectively. The HFCD obtained from Research Diets Inc. (New Brunswick, NJ, USA, D12451 + 1% cholesterol) was known to induce obesity and dyslipidemia. It contained 4.77 kcal/g with 19.6, 34.4, and 46% calories from protein, carbohydrates, and fat, respectively. L-leucine (Luzhou Amino Acid Co., Ltd, Shandong, China) was directly mixed with the HFCD by percentage weight in supplemental diets. The animals had free access to food and water. The experiment lasted for 24 weeks. Body weight and food intakes were routinely recorded on a weekly basis. The average calorie intake was calculated by food intake.

Tissue sample and blood management

Blood samples were obtained from the angular vein after 12 h of fasting every 8 weeks including the start and end of the experiment (weeks 0, 8, 16, and 24). Serum was separated and stored at −80°C in a freezer until analysis. At the 24th week of the experiment, the animals were sacrificed under mild ether anesthesia. Peritoneal adipose tissue (excepting mesenteric) was removed and weighted. The liver, epididymal WAT, and interscapular BAT were immediately collected, frozen in liquid nitrogen, and stored at −80°C in a freezer for further analyses.

Histological examination

Histological examination of livers and WAT samples was carried out using the HE staining method. The samples were fixed in 10% neutral buffered formalin for 6 h and dehydrated as standard before embedding in paraffin wax. Sections were cut into 4-μm slices and mounted on polylysine-handled glass slides, and HE staining was performed.

Biochemical analysis in serum and liver

Serum levels of total cholesterol (TC) and triglyceride (TG) at each time point were determined by enzymatic methods using commercial kits (Applygen Technologies Inc., Beijing, China). The serum sample at the end of the experiment was also used to determine glucose (Applygen Technologies Inc., Beijing, China), insulin (Mercodia AB, Sweden), and adipocytokines including interleukin-6 (IL-6), leptin, tumor necrosis factor-alpha (TNF-α), and adiponectin with Luminex® xMAP Technology (Merck Millipore Bioscience, USA). The insulin resistance was estimated by homeostasis model assessment-insulin resistance (HOMA-IR) using the following formula: HOMA-IR = fasting glucose (mmol/L) × insulin (pmol/L)/22.5. Parts of the liver tissue were homogenated. The hepatic levels of TG and TC were analyzed with commercialized kits (Applygen Technologies Inc., Beijing, China) and normalized to protein levels.

Western blot analysis

The hepatic tissue and epididymal and interscapular adipose tissue samples were homogenized in lysis buffer (Beyotime Institute of Biotechnology, Nantong, China). Protein concentration was determined according to the bicinchoninic acid assay (BCA) protein assay (Beyotime

Institute of Biotechnology, Nantong, China). Equal amounts of protein (30–50 μg) were loaded to a 12% sodium dodecylsulfate (SDS)-polyacrylamide gel and then transferred to a polyvinylidene fluoride (PVDF) membrane (EMD Millipore Corporation, CA, USA) through electrophoretic transfer. Subsequently, non-specific binding sites were blocked with 5% fat-free dry milk in phosphate-buffered saline containing 0.1% Tween-20 for 1 h at room temperature. The blots were incubated overnight at 4°C with primary antibodies according to the recommendation of the manufacturer. The antibodies for hepatic tissues included fatty acid synthase (FAS, Cell Signaling Technology, CST3180, 1:1000), acetyl-coenzyme A carboxylase (ACC, CST3676, 1:1000), sterol regulatory element binding protein-1 (SREBP-1, Abcam ab28481, 1:500), and liver X receptorα (LXRα, Abcam ab176323, 1:1000). Hormone-sensitive lipase (HSL, Abcam ab45422, 1:1000), p-HSL (Ser563, CST4139, 1:1000), p-HSL (Ser660, CST4139, 1:1000), adipose triglyceride lipase (ATGL, CST2138, 1:1000), and cAMP-dependent protein kinase (PKA, YT 374, 1:1000) were used in epididymal adipose tissues. Meanwhile, uncoupling protein 1 (UCP1, Abcamab10983), β3 adrenergic receptors (β3AR, YT 0363, 1:1000), peroxisome proliferator-activated receptor g coactivator-1α + β (PGC-1α + β, Abcam ab72230, 1:1000), and fibroblast growth factor 21 (FGF-21, Abcam ab171941, 1:1000) were used in epididymal and interscapular adipose tissues. After washing for three times, the antigen–antibody complexes were visualized for 1–1.5 h at room temperature with Peroxidase AffiniPure goat anti-mouse or anti-rabbit IgG antibody (Jackson ImmunoResarch Laboratories, Inc., Canada). Antibody reactivity was detected by chemiluminescence using enhanced chemiluminescent (ECL) Detection Systems (EMD Millipore Corporation, CA, USA). Blots were performed at least three times to confirm the reproducibility of the results. The intensity of the bands was normalized using each corresponding β-actin density as an internal control.

Statistical analysis

Data are expressed as the mean ± standard deviation. All the analyses were performed using SPSS version 16.0 statistical analysis package (SPSS Inc., Chicago, IL, USA). The significance of differences among the four dietary groups was assessed by one-way ANOVA, followed by Fisher's least significant difference (LSD) *post hoc* test. Differences were considered significant when $p < 0.05$.

Results

Mice in the HFCD group grew fast during the entire study course and exhibited increased body weight of 71.89% higher than those in the CD group at the end of the experiment. The mice in the two leucine groups had comparable body weights, but they were heavier than

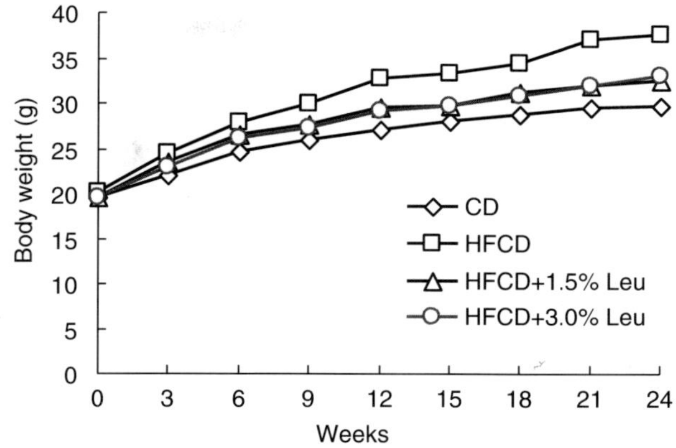

Fig. 1. Chronic leucine supplementation decreases the body weight in HFCD-fed mice from week 9. ($n = 14$ for each group). CD, chow diet; HFCD, high-fat/cholesterol diet; Leu, leucine.

those in the CD group and significantly lower than those in the HFCD group from week 9 (Fig. 1). At the end of the experiment, the weight gain of the mice was 9.21 ± 1.46, 17.55 ± 2.60, 12.94 ± 2.22, and 13.78 ± 2.50 g in the CD group, HFCD group, HFCD + 1.5% Leu group, and HFCD + 3.0% Leu group, respectively. Weight gain was significantly lower in the supplemented leucine groups than in the HFCD group. The mice fed with HFCD with and without leucine ingested less food than the mice in the CD group. However, when expressed in kcal/day, energy intake by the four groups was comparable. HFCD feeding significantly increased peritoneal adipose tissue and liver weights. Supplemental leucine significantly decreased their weights compared with the HFCD group; however, there were no significant differences in the ratios of fat and liver weights to body weight between HFCD with and without leucine (Table 1).

As expected, serum TC and TG were significantly higher in the HFCD group than in the CD group. Serum TC was significantly lower in the two leucine groups than in the HFCD group at weeks 16 and 24. At the end of the experiment (week 24), the serum TC levels were 1.71 ± 0.20, 2.69 ± 0.45, 2.15 ± 0.54, and 2.12 ± 0.60 mmol/L. Leucine supplementation mitigated serum TG compared with the HFCD group, but no significant difference was observed. For hepatic lipids, TC levels in the liver homogenate were significantly increased by HFCD (0.31 ± 0.19 μmol/g vs. 0.52 ± 0.19 μmol/g) and significantly decreased to a level similar to the CD group by supplemental 1.5% leucine (0.39 ± 0.11 μmol/g) and 3.0% leucine (0.31 ± 0.09 μmol/g). Meanwhile, hepatic TG was slightly increased by HFCD, and its decrease through leucine supplementation was not significant. The levels of TC and TG in circulation and in the liver were comparable in both leucine supplementation groups (Fig. 2).

HFCD resulted in a significant increase in fasting glucose and insulin. Although fasting glucose levels were

Table 1. Effects of leucine supplementation on food and energy intake, body and organ weight in C57BL/6J mice

	Food intake (g/day)	Energy (kcal/day)	Weight gain (g)	Fat weight[a] (g)	Fat weight/BW (%)	Liver weight (g)	Liver weight/BW (%)
CD	3.14±0.23	12.26±0.89	9.21±1.46	0.57±0.22	1.89±0.70	1.16±0.10	3.89±0.26
HFCD	2.57±0.22**	12.25±1.08	17.55±2.60**	2.29±0.62**	6.02±1.26**	1.44±0.15*	3.80±0.17
HFCD + 1.5% leucine (Leu)	2.52±0.30**	11.98±1.41	12.94±2.22*,#	1.70±0.84**,#	5.24±1.79**	1.29±0.11*,#	3.89±0.39
HFCD + 3% Leu	2.59±0.30**	12.31±1.44	13.78±2.50*,#	1.71±0.85**,#	4.74±1.72**	1.24±0.09#	3.53±0.50

Values are mean ± SD ($n = 14$).
*$p < 0.05$ versus CD group; **$p < 0.01$ versus CD group; #$p < 0.05$ versus HFCD group.
[a]Peritoneal adipose tissue (excepting mesenteric).
CD, chow diet; HFCD, high-fat/cholesterol diet; BW, body weight.

comparable regardless of whether leucine was supplemented, leucine supplementation caused significantly lower fasting plasma insulin, leading to a decreased HOMA index in the leucine-supplemented group compared with the HFCD group. We also determined several notable adipokines implicated in obesity and obesity-related metabolic disorders, which included leptin, IL-6, TNF-α, and adiponectin. HFCD significantly increased serum levels of leptin, IL-6, and TNF-α and decreased adiponectin. Compared with the HFCD group, leptin level was significantly decreased in the HFC + 1.5% Leu and HFC + 3.0% Leu groups, and IL-6 and TNF-α levels were significantly decreased in the HFC + 3.0% Leu group. However, no difference in adiponectin level was observed between HFCD group and HFCD groups supplemented with leucine (Table 2).

Histological examination showed that HFCD enlarged the adipocyte size of WAT and caused the hepatic lipids to accumulate. However, adipocyte size was markedly reduced, and hepatic lipid accumulation was alleviated after leucine supplementation (Fig. 3).

To provide molecular evidence for the role of leucine in hepatic lipid metabolism, protein expression of lipogenic enzymes, including FAS and ACC, was measured. As a

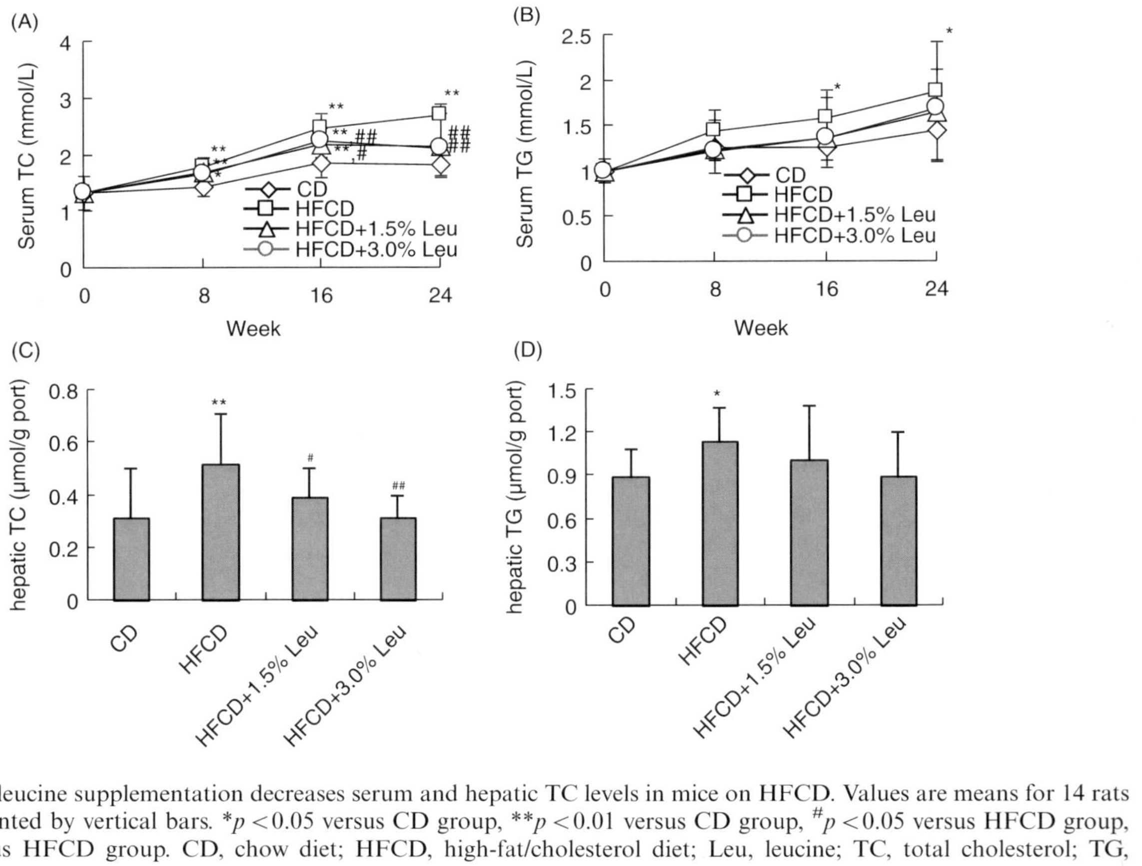

Fig. 2. Chronic leucine supplementation decreases serum and hepatic TC levels in mice on HFCD. Values are means for 14 rats with SD represented by vertical bars. *$p < 0.05$ versus CD group, **$p < 0.01$ versus CD group, #$p < 0.05$ versus HFCD group, ##$p < 0.01$ versus HFCD group. CD, chow diet; HFCD, high-fat/cholesterol diet; Leu, leucine; TC, total cholesterol; TG, triglyceride.

Table 2. Effects of leucine supplementation on glucose metabolism and serum adipokines in C57BL/6J mice

	Insulin (μg/L)	Glucose (mmol/L)	HOMA-IR	Leptin (ng/mL)	Adiponectin (ng/mL)	IL-6 (pg/mL)	TNF-α (pg/mL)
CD	0.55 ± 0.09	6.66 ± 1.18	3.43 ± 0.80	0.73 ± 0.42	16.71 ± 1.66	3.64 ± 1.80	2.67 ± 0.86
HFCD	0.75 ± 0.22*	8.21 ± 2.06*	6.41 ± 2.00**	7.14 ± 3.44**	13.88 ± 1.51**	7.93 ± 3.16**	3.86 ± 1.45**
HFCD + 1.5% leucine (Leu)	0.55 ± 0.11##	7.98 ± 1.91	3.65 ± 1.32##	4.21 ± 2.37**,##	15.34 ± 2.03	6.93 ± 1.52**	3.22 ± 0.82
HFCD + 3% Leu	0.61 ± 0.16#	7.94 ± 1.22	4.72 ± 1.76*,##	4.24 ± 2.22**,##	14.89 ± 2.41	6.15 ± 1.87**,#	2.85 ± 0.76#

Values are mean ± SD ($n = 14$). *$p < 0.05$ versus CD group, **$p < 0.01$ versus CD group, #$p < 0.05$ versus HFCD group, ##$p < 0.05$ versus HFCD group.

CD, chow diet; HFCD, high-fat/cholesterol diet; HOMA-IR, homeostasis model assessment-insulin resistance; TNF-α, tumor necrosis factor-alpha.

result, HFCD increased FAS and ACC expression, and the overexpression was retarded by additional leucine supplementation. On the contrary, ACC and FAS were regulated by SREBP-1, which is strongly activated by LXRα. Similarly, the overexpression of LXRa and SREBP-1 by HFCD was reverted by leucine supplementation. The protein expression was even lower in the HFCD + 3.0 Leu group than in the CD group (Fig. 4).

HSL and ATGL are two major lipases in adipocyte lipolysis. Their protein expression levels were measured in the epididymal WAT. Although total HSL expression had no effect, phosphorylated HSL was significantly decreased by HFCD. The protein expression of phosphorylated HSL and ATGL was markedly increased by leucine supplementation, even exceeding the CD group in the HFC + 3.0% Leu group. Compared with the HFCD group, the protein expression of p-HSL(563), p-HSL(660), and ATGL increased by 2.80, 2.99, and 1.87 times in the HFC-3.0% Leu group. The abovementioned lipolysis mainly involves the PKA pathway. We also analyzed the expression of PKA in WAT and found that the decreased expression by HFCD was restored by additional leucine supplementation (Fig. 5).

UCP1, β3AR, PGC-1, and FGF-21 were involved in the thermogenic program and WAT browning. In BAT, HFCD had no effect or even slightly upregulated their expression. Leucine supplementation remarkably increased the expression of the four proteins in a dose-response manner. Compared with the HFCD group, the protein expression levels of UCP1, β3AR, PGC-1, and FGF-21 in HFCD + 3.0% Leu group increased by 1.34, 3.94, 1.54, and 1.45 times, respectively. Unlike BAT, HFCD caused the decreased expression of these proteins in WAT. However, leucine supplementation still increased their expression in a dose-response manner. Compared with the HFCD group, the expression of these proteins in the HFCD + 3.0% Leu group increased by 3.06, 4.70, 1.20, and 1.69 times (Fig. 6).

Discussion

In modern times, consuming high cholesterol in a HFD is increasingly popular worldwide and is strongly associated with conditions of obesity and other lifestyle diseases (22). This study demonstrated that dietary leucine prevents obesity induced by a HFD supplemented with additional

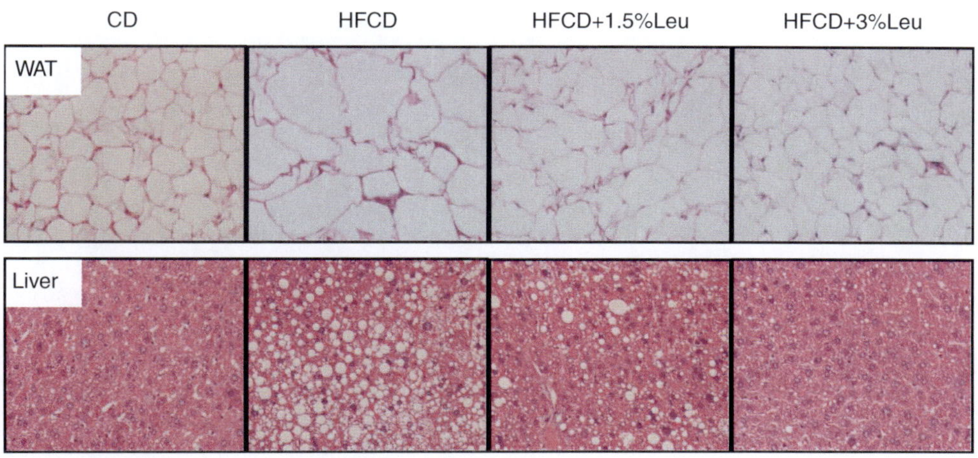

Fig. 3. Histological examination (400 ×) showed that adipocyte size was markedly reduced, and hepatic lipid accumulation was alleviated after leucine supplementation. CD, chow diet; HFCD, high-fat/cholesterol diet; Leu, leucine; WAT, white adipose tissue.

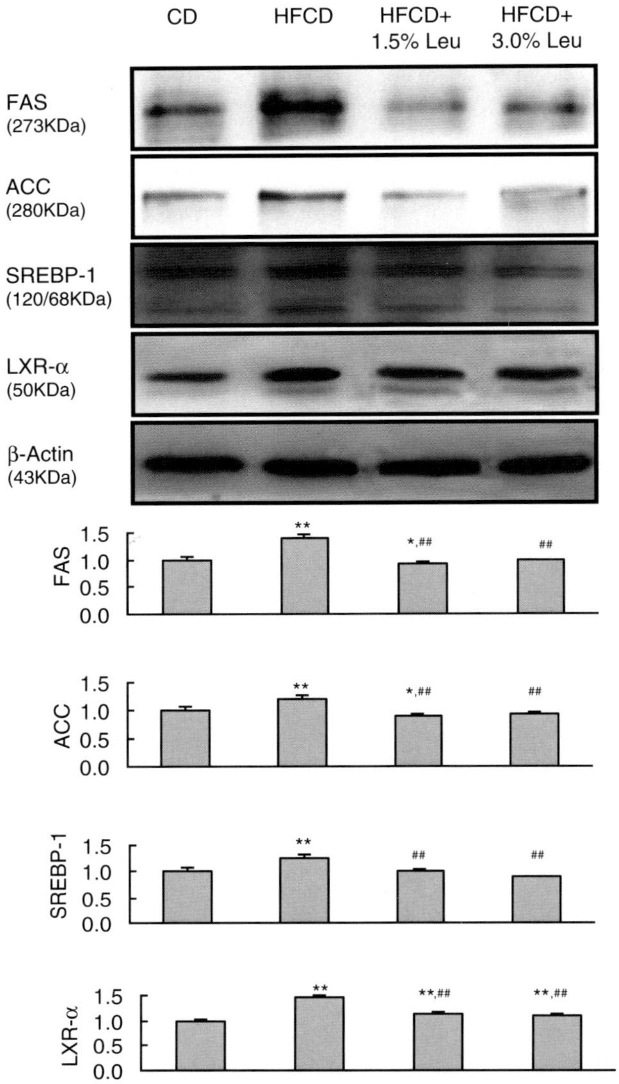

Fig. 4. Chronic leucine supplementation improves lipid metabolism by decreased hepatic lipogenesis in mice fed with HFCD. Values are means for three rats with SD represented by vertical bars. $^{*}p < 0.05$ versus CD group, $^{**}p < 0.01$ versus CD group, $^{\#\#}p < 0.01$ versus HFCD group. CD, chow diet; HFCD, high-fat/cholesterol diet; Leu, leucine; FAS, fatty acid synthase; ACC, acetyl-coenzyme A carboxylase; SREBP-1, sterol regulatory element binding protein-1; LXRα, liver X receptor α.

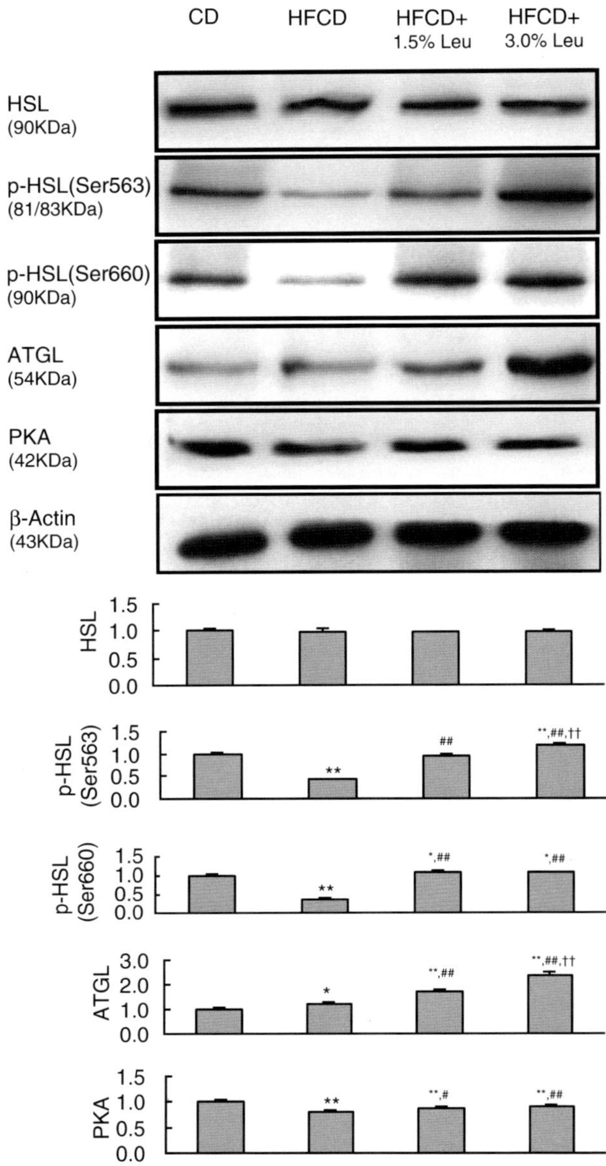

Fig. 5. Chronic leucine supplementation improves lipid metabolism by increased adipocyte lipolysis in WAT of mice fed with HFCD. Values are means for three rats with SD represented by vertical bars. $^{*}p < 0.05$ versus CD group, $^{**}p < 0.01$ versus CD group, $^{\#}p < 0.05$ versus HFCD group, $^{\#\#}p < 0.01$ versus HFCD group, $^{\dagger\dagger}p < 0.01$ versus HFCD + 1.5% Leu group. WAT, white adipose tissue; CD, chow diet; HFCD, high-fat/cholesterol diet; Leu, leucine; HSL, hormone-sensitive lipase; Ser, serine; ATGL, adipose triglyceride lipase; PKA, cAMP-dependent protein kinase.

cholesterol. The reduced obesity can be explained by improving lipid metabolism in the liver and adipose tissues.

In this study, leucine supplementation retarded weight gain without reducing energy intake, thereby suggesting a leucine-mediated increase in energy expenditure. Our observation was consistent with Zhang's and Binder's studies, in which leucine was consumed in drinking water along with a HFD (11, 17). Besides the decrease of fat and liver weights, histological examination also showed that HFCD-induced lipid accumulation in WAT and liver was markedly reduced by leucine supplementation. In fact, HFD feeding in rats for 3 weeks successfully reproduced the key features of non-alcoholic steatohepatitis, (23) and leucine supplementation improved this hepatic steatosis (13). Even in middle-aged adults during 14 days of bed rest, leucine prevented an increase in body fat percentage (24). Obesity results in dyslipidemia and dysglycemia. The beneficial effect of leucine supplementation on the lipid profile and circulating glucose/insulin levels has been extensively investigated in several obese animal models induced by a HFD (11–18). To better mimic

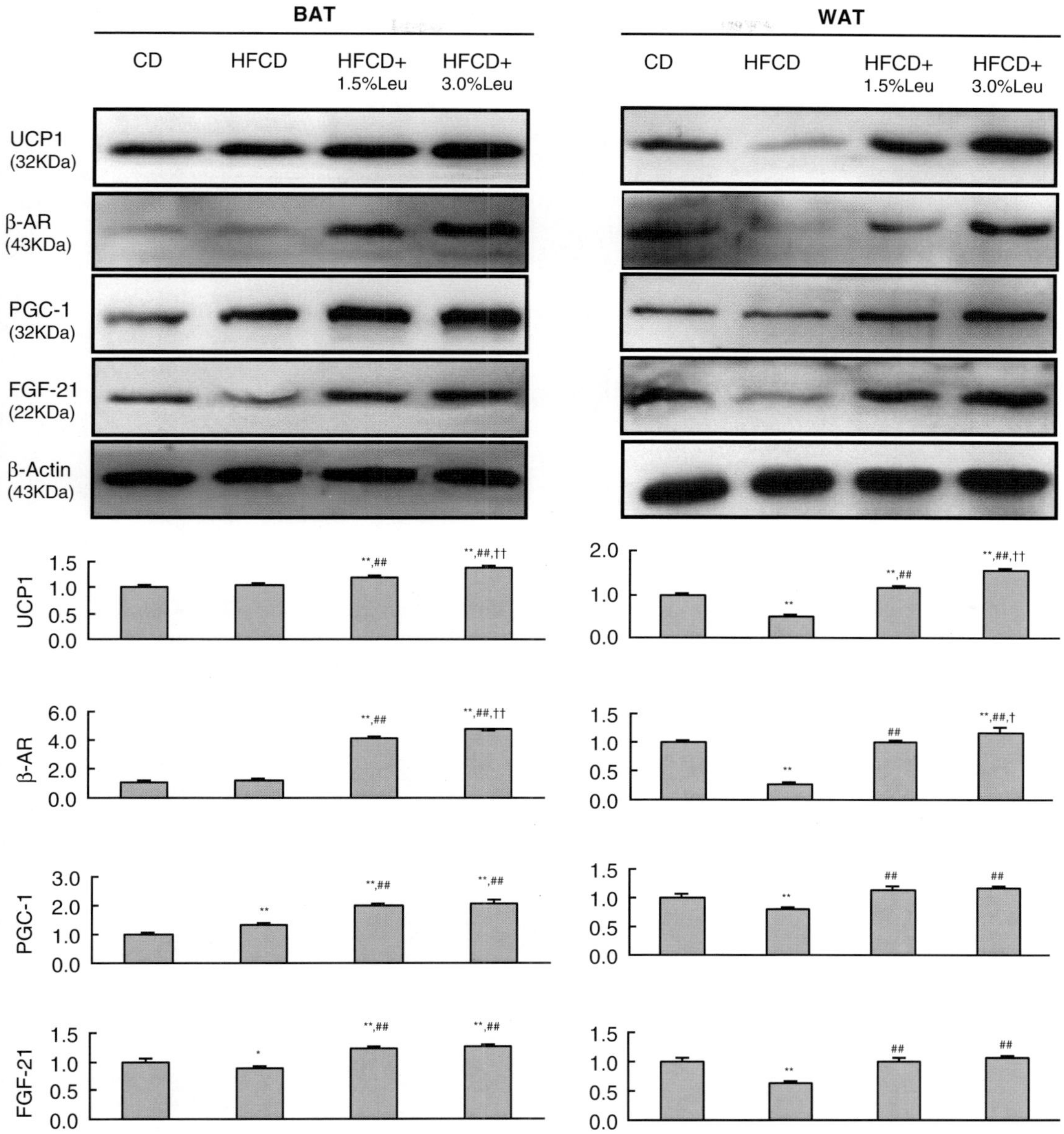

Fig. 6. Chronic leucine supplementation improves lipid metabolism through thermogenic program and WAT browning in mice fed with HFCD. Values are means for three rats with SD represented by vertical bars. $^{*}p < 0.05$ versus CD group, $^{**}p < 0.01$ versus CD group, $^{\#\#}p < 0.01$ versus HFCD group, $^{\dagger}p < 0.05$ versus HFCD + 1.5% Leu group, $^{\dagger\dagger}p < 0.01$ versus HFCD + 1.5% Leu group. BAT, brown adipose tissue; WAT, white adipose tissue; CD, chow diet; HFCD, high-fat/cholesterol diet; Leu, leucine; UCP1, uncoupling protein 1; β3AR, β3 adrenergic receptors; PGC-1, peroxisome proliferator-activated receptor g coactivator-1; FGF-21, fibroblast growth factor 21.

hypercholesterolemia, additional cholesterol was contained in HFD to make HFCD in this study. As a result, leucine supplementation decreased the serum and hepatic TC and HOMA index. Therefore, with the reduced body weight and lipid accumulation, leucine supplementation generally improved lipid and glucose metabolism in this study. However, not all studies showed consistent results between body weight and glucose/lipid metabolism. For example, Macotela found that leucine supplementation causes a marked improvement in glucose tolerance and insulin signaling without altering weight gain and serum cholesterol in HFD-induced obese mice (13). Li even observed that leucine supplementation improves the insulin signaling pathway, while increasing the body weight and hepatic lipid accumulation in HFD-induced obese rats (16).

WAT is no longer considered a tissue mainly devoted to energy storage but is emerging as an active participant in regulating physiologic and pathologic processes through the synthesis and secretion of various adipokines. Excessive intake of dietary fat promotes adipocyte hypertrophy, altering their normal endocrine function (25). In this study, the inflammatory pathologic condition was found in HFCD-induced obese mice, in which increased levels of serum leptin, TNF-α, and IL-6 (proinflammatory adipokines) and reduced levels of adiponectin (main anti-inflammatory factor) were observed. Leucine supplementation decreased leptin, TNF-α, and IL-6, suggesting that inflammatory stress was attenuated. TNF-α is central to the chronic inflammatory state present in obesity (25). Reduced plasma TNF-α levels were observed in 20 overweight and obese subjects that received leucine-containing nutraceutical for 4 weeks (26). The mRNA level of TNF-α was also significantly reduced in perigonadal and subcutaneous adipose tissues of HFD-induced obese mice simultaneously supplemented with leucine for 8 weeks (13). Consistent with our study, Zhang also found that leucine intake decreases plasma leptin levels in obese mice (11). Our previous study further confirmed that chronic leucine supplementation improves HFD-induced leptin resistance by decreasing the circulating leptin level (19). Besides inflammation, oxidative stress is inextricably linked and plays major roles in the onset and development of obesity (27). In our previous study, leucine supplementation for 8 weeks resulted in a significant increase in the levels of total antioxidant capacity, superoxide dismutase (SOD), and glutathione, as well as a decrease in the malondialdehyde (MDA) level in insulin-resistant rats (28). Other studies also found that leucine supplementation inhibits the HFD-induced expression of manganese SOD in the liver and decreases the MDA level in the blood of animals fed with a HFD, which indicates that a chronic leucine supplementation may prevent HFD-induced oxidative stress (16). Together, the overall beneficial effect of leucine supplementation on lipid/glucose metabolism and adipokine inflammatory stress promoted us to investigate liver lipogenesis and adipose tissue lipolysis at the protein level.

HFD is known to upregulate LXRa, which then upregulates SREBP-1 to increase the activity of lipogenic enzymes, such as FAS and ACC, and accumulate TG in hepatocytes (29). Except through SREBP-1, LXRα directly regulates FAS and ACC (30). For the first time, we found that leucine reduced the expression of these two proteins in the liver, which was supported by the downregulation of their upstream proteins (LXRα and SREBP-1). Some studies observed FAS and ACC at the mRNA level in different tissues. In the study by Macotela, the expression levels of FAS and ACC mRNA increased in livers of HFD mice, and they were reverted to control levels when additional leucine was added (13). However, in already obese mice, leucine supplementation increased the FAS mRNA level, but not the FAS protein level in WAT (17). Interestingly, the downregulation of lipogenic enzyme at the mRNA level by leucine or other two BCAAs (isoleucine and valine) was also observed in the human intestinal cell line, NCI-H716 (31).

Catalytically active PKA phosphorylates downstream targets-HSL, which contribute to the initiation of ATGL, ultimately leading to the breakdown of TG (32). The effect of leucine on lipase-related protein has not been investigated. However, leucine is a potent activator of mTORC1 signaling (11, 16), which promotes lipolysis by acting on common lipolytic targets (e.g. HSL) through a pathway parallel to PKA (33). Whey protein is rich in leucine. Freudenberg found that high amounts of whey protein lead to increased lipolysis in white fat as indicated by increased gene expression of ATGL and HSL in mice fed with semisynthetic HFD for 20 weeks (34). In this study, leucine supplementation upregulated the expression of PKA, following the increase in HSL phosphorylation on Ser563, which is thought to promote the intrinsic catalytic activity of HSL, and HSL phosphorylation on Ser660, which is thought to promote the translocation of cytosolic HSL to the surface of the lipid droplet (32).

In rodents, BAT is the major organ responsible for adaptive thermogenesis during cold exposure (20). The UCP1 gene is known to be specifically expressed in BAT and is regarded as a BAT marker (35). The expression of UCP1 is driven by several transcriptional components, including the coactivator of PGC-1, which is strongly induced by β-adrenegic signaling (36). In addition, adipose-derived FGF21 acts to increase UCP1 expression by enhancing the PGC-1 protein level of adipose tissues (37). In this study, the expression levels of these proteins were detected in BAT and WAT. Interestingly, HFCD did not affect their expression in BAT, but remarkably decreased their expression in WAT. This finding suggested that high fat in diet had more profound effects on fat deposit in WAT. Recently, WAT browning in response to appropriate stimulation has become the target of numerous obesity therapeutics (20). An important characteristic of WAT browning is the overexpression of UCP1 in WAT. In fact, earlier studies showed that enhanced expression of UCP1 in WAT of mice can reduce obesity (38). Meanwhile, FGF21 is considered a novel adipokine that has recently been demonstrated to stimulate the browning of WAT in obese mice, even in healthy human (39, 40). Wang further found that the injection of recombinant murine FGF21 reduces IL-6, TNF-α, and leptin mRNA levels in WAT of monosodium glutamate-induced obese rats, with the improvement of glucose tolerance, lipid metabolic spectrum, and hepatic steatosis (41).

Until now, the effect of leucine on the expression of these proteins in adipose tissue has not been investigated. In Binder's previous study on already obese mice, leucine-supplemented mice exhibited a significant increase in mRNA expression of UCP1 in WAT, but not in BAT and muscle tissues (17). Vaughan found that leucine treatment induces a significant dose-dependent expression of PGC-1 in human rhabdomyosarcoma cells and mouse myoblast (C2C12) cells (42). This study demonstrated that leucine supplementation upregulated the expression levels of UCP1, β3AR, PGC-1, and FGF-21 in WAT, in addition to their overexpression in BAT in a dose-dependent manner. Thus, leucine supplementation both enhanced energy transformation from nutrients to heat directly in BAT and promoted WAT browning in WAT, thereby reducing obesity.

In conclusion, the present findings strengthen current evidence suggesting a beneficial role for leucine in the prevention of diet-induced obesity. Unlike previous studies, additional cholesterol in HFD and the beneficial effects of leucine on the lipid profile, glucose metabolism, and adipokine inflammatory stress were observed. This study focused on the systemic determination of protein expression related to lipid metabolism. This beneficial effect was ascribed to hepatic lipogenesis, adipocyte lipolysis, and WAT browning.

Conflict of interest and funding

The authors declare no competing financial interest. This work was supported by grants from the National Natural Science Foundation of China (No. 81472974, 81273067, 31400091) and the 'Blue Project' of Jiangsu Province. Further support was obtained from the Priority Academic Program Development of Jiangsu Higher Education Institutions (PAPD).

References

1. Seidell JC, Halberstadt J. The global burden of obesity and the challenges of prevention. Ann Nutr Metab 2015; 66: 7–12.
2. Schelbert KB. Comorbidities of obesity. Prim Care 2009; 36: 271–85.
3. Surani SR. Diabetes, sleep apnea, obesity and cardiovascular disease: why not address them together? World J Diabetes 2014; 5: 381–4.
4. Swinburn B, Kraak V, Rutter H, Vandevijvere S, Lobstein T, Sacks G, et al. Strengthening of accountability systems to create healthy food environments and reduce global obesity. Lancet 2015; 385: 2534–45.
5. Schutz Y. Macronutrients and energy balance in obesity. Metabolism 1995; 44: 7–11.
6. Morrison CD, Laeger T. Protein-dependent regulation of feeding and metabolism. Trends Endocrinol Metab 2015; 26: 256–62.
7. Cota D, Proulx K, Smith KA, Kozma SC, Thomas G, Woods SC, et al. Hypothalamic mTOR signaling regulates food intake. Science 2006; 312: 927–30.
8. McAllan L, Cotter PD, Roche HM, Korpela R, Nilaweera KN. Impact of leucine on energy balance. J Physiol Biochem 2013; 69: 155–63.
9. Pedroso JA, Zampieri TT, Donato J, Jr. Reviewing the effects of L-Leucine supplementation in the regulation of food intake, energy balance, and glucose homeostasis. Nutrients 2015; 7: 3914–37.
10. Qin LQ, Xun P, Bujnowski D, Daviglus ML, Van Horn L, Stamler J, et al. Higher branched-chain amino acid intake is associated with a lower prevalence of being overweight or obese in middle-aged East Asian and Western adults. J Nutr 2011; 141: 249–54.
11. Zhang Y, Guo K, LeBlanc RE, Loh D, Schwartz GJ, Yu YH. Increasing dietary leucine intake reduces diet-induced obesity and improves glucose and cholesterol metabolism in mice via multimechanisms. Diabetes 2007; 56: 1647–54.
12. Nairizi A, She P, Vary TC, Lynch CJ. Leucine supplementation of drinking water does not alter susceptibility to diet-induced obesity in mice. J Nutr 2009; 139: 715–19.
13. Macotela Y, Emanuelli B, Bång AM, Espinoza DO, Boucher J, Beebe K, et al. Dietary leucine – an environmental modifier of insulin resistance acting on multiple levels of metabolism. PLoS One 2011; 6: e21187.
14. Torres-Leal FL, Fonseca-Alaniz MH, Teodoro GF, de Capitani MD, Vianna D, Pantaleão LC, et al. Leucine supplementation improves adiponectin and total cholesterol concentrations despite the lack of changes in adiposity or glucose homeostasis in rats previously exposed to a high-fat diet. Nutr Metab 2011; 8: 62.
15. Binder E, Bermúdez-Silva FJ, André C, Elie M, Romero-Zerbo SY, Leste-Lasserre T, et al. Leucine supplementation protects from insulin resistance by regulating adiposity levels. PLoS One 2013; 8: e74705.
16. Li X, Wang X, Liu R, Ma Y, Guo H, Hao L, et al. Chronic leucine supplementation increases body weight and insulin sensitivity in rats on high-fat diet likely by promoting insulin signaling in insulin-target tissues. Mol Nutr Food Res 2013; 57: 1067–79.
17. Binder E, Bermu′dez-Silva FJ, Elie M, Leste-Lasserre T, Belluomo I, Clark S, et al. Leucine supplementation modulates fuel substrates utilization and glucose metabolism in previously obese mice. Obesity 2014; 22: 713–20.
18. Fu L, Bruckbauer A, Li F, Cao Q, Cui X, Wu R, et al. Leucine amplifies the effects of metformin on insulin sensitivity and glycemic control in diet-inducedobese mice. Metabolism 2015; 64: 845–56.
19. Yuan XW, Han SF, Zhang JW, Xu JY, Qin LQ. Leucine supplementation improves leptin sensitivity in high-fat diet fed rats. Food Nutr Res 2015; 59: 27373, doi: http://dx.doi.org/10.3402/fnr.v59.27373
20. Kozak LP. Brown fat and the myth of diet-induced thermogenesis. Cell Metab 2010; 11: 263–7.
21. Nedergaard J, Cannon B. The browning of white adipose tissue: some burning issues. Cell Metab 2014; 20: 396–407.
22. Veghari G, Sedaghat M, Maghsodlo S, Banihashem S, Moharloei P, Angizeh A, et al. The association between abdominal obesity and serum cholesterol level. Int J Appl Basic Med Res 2015; 5: 83–6.
23. Lieber CS, Leo MA, Mak KM, Xu Y, Cao Q, Ren C, et al. Model of nonalcoholic steatohepatitis. Am J Clin Nutr 2004; 79: 502–9.
24. English KL, Mettler JA, Ellison JB, Mamerow MM, Arentson-Lantz E, Pattarini JM, et al. Leucine partially protects muscle mass and function during bed rest in middle-aged adults. Am J Clin Nutr 2016; 103: 465–73.
25. Khan M, Joseph F. Adipose tissue and adipokines: the association with and application of adipokines in obesity. Scientifica (Cairo) 2014; 2014: 328592.
26. Zemel MB, Bruckbauer A. Effects of a leucine and pyridoxine-containing nutraceutical on fat oxidation, and oxidative and inflammatory stress in overweight and obese subjects. Nutrients 2012; 4: 529–41.
27. Camps J, García-Heredia A. Introduction: oxidation and inflammation, a molecular link between non-communicable diseases. Adv Exp Med Biol 2014; 824: 1–4.
28. Tong X, Li W, Xu JY, Han S, Qin LQ. Effects of whey protein and leucine supplementation on insulin resistance in non-obese insulin-resistant model rats. Nutrition 2014; 30: 1076–80.
29. Ai ZL, Zhu CH, Min M, Wang J, Lan CH, Fan LL, et al. The role of hepatic liver X receptor α-and sterol regulatory element

binding protein-1c-mediated lipid disorder in the pathogenesis of non-alcoholic steatohepatitis in rats. J Int Med Res 2011; 39: 1219–29.
30. Joseph SB, Laffitte BA, Patel PH, Watson MA. Direct and indirect mechanisms for regulation of fatty acid synthase gene expression by liver X receptors. J Biol Chem 2002; 277: 11019–25.
31. Chen Q, Reimer RA. Dairy protein and leucine alter GLP-1 release and mRNA of genes involved in intestinal lipid metabolism *in vitro*. Nutrition 2009; 25: 340–9.
32. Lafontan M, Langin D. Lipolysis and lipid mobilization in human adipose tissue. Prog Lipid Res 2009; 48: 275–97.
33. Ricoult SJ, Manning BD. The multifaceted role of mTORC1 in the control of lipid metabolism. EMBO Rep 2013; 14: 242–51.
34. Freudenberg A, Petzke KJ, Klaus S. Comparison of high-protein diets and leucine supplementation in the prevention of metabolic syndrome and related disorders in mice. J Nutr Biochem 2012; 3: 1524–30.
35. Ocloo A, Shabalina IG, Nedergaard J, Brand MD. Cold-induced alterations of phospholipid fatty acyl composition in brown adipose tissuemitochondria are independent of uncoupling protein-1. Am J Physiol Regul Integr Comp Physiol 2007; 293: R1086–93.
36. Barbera MJ, Schluter A, Pedraza N, Iglesias R, Giralt M. Peroxisome proliferator-activated receptor alpha activates transcription of the brown fat uncoupling protein-1 gene. A link between regulation of the thermogenic and lipid oxidation pathways in the brown fat cell. J Biol Chem 2001; 276: 1486–93.
37. Fisher FM, Kleiner S, Douris N, Fox EC, Mepani RJ, Verdeguer F, et al. FGF21 regulates PGC-1α and browning of white adipose tissues in adaptive thermogenesis. Genes Dev 2012; 26: 271–81.
38. Kopecky J, Clarke G, Enerbäck S, Spiegelman B, Kozak LP. Expression of the mitochondrial uncoupling protein gene from the aP2 gene promoter prevents genetic obesity. J Clinl Invest 1995; 96: 2914–23.
39. Coskun T, Bina HA, Schneider MA, Dunbar JD, Hu CC, Chen Y, et al. Fibroblast growth factor 21 corrects obesity in mice. Endocrinology 2008; 149: 6018–27.
40. Hanssen MJ, Broeders E, Samms RJ, Vosselman MJ, van der Lans AA, Cheng CC, et al. Serum FGF21 levels are associated with brown adipose tissue activity in humans. Sci Rep 2015; 5: 10275.
41. Wang WF, Li SM, Ren GP, Zheng W, Lu YJ, Yu YH, et al. Recombinant murine fibroblast growth factor 21 ameliorates obesity-related inflammation in monosodium glutamate-induced obesity rats. Endocrine 2015; 49: 119–29.
42. Vaughan RA, Garcia-Smith R, Gannon NP, Bisoffi M, Trujillo KA, Conn CA. Leucine treatment enhances oxidative capacity through complete carbohydrate oxidation and increased mitochondrial density in skeletal muscle cells. Amino Acids 2013; 45: 901–11.

***Li-Qiang Qin**
Department of Nutrition and Food Hygiene
School of Public Health
Soochow University, 199 Renai Road
Suzhou, 215123
Jiangsu, China
Email: qinliqiang@suda.edu.cn

Plasma phospholipid pentadecanoic acid, EPA, and DHA, and the frequency of dairy and fish product intake in young children

Nicolai A. Lund-Blix[1,2,3]*, Kjersti S. Rønningen[1], Håkon Bøås[3], German Tapia[3] and Lene F. Andersen[2]

[1]Department of Pediatric Research, Oslo University Hospital, Rikshospitalet, Oslo, Norway; [2]Department of Nutrition, Institute of Basic Medical Sciences, University of Oslo, Oslo, Norway; [3]Division of Epidemiology, Norwegian Institute of Public Health, Oslo, Norway

Abstract

Background: There is a lack of studies comparing dietary assessment methods with the biomarkers of fatty acids in children.

Objective: The objective was to evaluate the suitability of a food frequency questionnaire (FFQ) to rank young children according to their intake of dairy and fish products by comparing food frequency estimates to the plasma phospholipid fatty acids pentadecanoic acid, eicosapentaenoic acid (EPA), and docosahexaenoic acid (DHA).

Design: Cross-sectional data for the present study were derived from the prospective cohort 'Environmental Triggers of Type 1 Diabetes Study'. Infants were recruited from the Norwegian general population during 2001–2007. One hundred and ten (age 3–10 years) children had sufficient volumes of plasma and FFQ filled in within 2 months from blood sampling and were included in this evaluation study. The quantitative determination of plasma phospholipid fatty acids was done by fatty acid methyl ester analysis. The association between the frequency of dairy and fish product intake and the plasma phospholipid fatty acids was assessed by a Spearman correlation analysis and by investigating whether participants were classified into the same quartiles of distribution.

Results: Significant correlations were found between pentadecanoic acid and the intake frequency of total dairy products ($r = 0.29$), total fat dairy products ($r = 0.39$), and cheese products ($r = 0.36$). EPA and DHA were significantly correlated with the intake frequency of oily fish ($r = 0.26$ and 0.37, respectively) and cod liver/fish oil supplements ($r = 0.47$ for EPA and $r = 0.50$ DHA). To a large extent, the FFQ was able to classify individuals into the same quartile as the relevant fatty acid biomarker.

Conclusions: The present study suggests that, when using the plasma phospholipid fatty acids pentadecanoic acid, EPA, and DHA as biomarkers, the FFQ used in young children showed a moderate capability to rank the intake frequency of dairy products with a high-fat content and cod liver/fish oil supplements.

Keywords: *biomarkers*; *dietary assessment*; *food frequency questionnaire*; *fatty acids*; *plasma phospholipids*

Assessing dietary intake in epidemiological studies is a complex undertaking. Valid methods for assessing food intake in children are essential for monitoring dietary habits in early life and studying the implications of dietary factors on health outcomes in childhood and later in life. Methods like food frequency questionnaires (FFQ) allow the collection of data in large samples of individuals. They are easy and relatively inexpensive to administer and can estimate the frequency and sometimes also the amount of the intake of foods and beverages over a defined period of time (1). Other methods, such as 24-h recall and diet record, are usually more expensive and demanding for both the participant and the researcher, and are unrepresentative of the usual intake because the data assessed covers a limited time (1).

It is important to evaluate the dietary assessment methods used in epidemiological studies. Objective biomarkers could be useful for this purpose as their errors are essentially uncorrelated with errors in any dietary assessment method (1). Plasma phospholipid fatty acids are considered good markers of dietary fatty acid intake over a short to medium time period (1–3), show good long-term reproducibility (4, 5), and are considered to be less affected by recent meal intake than plasma triglycerides (1–3).

Polyunsaturated fatty acids and odd-numbered saturated fatty acids are considered optimal fatty acid biomarkers as there is a limited or no endogenous synthesis (6, 7). Eicosapentaenoic acid (EPA, 20:5n-3) and docosahexaenoic acid (DHA, 22:6n-3) from oily fish and pentadecanoic acid (15:0) from dairy products are examples of such fatty acids. Several studies in adults have used these biomarkers to evaluate the dietary intake of fish and dairy products or specific fatty acids estimated with an FFQ (8–18). However, among children, there is a lack of studies comparing dietary assessment methods with biomarkers of fatty acids in general (19–23); and, to our knowledge, no studies compare plasma phospholipid pentadecanoic acid, EPA, and DHA, and the frequency of dairy and fish product intake estimated with an FFQ.

In the present study, a simple FFQ was developed to estimate the usual intake frequency of common foods and beverages. The objective was to evaluate the suitability of the FFQ to rank young children according to their intake of dairy and fish products by comparing food frequency estimates to the plasma phospholipid fatty acids pentadecanoic acid, EPA, and DHA.

Methods

Subjects and design

Cross-sectional data for the present study were derived from the 'Environmental Triggers of Type 1 Diabetes Study' (MIDIA), a prospective ongoing cohort study conducted by the Norwegian Institute of Public Health. The MIDIA study is described in more detail elsewhere (24). Briefly, nearly 50,000 infants from the general population were screened, and 1,003 infants carrying the HLA genotype DRB1*04:01-DQA1*03-DQB1*03:02/DRB1*03-DQA1*05-DQB1*02, conferring the highest risk of type 1 diabetes, were identified during the inclusion period (2001–2007). Questionnaires were filled out by the parents if the child was 3, 6, 9, or 12 months of age, and repeated annually thereafter. Blood samples were obtained from children at the same intervals. In total, 908 subjects (Fig. 1) returned at least one blood sample and questionnaire. The blood samples were sent to the Norwegian Institute of Public Health by ordinary mail and stored at -80°C until further use.

Out of the 908 subjects, 292 subjects were invited to a dietary project, in which 110 subjects were included in this evaluation study in January 2013 (Fig. 1). To be included, the FFQ had to be answered within 2 months of the date of blood sampling, and the volume of plasma accessible from each subject had to be sufficient for the determination of plasma phospholipid fatty acids. Five of the subjects included in the study had blood autoantibodies showing islet autoimmunity, but none had developed type 1 diabetes.

The food frequency questionnaire

The questionnaire was not quantitative and included questions about the dietary habits of the mother and the child. In the present study, the dietary information about the child's intake frequency of fish and dairy products has been used. This information was derived from three main questions included in the questionnaires used for all age levels, which concerned the intake frequency of (1) oily fish, other fish, fish spread, white cheese, brown cheese, yoghurt, and dairy ice cream; (2) whole fat milk, semi-skimmed milk, skimmed milk, chocolate milk, and yoghurt drink; and (3) cod liver/fish oil supplements (hereinafter referred to as cod liver oil).

The quantitative determination of fatty acids in the phospholipid fraction of human plasma

An analysis of plasma phospholipid fatty acids was performed at a commercial laboratory in Oslo, Norway (AS Vitas). Plasma stored at -80°C were thawed overnight at 4°C and vortexed for 5 sec. Dichloromethane/methanol was added to 100-µL plasma and 100-µL internal standard (1,2 diheptadecaonyl-*sn*-glycero-3-phosphatidylcholin). After shaking and centrifugation, the supernatants were transferred to new glasses and washed in a 0.9% NaCl solution. The lower phase was transferred to solid-phase extraction columns. Neutral lipids were washed out with dichloromethane/isopropanol and methyl tertiary butyl ether/formic acid. Phospholipids were eluted with methanol. After evaporation to dryness in a vacuum centrifuge, phospholipids were transmethylated with sodium methoxide and fatty acid methyl esters were extracted to hexane before gas chromatography analysis. Analysis was performed on a 7890A Gas Chromatography system with a split/split less injector, a 7683B automatic liquid sampler, and flame ionization detection (Agilent Technologies, Palo Alto, CA). Separation was performed on an SP 2380 (30 m $\times$ 0.22 mm i.d. $\times$ 0.25-µm film thickness) column (Supelco, Inc., Bellefonte, PA). The coefficient of variation was 4% for the main fatty acids and 6% for EPA and DHA (AS Vitas, Oslo). Plasma phospholipid fatty acids were expressed as µg/mL and in weight percentage.

Data analysis

Intake frequency of food items (oily fish, other fish, fish spread, cod liver oil, whole fat milk, semi-skimmed milk, 0.7% fat milk, skimmed milk, chocolate milk, white cheese, brown cheese, yoghurt, yoghurt drink, and dairy ice cream) was reported as frequency per week and recalculated into frequency per day. In addition, different food items were combined into groups, which were *Cheese* (white cheese and brown cheese), *Total milk* (whole fat milk, semi-skimmed milk, 0.7% fat milk, skimmed milk, and chocolate milk), *Total milk/yoghurt* (total milk, yoghurt, and yoghurt drink), *Total fat dairy* (cheese, whole fat milk, yoghurt, and dairy ice cream), *Total dairy* (cheese, total

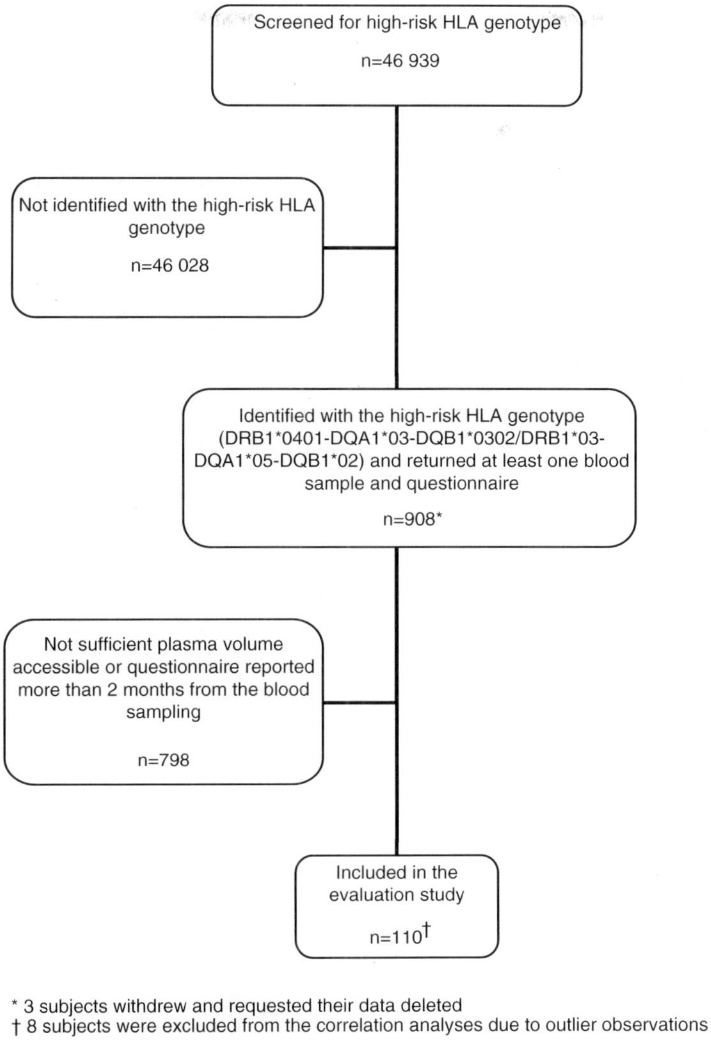

Fig. 1. Flow-chart showing 'Environmental Triggers of Type 1 Diabetes Study' (MIDIA) participants included in the evaluation study.

milk/yoghurt, and dairy ice cream), *Total oily fish* (oily fish and fish spread), *Total fish* (other fish and total oily fish), *Cod liver oil/total oily fish*, and *Cod liver oil/total fish*.

Intake frequency estimates and plasma phospholipid acids were presented as mean values and SD, and median values and interquartile range (IQR), since not all of the data were normally distributed. To check for potential outliers, the data were visualized with box and scatter plots, and observations deemed to be outliers were removed from the main analysis. The suitability of the FFQ for ranking participants was assessed by conducting a Spearman correlation analysis and by investigating whether participants are classified into the same quartiles of distribution, based on the reported frequency of dairy product intake and plasma phospholipid pentadecanoic acid, and the frequency of fish product intake and plasma phospholipid EPA and DHA, respectively. The correlation coefficients were calculated for both μg/mL and weight percentage of plasma phospholipid fatty acids, and presented with 95% CI based on 1,000 bootstrap samples. Individuals classified into the same quartile, based on intake frequency and concentration of plasma phospholipids, were defined as 'correctly classified', and individuals classified into opposite quartiles were defined as 'grossly misclassified'. The Spearman correlation analysis of the intake frequency of total oily fish and the plasma phospholipid DHA concentration was also conducted for the subpopulations that consumed or did not consume cod liver oil. Due to concerns regarding the use of pentadecanoic acid as a biomarker in populations with a high fish consumption (25), an additional Spearman correlation analysis of the frequency of fish product intake and plasma phospholipid pentadecanoic acid was conducted. Separate analyses of those who filled in the FFQ before and after the date of blood sampling and an analysis excluding the children with islet autoimmunity were also performed. Statistical analyses were performed with the Statistical Package for Social

Sciences statistical software package version 20.0 (SPSS, Inc., Chicago, IL) and STATA version 13 (Statacorp, TX). The chosen level of statistical significance was 5%. Based on previous studies in adults, a correlation of $r=0.30$ was expected. With a significance level of 5% ($\alpha=0.05$) and power 80% ($\beta=0.20$), the required sample size was estimated to be $n=85$.

Results

The study included children ($n=110$, 59 boys and 51 girls) with a mean age of 5.6 years (SD 1.6) ranging from 3 to 10 years of age. The median frequency intake of total dairy products was 1.9 times/day and 1.1 times/day for total fat dairy products. The median frequency intake of total fish was 0.6 times/day, and cod liver oil was consumed with a median frequency intake of 0.1 times/day (Table 1). Cod liver oil was consumed by 55.5% of the children ($n=61$). Of the measured plasma phospholipid fatty acids, DHA was found to have the highest mean plasma concentration with 55.3 µg/mL (Table 2). In total, eight observations were considered outliers and excluded in the subsequent analyses.

Spearman correlation analysis

Using absolute values (µg/mL) of plasma phospholipid fatty acids, significant correlations ($p \leq 0.01$) were found between pentadecanoic acid and the intake frequency of total dairy products ($r=0.29$), and total fat dairy products ($r=0.39$) and cheese products ($r=0.36$). There was no significant correlation between pentadecanoic acid and the intake frequency of total milk and yoghurt (Table 3). Significant correlations were observed between the intake frequency of total oily fish and EPA and DHA ($r=0.26$ and 0.37, respectively). Similarly, cod liver oil was significantly correlated with the long chained omega-3 fatty acids ($r=0.47$ for EPA and $r=0.50$ DHA). No significant correlations were observed for the food group other fish (Table 4). The correlation between the intake frequency of total oily fish and DHA was lower for the subpopulation that did not consume cod liver oil ($r=0.22$), than for the group that did ($r=0.36$) (Fig. 2). There was no significant correlation between pentadecanoic acid and the intake frequency of total oily fish ($r=0.04$) or cod liver oil ($r=-0.07$). Using the relative distribution of fatty acids instead of absolute values in the analysis did not give any major differences in the Spearman's rank correlation coefficients (Tables 3 and 4).

In comparison to the date of blood sampling, the FFQ was completed at the same date or up to 2 months after for 63.6% ($n=70$) of the participating children, and until 2 months before for 36.4% ($n=40$). A separate analysis showed that there were no major differences between the correlation coefficients of those who filled in the FFQ after or before the blood sampling (data not shown).

Five of the children had blood autoantibodies showing islet autoimmunity, but none had developed type 1 diabetes. An analysis excluding the children with islet autoimmunity ($n=5$), showed unchanged results (data not shown).

Table 1. The mean (SD) and median (IQR) frequency of dairy and fish product intake estimated with a food frequency questionnaire ($n=110$)[a]

	Frequency (Times per Day)			
Food Items/Groups	Mean	SD	Median	IQR
White cheese	0.56	0.55	0.29	0.42
Brown cheese	0.32	0.30	0.29	0.64
Whole fat milk	0.02	0.08	0.00	0.00
Semi-skimmed milk	0.38	0.32	0.29	0.71
Yoghurt	0.21	0.23	0.07	0.22
Cheese	0.89	0.68	0.71	0.77
Total milk	0.60	0.38	0.71	0.49
Total milk/yoghurt	0.89	0.49	0.85	0.58
Total fat dairy	1.30	0.76	1.14	0.81
Total dairy	1.97	0.88	1.92	1.25
Total oily fish	0.38	0.38	0.29	0.44
Other fish	0.23	0.12	0.29	0.22
Total fish	0.61	0.41	0.58	0.32
Cod liver oil	0.35	0.42	0.07	0.64
Cod liver oil/total oily fish	0.73	0.62	0.58	0.95
Cod liver oil/total fish	0.96	0.64	0.82	1.00

[a]All observations were included.

Quartiles of distribution

Based on the intake frequency of dairy and fish products and the concentration of plasma phospholipid pentadecanoic acid, EPA, and DHA, the proportion of subjects appearing in the same quartile varied from 22.6% for the food group, other fish, and DHA, to 42.2% for cod liver oil/total fish and DHA (Table 5). The percentage of subjects grossly misclassified varied from 14.7% for total milk and pentadecanoic acid to 3.9% for cod liver oil/total fish and cod liver oil/total oily fish and EPA and DHA, cod liver oil and DHA, and total fat dairy and pentadecanoic acid (Table 5).

Discussion

In the present study, the reported frequency of high-fat dairy product intake was weakly to moderately correlated with plasma phospholipid pentadecanoic acid. The reported intake frequency of total oily fish was weakly correlated, and cod liver oil was moderately to strongly correlated with the long-chain omega 3 fatty acids EPA and DHA.

A strength of the study is that we could choose blood samples close to the time period of the completion of the questionnaire. As plasma phospholipid fatty acids are considered to reflect dietary fatty acid intake over a short

Table 2. The mean (SD) and median (IQR) concentration and weight percentage of plasma phospholipid pentadecanoic acid, EPA, and DHA ($n=110$)[a]

Plasma Phospholipids	Mean (µg/mL)	SD	Mean Weight Percentage	SD	Median (µg/mL)	IQR	Median Weight Percentage	IQR
Pentadecanoic acid	2.20	0.46	0.24	0.04	2.16	0.65	0.23	0.05
EPA	15.8	10.8	1.69	1.07	11.6	10.2	1.30	1.18
DHA	55.3	17.3	5.95	1.71	52.1	20.7	5.77	2.10

[a]All observations were included.

to medium time period (1–3), one could assume that the most appropriate design would be to study those who filled in the FFQ in the time period from 2 months before and up to the date of blood sampling. However, a separate analysis showed that there were no major differences between the correlation coefficients of those who reported the FFQ at the date of blood sampling or up to 2 months after and those who reported the FFQ until 2 months before the blood sampling.

We have studied children genetically susceptible to type 1 diabetes, and the results are not necessarily generalizable to the whole population, but to the study population. Nevertheless, it is unlikely that the specific HLA genotype of these children would directly influence their lipid concentrations. In our study, only five children had developed islet autoimmunity, and excluding these did not influence the conclusions. Participation in the study might select for a perceived healthier diet, and there was a higher percentage of cod liver oil users in our study compared to those of a Norwegian national survey among 4-, 9-, and 13-year-olds (26, 27).

It could be considered a limitation that we do not have multiple measures of the food intake or another dietary assessment method, such as 24-h recall or diet record, to compare with the methods we used. However, these self-reporting methods share some of the same sources of error that occur in the reporting of any FFQ for which a biomarker is uncorrelated to errors in any dietary questionnaire (1). A limitation to the study is that there were no specific restrictions on diet in relation to the sampling of blood. The plasma phospholipid fraction could be influenced by a recent meal, although less than the plasma triglyceride fraction would be affected (1–3).

Table 3. Spearman's rank correlation coefficients (95% CI[a]) between the frequency of dairy product intake estimated with a food frequency questionnaire (FFQ) and the µg/mL and weight percentage of plasma phospholipid pentadecanoic acid ($n=102$[b])

	Pentadecanoic Acid	
Dairy Product	µg/mL	Weight Percentage
Cheese	0.36 (0.18, 0.52)*	0.39 (0.21, 0.54)*
Whole fat milk	0.12 (−0.11, 0.34)	0.15 (−0.07, 0.33)
Total milk	0.08 (−0.12, 0.27)	0.08 (−0.11, 0.27)
Total milk/yoghurt	0.07 (−0.13, 0.27)	0.09 (−0.12, 0.28)
Total fat dairy	0.39 (0.20, 0.56)*	0.43 (0.26, 0.58)*
Total dairy	0.29 (0.11, 0.47)*	0.31 (0.11, 0.48)*

[a]Presented with 95% CI based on 1,000 bootstrap samples.
[b]Eight observations were considered as outliers and excluded from the analysis.
*$P \leq 0.01$.

Pentadecanoic acid has been used as a biomarker for the dairy intake in several studies, but since this fatty acid is also present at low amounts in fish, some concerns have been raised regarding its use as a biomarker in populations with a high fish consumption (25). In our population, the intake of both fat dairy and fish products was relatively high, and we found no correlation between pentadecanoic acid and fish products.

Our results in children are in line with those from studies in adults that have correlated the fish intake estimated from FFQ with plasma phospholipid EPA and DHA, with correlations ranging from 0.1 to 0.3 for total fish and 0.4 to 0.5 for cod liver oil (11–13). One study did not report correlation coefficients but showed increased plasma phospholipid EPA and DHA with an increased intake of fish, and higher levels of plasma phospholipid EPA and DHA in people taking cod liver and fish oil supplements (13). In concurrence with our results, similar correlations for absolute and relative measures of plasma phospholipid EPA and DHA have previously been shown in adults (11). Studies in the adult population mainly show significant correlations between the reported intake of fat dairy products or total diary fat and pentadecanoic acid in different blood fractions but not for low-fat dairy products (8–10).

In line with our results, a study on Finnish children, adolescents, and young adults aged 9–24 years ($n=759$) showed significant correlations between the intake of fish reported by 48-h recall and serum phospholipid EPA and DHA, with correlation coefficients of $r=0.42$ and 0.28, respectively (20). A recent study among Finnish children aged 6–8 years reported a significant correlation of $r=0.15$ between the intake of fish reported by 3-day dietary records and plasma phospholipid DHA, but not for EPA (21). A significant correlation of $r=0.22$ between the intake of fatty milk and pentadecanoic acid was reported, but not for the intake of cheese (21). A Finnish study among 1- to 3-year-old toddlers found a

Table 4. Spearman's rank correlation coefficients (95% CI[a]) between the frequency of fish product intake estimated with a food frequency questionnaire (FFQ) and the μg/mL and weight percentage of plasma phospholipid EPA and DHA ($n = 102$[b])

	EPA	DHA	EPA	DHA
Fish product	μg/mL	μg/mL	Weight Percentage	Weight Percentage
Total oily fish	0.26 (0.07, 0.43)*	0.37 (0.18, 0.54)*	0.28 (0.10, 0.45)*	0.40 (0.23, 0.55)*
Other fish	0.07 (−0.11, 0.27)	−0.12 (−0.31, 0.06)	0.07 (−0.11, 0.25)	−0.14 (−0.33, 0.05)
Total fish	0.25 (0.06, 0.42)*	0.29 (0.09, 0.47)*	0.27 (0.08, 0.42)*	0.30 (0.10, 0.47)*
Cod liver oil	0.47 (0.30, 0.61)*	0.50 (0.31, 0.64)*	0.46 (0.28, 0.61)*	0.46 (0.27, 0.61)*
Cod liver oil/total oily fish	0.48 (0.29, 0.62)*	0.51 (0.32, 0.66)*	0.47 (0.30, 0.63)*	0.49 (0.31, 0.64)*
Cod liver oil/total fish	0.46 (0.27, 0.62)*	0.45 (0.26, 0.62)*	0.45 (0.26, 0.60)*	0.43 (0.23, 0.59)*

[a]Presented with 95% CI based on 1,000 bootstrap samples.
[b]$n = 8$ observations were considered outliers and excluded from the analysis.
*$P \leq 0.01$.

positive correlation between the intake of fatty milk reported by 3-day dietary records and pentadecanoic acid in whole serum, but found no consistent correlation between the intake of fish and EPA or DHA (22). Neither of these studies among children analysed the intake of oily and other fish separately, and the authors state that the frequency intake of fish was low, which may affect the correlations. As for dairy, this discrepancy may be due to the low frequency intake of fatty milk and the relatively high intake of cheese reported in our study. Although we did not differentiate between regular (25–40% fat) and low-fat cheese (15–20% fat) in the FFQ, these products are generally high in fat content. An American study among young children, 1–11 years of age with high-risk of developing type 1 diabetes, found a positive correlation of $r = 0.42$ between the estimated intake of total marine fatty acids reported by FFQ, and EPA and DHA in the erythrocyte membrane (23). However, they did not investigate the frequency intake of specific food groups.

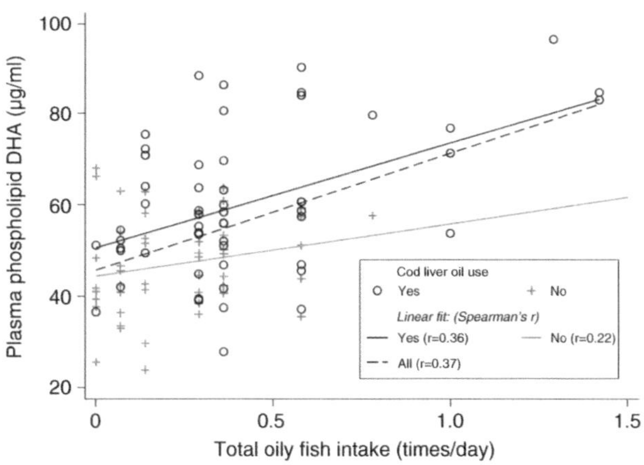

Fig. 2. Intake frequency of total oily fish and plasma phospholipid docosahexaenoic acid (DHA) concentration (μg/mL). Distribution of the intake frequency of total oily fish estimated with a food frequency questionnaire (FFQ) and the plasma phospholipid DHA (μg/mL), and Spearman's correlation coefficients for the whole sample ($n = 102$), and subpopulations that used cod liver oil ($n = 55$) and those that did not ($n = 47$). In total, 8 observations were considered outliers and are not shown nor used in the correlation analyses.

By classifying individuals into quartiles, we expect, by chance, 25.0% to fall in the same quartile and 12.5% in the other quartiles (12). The FFQ was, to a large extent, able to classify individuals into the same quartile as the relevant biomarker. A higher percentage of correct classification and a lower percentage of misclassification of individuals were found for the intake frequency of dairy products with a high-fat content, compared to dairy products with a low-fat content. The findings from the cross-classification analyses correspond well with the correlations between the reported frequency of dairy product intake and plasma phospholipid pentadecanoic acid. As for dairy products, a higher percentage of correct classification and a lower percentage of misclassification of individuals was found for the intake frequency of fish products high in fat content, compared to fish with a lower fat content. This is in line with the correlations between the reported frequency of fish product intake and plasma phospholipid EPA and DHA.

Of all dairy products, cheese had the strongest correlation with the concentration of plasma pentadecanoic acid. The moderate correlation between the intake frequency of total fat dairy and pentadecanoic acid was mainly explained by the contribution from cheese. The correlation between total oily fish and DHA, stronger than for total oily fish and EPA, reflects the relative content of these marine fatty acids in oily fish. The intake of other fish did not correlate with either EPA or DHA, which could be explained by a lower content of marine fatty acids in lean fish and fish products. There was a lower correlation

Table 5. Cross-classification of subjects by quartiles of the frequency of dairy and fish product intake estimated with a food frequency questionnaire (FFQ) and the μg/mL of plasma phospholipid pentadecanoic acid, EPA, and DHA ($n = 102^{a}$)

	Correctly classified (%)	Correct plus adjacent quartiles (%)	Grossly misclassified[b] (%)
Dairy intake and pentadecanoic acid			
Cheese	38.2	73.5	4.9
Total milk	30.3	64.5	14.7
Total milk/yoghurt	27.4	65.6	11.8
Total fat dairy	31.4	75.6	3.9
Total dairy	30.4	70.7	5.9
Fish intake and EPA			
Total oily fish	31.4	71.6	5.8
Other fish	25.5	67.7	5.9
Total fish	29.4	69.4	5.9
Cod liver oil	38.1	72.4	5.9
Cod liver oil/total oily fish	42.1	81.3	3.9
Cod liver oil/total fish	41.1	82.2	3.9
Fish intake and DHA			
Total oily fish	33.3	76.4	4.0
Other fish	22.6	60.8	8.8
Total fish	32.3	74.5	6.9
Cod liver oil	41.1	76.4	3.9
Cod liver oil/total oily fish	42.1	80.4	3.9
Cod liver oil/total fish	42.2	82.4	3.9

[a]Eight observations were considered as outliers and excluded from the analysis.
[b]Classified into opposite quartiles.

between total oily fish and DHA for the subpopulation of those who did not use cod liver oil than for those who did, indicating that the correlation between total oily fish and DHA could in part be explained by the use of cod liver oil. However, these data have to be interpreted with caution because the number of participants was lower in the subpopulation analyses ($n = 47$ and $n = 55$, respectively), and, moreover, a majority of the children who consumed oily fish most frequently also consumed cod liver oil. Of all food items, cod liver oil had the strongest correlation with the concentration of plasma phospholipid fatty acids ($r = 0.47$ for EPA and $r = 0.50$ for DHA). The similar correlations could be explained by the high and more equally distributed content of EPA and DHA in cod liver oil compared to oily fish.

In conclusion, the present study suggests that when using the plasma phospholipid fatty acids pentadecanoic acid, EPA, and DHA as biomarkers, the FFQ used in young children showed a moderate capability to rank the intake frequency of dairy products with a high-fat content and cod liver oil.

Conflict of interest and funding

This project has been financially supported by the Norwegian Extra Foundation for Health and Rehabilitation through EXTRA fund 2010/2/0012 and by the Norwegian Diabetes Association. All authors declare no conflict of interest.

References

1. Willett W. Nutritional epidemiology. 3rd ed. New York: Oxford University Press; 2013.
2. Saadatian-Elahi M, Slimani N, Chajès V, Jenab M, Goudable J, Biessy C, et al. Plasma phospholipid fatty acid profiles and their association with food intakes: results from a cross-sectional study within the European Prospective Investigation into Cancer and Nutrition. Am J Clin Nutr 2009; 89(1): 331–46.
3. Arab L. Biomarkers of fat and fatty acid intake. J Nutr 2003; 133(Suppl 3): 925s–32s.
4. Lindberg M, Midthjell K, Bjerve KS. Long-term tracking of plasma phospholipid fatty acid concentrations and their correlation with the dietary intake of marine foods in newly diagnosed diabetic patients: results from a follow-up of the HUNT Study, Norway. Br J Nutr 2013; 109(6): 1123–34.
5. Ma J, Folsom AR, Eckfeldt JH, Lewis L, Chambless LE. Short- and long-term repeatability of fatty acid composition of human plasma phospholipids and cholesterol esters. The Atherosclerosis Risk in Communities (ARIC) Study Investigators. Am J Clin Nutr 1995; 62(3): 572–8.
6. Baylin A, Campos H. The use of fatty acid biomarkers to reflect dietary intake. Curr Opin Lipidol 2006; 17(1): 22–7.
7. Hodson L, Skeaff CM, Fielding BA. Fatty acid composition of adipose tissue and blood in humans and its use as a biomarker of dietary intake. Prog Lipid Res 2008; 47(5): 348–80.
8. Brevik A, Veierød MB, Drevon CA, Andersen LF. Evaluation of the odd fatty acids 15:0 and 17:0 in serum and adipose tissue as markers of intake of milk and dairy fat. Eur J Clin Nutr 2005; 59(12): 1417–22.
9. De Oliveira Otto MC, Nettleton JA, Lemaitre RN, Steffen LM, Kromhout D, Rich SS, et al. Biomarkers of dairy fatty acids and

risk of cardiovascular disease in the Multi-Ethnic Study of Atherosclerosis. J Am Heart Assoc 2013; 2(4): e000092.
10. Sun Q, Ma J, Campos H, Hu FB. Plasma and erythrocyte biomarkers of dairy fat intake and risk of ischemic heart disease. Am J Clin Nutr 2007; 86(4): 929–37.
11. Hjartåker A, Lund E, Bjerve KS. Serum phospholipid fatty acid composition and habitual intake of marine foods registered by a semi-quantitative food frequency questionnaire. Eur J Clin Nutr 1997; 51(11): 736–42.
12. Andersen LF, Solvoll K, Drevon CA. Very-long-chain n-3 fatty acids as biomarkers for intake of fish and n-3 fatty acid concentrates. Am J Clin Nutr 1996; 64(3): 305–11.
13. Hodge AM, Simpson JA, Gibson RA, Sinclair AJ, Makrides M, O'Dea K, et al. Plasma phospholipid fatty acid composition as a biomarker of habitual dietary fat intake in an ethnically diverse cohort. Nutr Metab Cardiovasc Dis 2007; 17(6): 415–26.
14. Sullivan BL, Williams PG, Meyer BJ. Biomarker validation of a long-chain omega-3 polyunsaturated fatty acid food frequency questionnaire. Lipids 2006; 41(9): 845–50.
15. Andersen LF, Solvoll K, Johansson LR, Salminen I, Aro A, Drevon CA. Evaluation of a food frequency questionnaire with weighed records, fatty acids, and alpha-tocopherol in adipose tissue and serum. Am J Epidemiol 1999; 150(1): 75–87.
16. Ma J, Folsom AR, Shahar E, Eckfeldt JH. Plasma fatty acid composition as an indicator of habitual dietary fat intake in middle-aged adults. The Atherosclerosis Risk in Communities (ARIC) Study Investigators. Am J Clin Nutr 1995; 62(3): 564–71.
17. Sun Q, Ma J, Campos H, Hankinson SE, Hu FB. Comparison between plasma and erythrocyte fatty acid content as biomarkers of fatty acid intake in US women. Am J Clin Nutr 2007; 86(1): 74–81.
18. McNaughton SA, Hughes MC, Marks GC. Validation of a FFQ to estimate the intake of PUFA using plasma phospholipid fatty acids and weighed foods records. Br J Nutr 2007; 97(3): 561–8.
19. Moilanen T, Räsänen L, Viikari J, Akerblom HK, Ahola M, Uhari M, et al. Fatty acid composition of serum cholesteryl esters in 3- to 18-year-old Finnish children and its relation to diet. Am J Clin Nutr 1985; 42(4): 708–13.
20. Moilanen T, Räsänen L, Viikari J, Akerblom HK, Nikkari T. Correlation of serum fatty acid composition with dietary intake data in children and young adults. Ann Med 1992; 24(1): 67–70.
21. Venäläinen T, Schwab U, Ågren J, de Mello V, Lindi V, Eloranta AM, et al. Cross-sectional associations of food consumption with plasma fatty acid composition and estimated desaturase activities in Finnish children. Lipids 2014; 49(5): 467–79.
22. Uusitalo L, Nevalainen J, Salminen I, Ovaskainen ML, Kronberg-Kippilä C, Ahonen S, et al. Fatty acids in serum and diet – a canonical correlation analysis among toddlers. Matern Child Nutr 2013; 9(3): 381–95.
23. Orton HD, Szabo NJ, Clare-Salzler M, Norris JM. Comparison between omega-3 and omega-6 polyunsaturated fatty acid intakes as assessed by a food frequency questionnaire and erythrocyte membrane fatty acid composition in young children. Eur J Clin Nutr 2008; 62(6): 733–8.
24. Stene LC, Witsø E, Torjesen PA, Rasmussen T, Magnus P, Cinek O, et al. Islet autoantibody development during follow-up of high-risk children from the general Norwegian population from three months of age: design and early results from the MIDIA study. J Autoimmun 2007; 29(1): 44–51.
25. Lankinen M, Schwab U. Biomarkers of dairy fat. Am J Clin Nutr 2015; 101(5): 1101–2.
26. Norwegian Directorate of Health (2002). Ungkost-2000: Landsomfattende kostholdsundersøkelse blant 4-åringer (Ungkost-2000: Nationwide diet survey among four-year-olds). Oslo: Norwegian Directorate of Health.
27. Norwegian Directorate of Health (2002). Ungkost-2000: Landsomfattende kostholdsundersøkelse blant elever i 4.- og 8. klasse i Norge (Ungkost-2000: Nationwide diet survey among 4th and 8th grade pupils in Norway). Oslo: Norwegian Directorate of Health.

*Nicolai A. Lund-Blix
Department of Nutrition
Institute of Basic Medical Sciences
University of Oslo
PO Box NOR-1046, Blindern
NO-0316 Oslo, Norway
Email: n.a.lund@medisin.uio.no

13

Effects of stachyose on absorption and transportation of tea catechins in mice: possible role of Phase II metabolic enzymes and efflux transporters inhibition by stachyose

Wenfeng Li, Yalong Lu, Di Huang, Xiao Han and Xingbin Yang*

Shaanxi Engineering Laboratory for Food Green Processing and Safety Control, College of Food Engineering and Nutritional Science, Shaanxi Normal University, Xi'an, China

Abstract

Background: Nutritional and absorption-promoting properties of stachyose combined with tea catechins (TC) have been revealed. However, the mechanism involved in non-digestible oligosaccharides-mediated enhancement of flavonoid absorption has largely remained elusive.
Methods: This study was designed to investigate the molecular mechanism of stachyose in enhancing absorption and transportation of TC in mice. Mice were orally pre-treated with stachyose (50, 250, and 500 mg/kg·bw) for 0–8 weeks, and 1 h before sacrifice, mice were treated with TC (250 mg/kg·bw).
Results: Gas chromatography-mass spectrometry analysis showed that serum concentrations of epicatechin, epigallocatechin, epicatechin gallate, and epigallocatechin gallate were dose- and time-dependently elevated with stachyose pre-treatment in mice. Furthermore, pre-treatment with stachyose in mice reduced intestinal sulfotransferase and uridine diphosphate-glucuronosyltransferase levels by 3.3–43.2% and 23.9–30.4%, relative to control mice, respectively. Moreover, intestinal P-glycoprotein and multidrug resistance-associated protein-1 contents were decreased in mice by pre-administration of stachyose in dose- and time-dependent manner.
Conclusions: This is the first time to demonstrate that suppression of Phase II metabolic enzymes and efflux transporters of TC in the intestine can play a major role in increasing absorption of TC by stachyose feeding.

Keywords: *absorption*; *efflux transporter*; *Phase II metabolism*; *stachyose*; *tea catechins*

It is well recognized that tea is one of the most widely consumed beverages, next to water, in the world (1, 2). In the past few decades, tea has attracted much attention for its various physiological functions including anticancer, anti-arteriosclerosis, and hepatoprotective effects (3). These beneficial effects are associated with tea catechins (TC) closely, which consist primarily of four components, epicatechin (EC), epigallocatechin (EGC), epicatechin gallate (ECG), and epigallocatechin gallate (EGCG) (2, 4). However, extensive studies about the metabolism of TC suggest that bioavailability of TC *in vivo* is extremely poor by oral administration (3, 5, 6).

Interestingly, recent reports showed that non-digestible carbohydrates could promote absorption of diet polyphenols. For example, α-1,6-glucosaccharide promoted absorption of quercetin glycoside, and difructose anhydride III increased bioavailability of αG-rutin, and fructooligosaccharide enhanced absorption of α-glucosyl-isoquercitrin, genistein and daidzein, and chito-oligosaccharide improved absorption of phenolic acids of *Flos Lonicerae* extract (7–12). In addition, our recent research also revealed that stachyose, a non-digestible saccharide rich in soybean (*Glycine max*), *Rehmannia glutinosa* Libosch and *Lycopus lucidus* Turcz, could increase absorption and hepatoprotective effects of tea polyphenols in high fructose-fed mice (13). However, we still have a poor understanding of the mechanism that stachyose enhances absorption of TC.

It is interesting to note that intestinal and/or hepatic first-pass extraction via glucuronidation and sulphation, which are part of Phase II metabolism, can limit the oral bioavailability of flavonoids (14, 15). However, the activities of Phase II metabolic enzymes in the liver of rat were mediated by chitosan oligosaccharides and sulfated polysaccharide of *Monostroma nitidum*, suggesting that these non-digestible saccharides influenced Phase II detoxifying reactions in the liver (16, 17). In addition, the transport of ingested flavonoids across the intestinal barrier is also an important factor determining bioavailability upon oral intake (18). Previous reports suggest that the absorption extent of EC, ECG, and EGCG may be increased by inhibiting membrane transporters, mainly efflux transporters including P-glycoprotein (P-gp) and multi-drug resistance proteins (19–21). Interestingly, some non-digestible saccharides, such as hyaluronan oligosaccharides and astragalus polysaccharides, have recently been shown to down-modulate P-gp and multidrug resistance-associated protein-1 (MRP1) expression, thereby increasing the intracellular concentration of chemotherapeutic drugs (22, 23). In this regard, stachyose-elevated absorption of TC is likely associated with inhibition of first-pass metabolism of TC *in vivo*.

Therefore, the aim of the present study was to provide evidence that the feeding of stachyose actually inhibited the expression of efflux transporters and Phase II enzymes in the intestine and/or liver, and these suppressions contributed to the promotion of TC absorption in mice. In addition, the characterization that stachyose-enhanced absorption of TC was also investigated by evaluation of serum TC concentrations.

Materials and methods

Materials and reagents

Stachyose (pure > 80%) was prepared in our laboratory (13). TC (pure > 70%), which consist primarily of 3.11% EC, 4.05% EGC, 11.74% ECG, and 52.24% EGCG, were purchased from Yongqi Biology Co. Ltd (Xi'an, China) (13). Pure standards of EC (98%), EGC (98%), ECG (98%), EGCG (98%), and genistein (IS, 98%) were obtained from Sigma-Aldrich (Steinheim, Germany). Enzyme-linked immuno sorbent assay (ELISA) kit of P-gp was purchased from R&D Systems, Inc. (Shanghai, China). ELISA kits of the MRP1, MRP2, uridine diphosphate-glucuronosyltransferase (UGT), and sulfotransferase (SULT) were purchased from Shanghai enzyme-linked biological technology Co., Ltd. (Shanghai, China). ELISA kit of cytochrome P450 enzymes (CYPs) was obtained from Jiancheng Bioengineering Institute (Nanjing, China). N,O-bis(trimethylsilyl)-trifluoroacetamide (BSTFA) was purchased from Adamas Reagent, Ltd. (Shanghai, China). β-Glucuronidase (G0251-100KU, EC 3.2.1.31) and sulfatase (S9626-10KU, EC 3.1.6.1) were purchased from Sigma-Aldrich (Shanghai, China). All other chemicals were of the highest grade available.

Animals

Male Kunming mice (15–20 g) and standard rodent chow were purchased from the Experimental Animal Center of the Fourth Military Medical University, China. They were housed in a controlled laboratory environment (22 ± 2°C, relative humidity of 60 ± 5%, and 12/12 h light–dark cycle). After 1-week acclimatization, the mice were divided randomly into seven groups with eight mice each (Table 1). Group I (normal group): mice were administered only intragastrically (i.g.) with physiological saline once daily during the experimental period for 8 weeks, and the serum EC, EGC, ECG, and EGCG were not detected in the normal mice. Control group II (Con. group): mice were treated with saline once daily for 8 weeks and were also administrated with TC at 250 mg/kg·bw (i.g., 0.4 mL) onetime 1 h before sacrifice.

Groups III, IV, and V (dose-dependent test groups): mice were pre-treated with saline once daily for a continuous 4-week period and subsequently pre-treated with stachyose at 50, 250, and 500 mg/kg·bw (i.g., 0.4 mL) once daily for another 4 weeks, respectively; and finally, the mice of Groups III–V were also administrated with TC at 250 mg/kg·bw one time 1 h before sacrifice. To evaluate time-dependent effects of stachyose pre-treatment on absorption of TC, the mice in Groups VI and VII were administrated with stachyose at 250 mg/kg·bw once daily for 2 and 8 weeks, which began from the 7th and 1st week, respectively, and before the treatment of stachyose, the mice in Groups VI and VII were administrated with saline once daily. Meanwhile, the mice of Groups VI and VII were also administrated with 250 mg/kg·bw TC one time 1 h before sacrifice. During the administration period, all the mice were allowed free access to food and tap water. The animals were fully anesthetized by the inhalation of isoflurane and sacrificed to obtain plasma, liver, and small intestine samples.

Table 1. Experimental design

	Groups						
Administration	I	II	III	IV	V	VI	VII
Time for pre-treatment of stachyose (week)	–	–	5th ~ 8th	5th ~ 8th	5th ~ 8th	7th ~ 8th	1th ~ 8th
Duration for pre-treatment of stachyose	–	–	4 weeks	4 weeks	4 weeks	2 weeks	8 weeks
Time for treatment of saline (week)	1th ~ 8th	1th ~ 8th	1th ~ 4th	1th ~ 4th	1th ~ 4th	1th ~ 6th	–
Stachyose (mg/kg·bw)[a]	–	–	50	250	500	250	250
TC (mg/kg·bw)[b]	–	250	250	250	250	250	250

[a]The treatment of stachyose at the last time was combined together with the administration of TC; [b]the administration of TC was performed for mice 1 h before sacrifice. In addition, the TC was dissolved in water together with stachyose at relevant doses.

All the experiments were conducted according to the Guidelines of Experimental Animal Administration published by the State Committee of Science and Technology of People's Republic of China. The experiment was approved by the Committee on Care and Use of Laboratory Animals of the University (XJYYLL-2015689), China.

Determination of serum catechins

Collected blood was centrifuged for 15 min at 1,500 × g to obtain serum. The serum EC, EGC, ECG, and EGCG concentrations were evaluated by a gas chromatography-mass spectrometry (GC-MS) analysis method, which was described in our previous work with a minor revision (13). A 100 μL serum was incubated with 5 μL internal standard (genistein, 38.33 μg/mL), 5 μL PBA (200 mg/mL vitamin C and 62.5 mg/mL NaH_2PO_4), 50 μL 66.59 mg/mL $CaCl_2$, 25 μL 20 UI/100 μL sulfatase, and 50 μL 200 UI/100 μL β-glucuronidase at 37°C for 90 min. After incubation, the serum was extracted twice with ethyl acetate (1.0 mL each time). The combined ethyl acetate extract was dried at 50°C for 50 min by a vacuum dryer (Rikakikai Co., Ltd, Tokyo, Japan), and then, the dried residue was redissolved in 60 μL pyridine and derivatized with 90 μL BSTFA at 70°C for 2 h.

One microliter derivatized extract was analyzed by a GC-MS 2010ultra (Shimadzu China Co., LTD., Shanghai, China) equipped with Rxi-5Sil MS Cap. column (30 m × 0.25 mm id, 0.25 μm film thickness; Risetech Technology Co., LTD, Beijing, China). The flow velocity of carrier gas (helium) is 1.0 mL/min. The initial column temperature was 70°C for 4 min, and then ramped to 100°C at 4°C/min where it was held for 3 min, and increased to 260°C at 30°C/min where it was held for 20 min and further increased at 10°C/min to 295°C where it remained for 30 min.

ELISA analysis

Intestinal tissue (0.5 g) or liver tissue (0.5 g) was homogenized with 4.5 mL saline and then centrifuged at 3,000 g for 10 min. In current work, the levels of P-gp, MRP1, MRP2, UGT, and SULT in intestinal tissue, and the levels of CYPs, UGT, and SULT in liver tissue were detected by commercial ELISA kits following the relevant manufacturer's instruction.

Statistical analysis

Analytical results of serum catechins were presented as the means ± SD. Statistical significance of difference between groups was performed by ANOVA followed by least significant difference test (LSD), which was performed by SPSS (20.0, IBM). $p < 0.05$ was considered to be statistically significant.

Results

Stachyose promotes intestinal absorption of TC in mice

To evaluate the effect of stachyose pre-treatment with different doses on absorption of TC, the mice were pre-treated with stachyose at 0, 50, 250, and 500 mg/kg·bw for 4 weeks and were subsequently administrated with TC at 250 mg/kg·bw 1 h before sacrifice. The serum levels of total TC and its monomer EC, EGC, ECG, and EGCG in the tested mice were determined by GC-MS, and the result is presented in Fig. 1a. Interestingly, the serum EC level was significantly increased by 57.5 and 71.3% in mice pre-treated with stachyose at 250 and 500 mg/kg·bw for 4 weeks, when compared with the control mice, respectively (Fig. 1a–A). Similarly, the serum EGC concentration was significantly elevated ($p < 0.05$) in mice by pre-administration of stachyose at 250 and 500 mg/kg·bw for 4 weeks, and this effect can be performed in a dose-dependent manner (Fig. 1a-B). The pre-treatment of stachyose at a low dose of 50 mg/kg·bw led to a slight increase in the level of serum EC and EGC, but statistical difference was not significant ($p > 0.05$). Furthermore, the pre-treatment with 250 and 500 mg/kg·bw stachyose in mice for 4 consecutive weeks notably elevated ($p < 0.05$) serum ECG levels by 48.4 and 53.8%, and serum EGCG contents by 56.9 and 73.0%, respectively, and the effect was dose-dependent (Fig. 1a-C, a-D). Although pre-administration of stachyose at 50 mg/kg·bw led to slight elevation in serum ECG and EGCG levels as compared to the control mice, there was no statistical significance ($p > 0.05$). As expected, pre-treatment of stachyose at 50, 250, and 500 mg/kg·bw for 4 weeks also dose-dependently elevated the total serum total TC level in mice (Fig. 1a-E).

To further test the time-dependent effect of stachyose ingestion on absorption of TC, mice were pre-treated with stachyose at 250 mg/kg·bw for 2, 4, and 8 weeks, and the mice were also orally administrated a single dose of TC (250 mg/kg·bw) 1 h before sacrifice. As can be seen in Fig. 1b-A and b-B, the serum EC and EGC levels in mice pre-treated with stachyose at 250 mg/kg·bw for 4 and 8 weeks were significantly higher ($p < 0.05$) than in control mice. In addition, serum EGC concentration was also significantly ($p < 0.05$) increased by 48.4 and 75.0% in mice pre-administrated with stachyose (250 mg/kg·bw) for 4 and 8 weeks, when compared to the control mice, respectively (Fig. 1b-C). It was noted that the EGCG concentration in the mice pre-treated with stachyose (250 mg/kg·bw) for 4 and 8 weeks was significantly ($p < 0.05$) augmented to 906.06 and 1267.64 ng/mL from 577.59 ng/mL of control mice, respectively (Fig. 1b-D). Furthermore, the serum total TC content was also elevated with the increase of pre-treatment time of stachyose in mice (Fig. 1b-E). Although the serum EC, EGC, ECG, EGCG, and total TC contents in mice pre-treated with stachyose at 250 mg/kg·bw for 2 weeks were higher than that in control

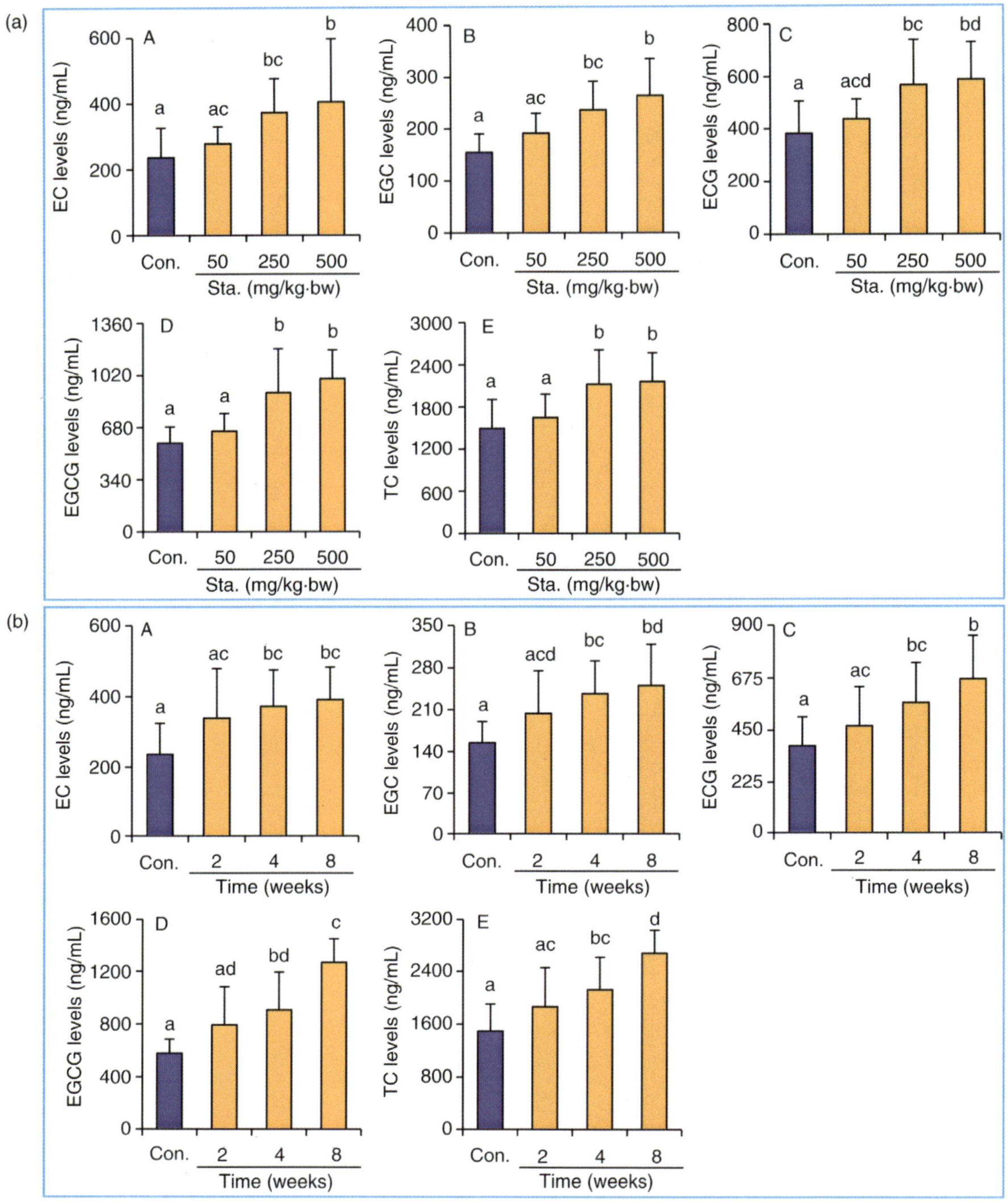

Fig. 1. Pre-treatment of stachyose at 50, 250, and 500 mg/kg·bw for 4 weeks (a) increased serum concentrations of epicatechin (EC, a-A), epigallocatechin (EGC, a-B), epicatechin gallate (ECG, a-C), epigallocatechin gallate (EGCG, a-D), and total tea catechins (TC, a-E) in mice, respectively. Pre-administration of stachyose at 250 mg/kg·bw for different time (b) elevated serum contents of EC (b–A), EGC (b–B), ECG (b-C), EGCG (b-D), and total TC (b-E) in mice. Each value is expressed as the means ± SD ($n = 8$). $^{a-d}$Mean values with different letters are significantly different from one another ($p < 0.05$). Sta., stachyose.

mice, it did not show statistical difference ($p > 0.05$). It was also observed that single administration of stachyose (250 mg/kg·bw) together with TC (250 mg/kg·bw) 1 h before sacrifice did not significantly elevate ($p > 0.05$) the serum catechins contents in mice, relative to control mice (data not shown). These results suggested that stachyose increased intestinal absorption of TC in a time-dependent manner.

Effects of stachyose on intestinal Phase II enzymes

In the enterocytes, the Phase II enzymes SULT and UGT are significant metabolic pathways for numerous

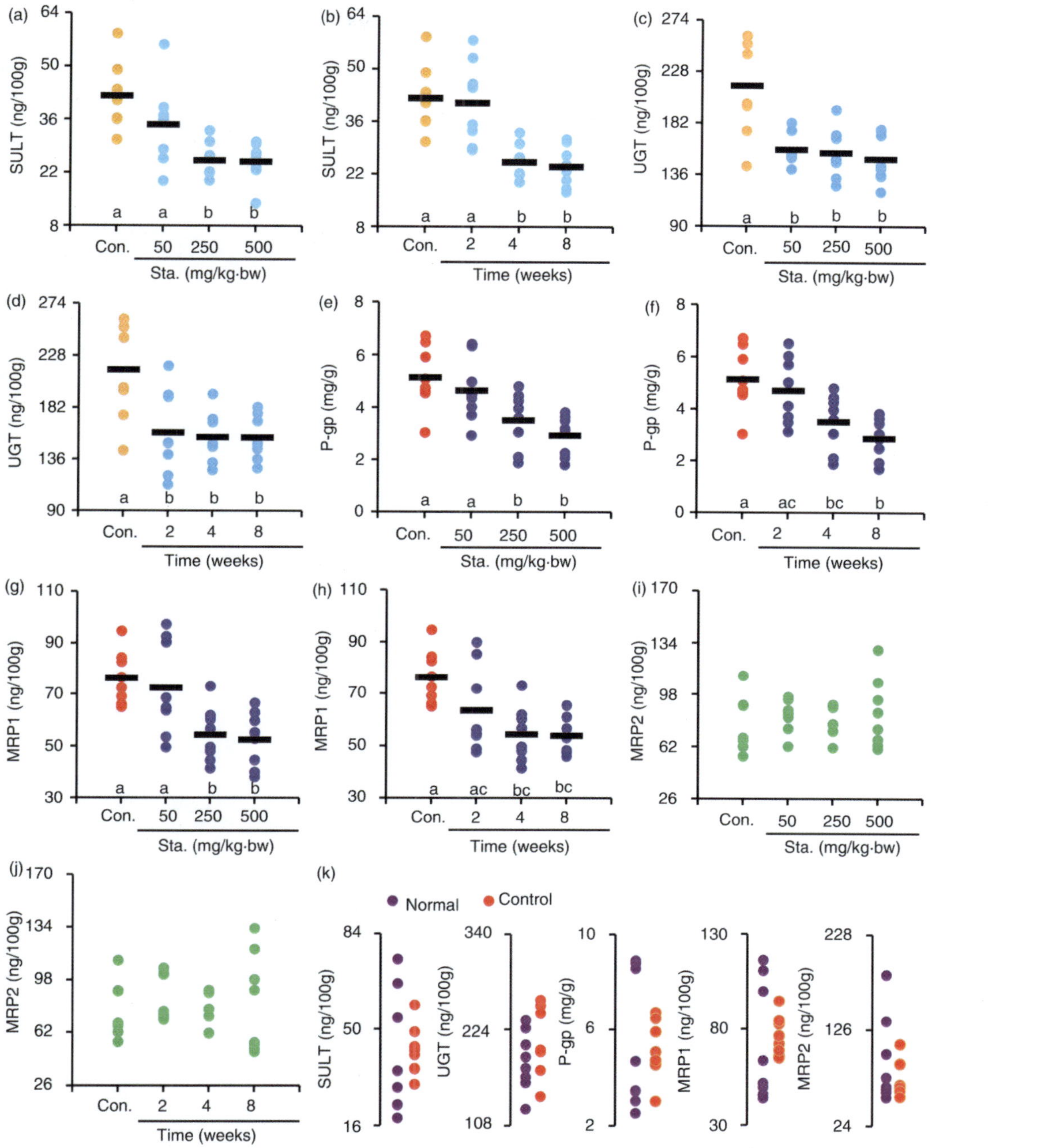

Fig. 2. Effects of pre-treatment of stachyose at different doses for 4 weeks on intestinal SULT (a), UGT (c), P-gp (e), MRP1 (g), and MRP2 (i) levels, respectively. The effects of pre-treatment of stachyose at 250 mg/kg·bw for different persistent periods on intestinal SULT (b), UGT (d), P-gp (f), MRP1 (h), and MRP2 (j) levels, respectively. Intestinal SULT, UGT, P-gp, MRP1, and MRP2 levels were also compared between untreated normal mice and TC alone-treated control mice (k). Each point in a group represents a value from a sample, and its average value was represented as a horizontal line. The letters (a–c), which are displayed on the abscissa, denote that the mean values with different letters are significantly different from one another ($p < 0.05$).

endo- and xenobiotics and are also known to interact with the ingested flavonoids, which may accelerate efflux transportation of flavonoids, and thereby reduce bioavailability of flavonoids (15, 24). As shown in Fig. 2a, the SULT levels of the mice pre-treated with stachyose at 250 and 500 mg/kg·bw for 4 weeks showed a dramatic ($p < 0.05$) decrease to 25.16 and 24.88 ng/100 g from 42.21 ng/100 g of control mice. Although the pre-treatment of stachyose at 250 mg/kg·bw for 2 weeks led to a slight decrease in the enteric SULT level ($p > 0.05$), administration of stachyose (250 mg/kg·bw) for 4 and 8 weeks significantly decreased intestinal SULT levels ($p < 0.05$) as compared to control mice (Fig. 2b). These findings suggest that the pre-treatment of stachyose can dose- and time-dependently inhibit intestinal SULT expression in mice. Besides, the intestinal UGT levels in mice were also analyzed by ELISA, and the results showed that the intestinal UGT level of mice pre-administrated with stachyose at all scheme was significantly lower than that of control mice ($p < 0.05$, Fig. 2c, d).

Stachyose inhibits expression of efflux transporters in mouse intestine

Flavonoids are known to interact with a number *of* membrane transporters, influencing *the* rate *of* intestinal nutrient *absorption, and* P-gp is a well-known efflux pump responsible for multiple drug resistance (25), and it plays a major role in the cells to transport catechins from intra-cell to outside (3). As depicted in Fig. 2e, the pre-administrations of stachyose at 50, 250, and 500 mg/kg·bw for 4 weeks and subsequent treatment of TC at 250 mg/kg·bw before sacrifice caused the dose-dependent decrease in P-gp expression of mouse intestinal tissue, showing the decrease by 9.6% ($p > 0.05$), 31.7% ($p < 0.05$), and 43.1% ($p < 0.05$), relative to control mice, respectively. In addition, the P-gp expression in intestinal tissue of mice pre-treated with stachyose at 250 mg/kg·bw for 2, 4, and 8 weeks was also reduced to 523.01 ($p > 0.05$), 389.71 ($p < 0.05$), and 317.99 μg/g ($p < 0.05$) from 570.82 μg/g of control mice, respectively (Fig. 2f).

MRP1 and MRP2 are also important membrane efflux transporters for Phase II metabolites of catechins (18, 26). As represented in Fig. 2g, the MRP1 levels in enterocytes of the mice pre-treated with stachyose at 50, 250, and 500 mg/kg·bw for 4 weeks were decreased to 72.43, 54.38, and 52.46 ng/100 g from 76.28 ng/100 g of control mice, respectively ($p > 0.05$, $p < 0.05$, $p < 0.05$). We also observed a time-dependent decrease in intestinal MRP1 levels in mice pre-treated with stachyose at 250 mg/kg·bw for 4 and 8 weeks, when compared to the control mice ($p < 0.05$, Fig. 2h). However, there were no prominent differences in the MRP2 levels in intestinal tissue among all mice ($p > 0.05$) (Fig. 2i, j). It was worth noting that the individual administration of TC did not significantly affect the expression of intestinal SULT, UGT, P-gp, MRP1, and MRP2 in control mice ($p > 0.05$ vs. the normal mice, Fig. 2k), indicating that the decrease of intestinal SULT, UGT, P-gp, and MRP1 levels in mice was not concerned with the administration of TC, and it was linked to pre-treatment of stachyose.

Effects of stachyose on hepatic Phase II enzymes and CYPs

The liver is an important organ for Phase I metabolism which is mainly catalyzed by CYPs, and also a major target for Phase II metabolism (glucuronidation and sulfation) of flavonoids (14, 24). Unexpectedly, our analysis showed that the hepatic SULT or UGT expression among all the tested mice showed no significant difference ($p > 0.05$) (Fig. 3a–d). However, pre-treatment of 50, 250, and 500 mg/kg·bw stachyose for 4 weeks and subsequent treatment with 250 mg/kg·bw TC once before sacrifice of mice dose-dependently decreased the CYPs contents by 12.6, 14.0, and 20.8%, relative to control mice, respectively (Fig. 3e). In addition, the hepatic CYPs levels in mice pre-treated with stachyose at 250 mg/kg·bw for 2, 4, and 8 weeks were time-dependently reduced ($p < 0.05$) by 1.1–15.4% as compared to control mice, respectively (Fig. 3f). Moreover, a dramatic decrease ($p < 0.05$) was also seen in the expression of liver CYPs following the individual administration of TC in control mice, relative to normal mice (Fig. 3g). The results obtained in this analysis clearly indicate that liver CYPs levels are decreased by the administration of TC, suggesting that non-digestible stachyose might inhibit liver CYPs via improving the absorption of TC.

Correlation analysis

To further understand the internal relation between serum catechin contents and the level of TC metabolism-related proteins, the identified data were assayed using correlation analysis, and the results are shown in Fig. 4. As expected, heat-map directly showed that negative correlations appeared between serum catechin contents and the level of TC metabolism-related proteins (SULT, UGT, P-gp and MRP1 in intestine, and SULT and CYPs in liver). This finding means that serum catechin concentrations increased with the decrease of intestinal SULT, UGT, P-gp and MRP1 levels, and hepatic SULT and CYPs levels in mice pre-treated with stachyose. It was also noticed that the levels of intestinal SULT, P-gp, and MRP1 were ($p < 0.05$) negatively correlated with serum total catechins, EC, EGC, ECG, and EGCG contents, respectively. In addition, one significant negative correlation ($p < 0.05$) was also presented between intestinal UGT level and serum EGC content, while the statistical significance was not found between intestinal UGT level and serum total catechins, EC, ECG, or EGCG concentrations, respectively. Moreover, liver SULT level was negatively ($p < 0.05$) correlated with serum total catechins, ECC and EGCG contents, respectively. Although the hepatic CYPs levels decreased with an increase of serum catechin contents, there was only one significant correlation appeared between hepatic CYPs levels and serum EGC level. According to the correlation matrix, the intimate connection existed between elevation of serum catechin contents and suppression of expression of TC metabolism-related proteins in stachyose-treated mice.

Discussion

Despite the abundant data revealing wide biological activities of dietary flavonoids, most flavonoids are poorly absorbed from the intestine and highly metabolized (27). Interestingly, previous research has suggested that non-digestible oligosaccharides can enhance intestinal absorption of polyphenols, which is possibly due to the fact that non-digestible oligosaccharides increase water-solubility of flavonoids and inhibit their degradation in gut (10, 28).

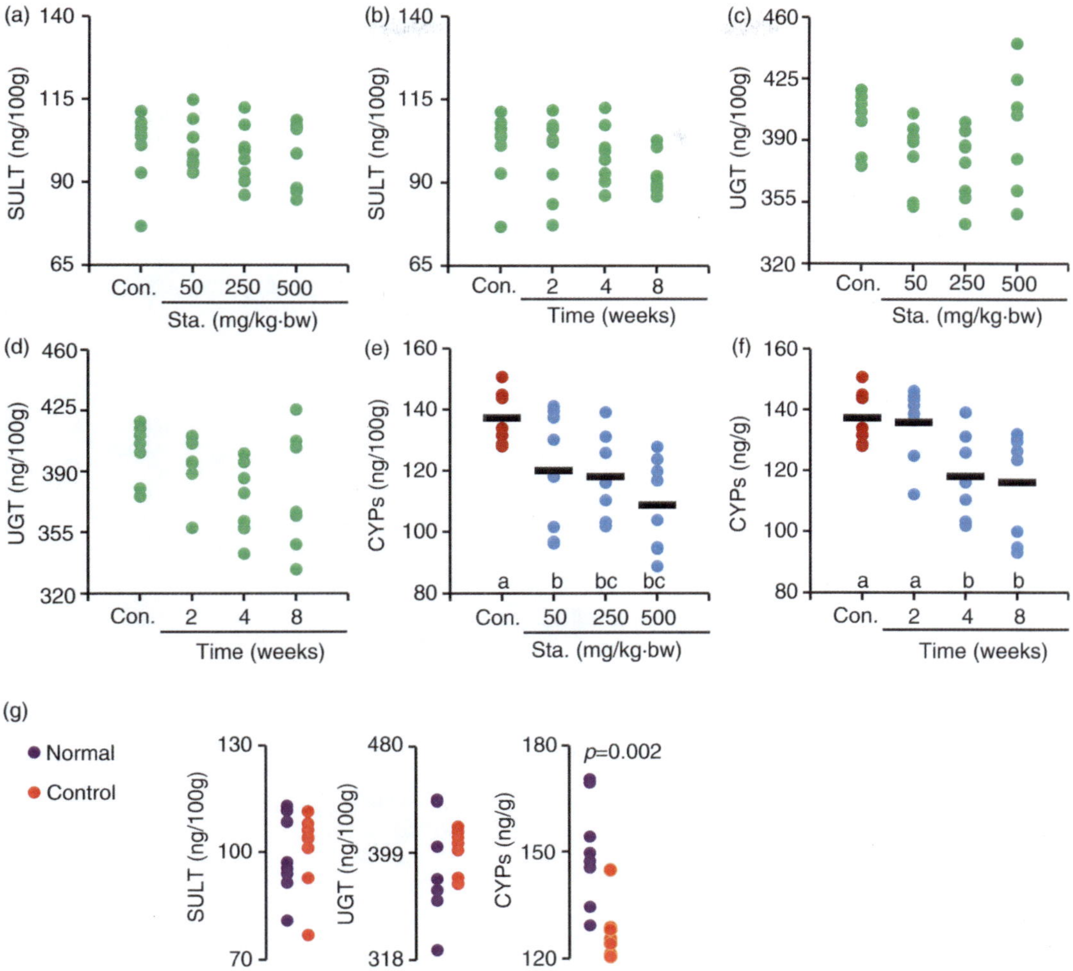

Fig. 3. Pre-treatment of stachyose at different doses for 4 weeks on hepatic SULT (a), UGT (c), and CYPs (e) levels in mice, respectively. Pre-treatment of stachyose at 250 mg/kg·bw for different persistent periods on hepatic SULT (b), UGT (d), and CYPs (f) levels, respectively. Liver SULT, UGT, and CYPs levels in normal mice and control mice were also compared (G). The letters (a–c), which are displayed on the abscissa, denote that the mean values with different letters are significantly different from one another ($p < 0.05$).

It is also widely recognized that TC can undergo Phase II biotransformation mainly including UGT and SULT in intestinal epithelial cells, which may greatly contribute to their first-pass metabolism (14, 27, 29). In our hands, the mice pre-treated with stachyose dose- and time-dependently presented the reduction of intestinal SULT levels in mice (Fig. 2a, b). Additionally, all the administration strategies of the tested stachyose also caused the dramatic decrease in intestinal UGT levels in mice (Fig. 2c, d). The present results for the first time suggested that glucuronidation and sulfonation of TC were limited in intestinal tissue by pre-administration of stachyose, which might contribute to an increase in absorption of TC.

Intestinal membrane-bound efflux pump transports proteins, such as P-gp, MRP1, and MRP2, which play an important role in efflux transportation of Phase II metabolites of polyphenols, which is a main factor for first-pass metabolism of TC (18). It is also reported that absorption extent of catechins is closely connected with efflux pump transporters, suggesting that inhibition for the efflux transporters may contribute to bioavailability improvement of polyphenols upon oral uptake (18). MRP2 is an important efflux transporter, and inhibition of MRP2 may contribute to cellular uptake of EC, ECG, and EGCG (20, 21, 30). However, this work demonstrated that pre-administrations of stachyose could not reduce intestinal MRP2 levels in mice (Fig. 2i, j), suggesting that the enhancing of TC absorption was irrelevant to MRP2 in mice with feeding of TC with stachyose. However, it was suggested that the cellular uptake of EC, ECG, EGC, and EGCG could be increased by inhibition of P-gp and MRP1 (19–21). Herein, pre-treatment of stachyose was clearly shown to be the dose- and time-dependent decrease in intestinal P-gp and MRP1 expression (Fig. 2e–h), strongly suggesting that stachyose caused the inhibition for efflux transportation of TC in mouse intestine, which might contribute to enhancing the absorption of TC. Although TC was the potent inhibitor for Phase II

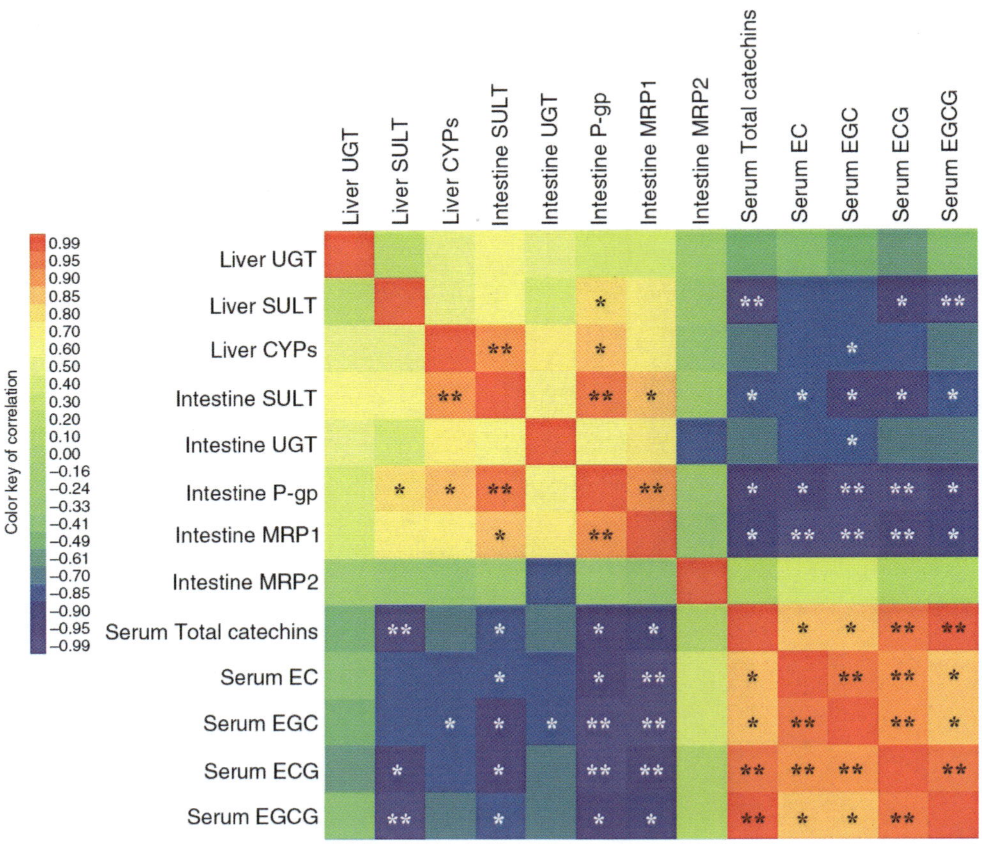

Fig. 4. A pairwise correlations analysis was performed to integrate intestinal and hepatic Phase II metabolic enzymes and transport proteins of TC expression values with relative serum TC concentration in mice. The heat-map represents the correlation structure of dataset, which is highlighted with red (positive correlations) or blue (negative correlations) according to the color key on the right. * and ** indicate statistically significant correlation at $p < 0.05$ and $p < 0.01$, respectively.

metabolizing enzymes and efflux transporters (21, 29), this study suggested that the sole administration of TC did not affect the expression of SULT, UGT, P-gp, and MRP1 in mouse intestine (Fig. 2k), and the decrease of intestinal SULT, UGT, P-gp, and MRP1 levels in mice was possibly due to the pre-treatment of stachyose. As a result, this was the first investigation with unequivocal evidence that stachyose could inhibit the expression of intestinal SULT, UGT, P-gp, and MRP1 in mice, which is responsible for the enhancement of TC transportation in enterocyte, and thereby contributed to the elevation in bioavailability of TC.

In this study, we have provided robust evidence that supplementation of stachyose can significantly enhance absorption of TC, which is confirmed by GC-MS analysis, revealing that the serum EC, EGC, ECG, and EGCG, and total catechins contents are increased with the increases of dose and time of stachyose pre-treatment in mice (Fig. 1). Further, correlation analysis indicated that there was an important interplay between enhancing absorption of TC and expression inhibition of Phase II metabolic enzymes and efflux pump transporters in intestine by stachyose consumption (Fig. 4). This finding for the first time demonstrated that non-digestible stachyose-enhanced absorption of TC was closely associated with the inhibition of Phase II metabolism and efflux transport of TC by stachyose ingestion, and this might be a novel molecular mechanism for non-digestible saccharides-elevated bioavailability of diet flavonoids. It is widely understood that flavonoids, which are absorbed and transferred to the blood, can be further metabolized by hepatic SULT, UGT, and CYPs, and the metabolites will be excreted via the kidney swiftly, which may aggravate the decreased bioavailability (24, 31). Herein, the hepatic SULT and UGT levels were not different among all the mice in this study (Fig. 3a–d), suggesting that pre-treatment of stachyose did not change Phase II biotransformation of TC in the liver. Most drugs undergo an initial Phase I metabolism, generally catalyzed by CYPs, to form more water-soluble metabolites, and the metabolites are then catalyzed by UGT and SULT (32). However, previous studies suggest that catechins are not likely to undergo Phase I metabolism by CYPs due to their molecular structure (3, 32). Although catechins are not the substrate of CYPs, it is well known that TC can exhibit the strong inhibition of CYPs, and this effect may decrease related nutrients metabolism (32). In our study, the pre-treatment of stachyose dose- and time-dependently decreased hepatic CYPs levels in the mice (Fig. 3e, f). The present study also showed that the individual administration of TC decreased hepatic CYPs levels in mice (Fig. 3g), suggesting that TC could inhibit the liver CYPs expression. For this reason, the elevation of circulating catechins concentration caused by stachyose pre-treatment was suggested to intensify the down-regulation in hepatic CYPs expression, which was confirmed by pairwise correlation analysis. It is well known that humans and monogastric animals do not possess the α-galactosidase enzyme to break down stachyose, and therefore, stachyose cannot be absorbed to enter blood circulation (13, 33). Interestingly, our finding in this work strongly indicated that a potential molecular mechanism of health-promoting property of non-digestible stachyose *in vivo* was due to the capacity of stachyose to increase absorption of flavonoids.

In summary, this is the first report to show that pre-treatment of stachyose time- and dose-dependently increases the absorption of TC in mice. It also demonstrates, for the first time, that the suppression of Phase II enzymes (SULT and UGT) and efflux transporters (P-gp and MRP1) expression in intestine has a key role for enhancing absorption of TC by stachyose ingestion. All these findings may supplement the mechanism that non-digestible oligosaccharide enhances bioavailability of dietary flavonoids, and provide a scientific basis for co-application of stachyose with TC for health effects.

Acknowledgements

This study was supported by grants from the National Natural Science Foundation of China (31671823), and the Development program for Innovative Research Team of Shaanxi Normal University, China (GK201501006), as well as Science and Technology Innovation as a Whole Plan Projects of Shaanxi Province, China (2015KTCQ02-01).

Conflict of interest and funding

The authors have not received any funding or benefits from industry or elsewhere to conduct this study.

References

1. Shim S-M, Yoo S-H, Ra C-S, Kim Y-K, Chung J-O, Lee S-J. Digestive stability and absorption of green tea polyphenols: influence of acid and xylitol addition. Food Res Int 2012; 45: 204–10.
2. Khan N, Mukhtar H. Tea polyphenols for health promotion. Life Sci 2007; 81: 519–33.
3. Feng WY. Metabolism of green tea catechins: an overview. Curr Drug Metab 2006; 7: 755–809.
4. Unno T, Sakuma M, Mitsuhashi S. Effect of dietary supplementation of (-)-epigallocatechin gallate on gut microbiota and biomarkers of colonic fermentation in rats. J Nutr Sci Vitaminol 2014; 60: 213–19.
5. Clifford MN, Van Der Hooft JJ, Crozier A. Human studies on the absorption, distribution, metabolism, and excretion of tea polyphenols. Am J Clin Nutr 2013; 98: 1619S–30S.
6. Manach C, Williamson G, Morand C, Scalbert A, Rémésy C. Bioavailability and bioefficacy of polyphenols in humans. I. Review of 97 bioavailability studies. Am J Clin Nutr 2005; 81: 230S–42S.
7. Matsumoto M, Matsukawa N, Chiji H, Hara H. Difructose anhydride III promotes absorption of the soluble flavonoid αG-rutin in rats. J Agric Food Chem 2007; 55: 4202–8.
8. Phuwamongkolwiwat P, Hira T, Hara H. A nondigestible saccharide, fructooligosaccharide, increases the promotive effect of a flavonoid, α-glucosyl-isoquercitrin, on glucagon-like peptide 1 (GLP-1) secretion in rat intestine and enteroendocrine cells. Mol Nutr Food Res 2014; 58: 1581–4.
9. Phuwamongkolwiwat P, Suzuki T, Hira T, Hara H. Fructooligosaccharide augments benefits of quercetin-3-O-β-glucoside on insulin sensitivity and plasma total cholesterol with promotion of flavonoid absorption in sucrose-fed rats. Eur J Nutr 2014; 53: 457–68.
10. Shinoki A, Lang W, Thawornkuno C, Kang HK, Kumagai Y, Okuyama M, et al. A novel mechanism for the promotion of quercetin glycoside absorption by megalo α-1,6-glucosaccharide in the rat small intestine. Food Chem 2013; 136: 293–6.
11. Uehara M, Ohta A, Sakai K, Suzuki K, Watanabe S, Adlercreutz H. Dietary fructooligosaccharides modify intestinal bioavailability of a single dose of genistein and daidzein and affect their urinary excretion and kinetics in blood of rats. J Nutr 2001; 131: 787–95.
12. Zhou W, Shan J, Tan X, Zou J, Yin A, Cai B, et al. Effect of chito-oligosaccharide on the oral absorptions of phenolic acids of *Flos Lonicerae* extract. Phytomedicine 2014; 21: 184–94.
13. Li W, Huang D, Gao A, Yang X. Stachyose increases absorption and hepatoprotective effect of tea polyphenols in high fructose-fed mice. Mol Nutr Food Res 2016; 60: 502–10.
14. Larkin T, Price WE, Astheimer L. The key importance of soy isoflavone bioavailability to understanding health benefits. Crit Rev Food Sci Nutr 2008; 48: 538–52.
15. Wu B, Kulkarni K, Basu S, Zhang S, Hu M. First-pass metabolism via UDP-glucuronosyltransferase: a barrier to oral bioavailability of phenolics. J Pharm Sci 2011; 100: 3655–81.
16. Yao HT, Luo MN, Hung LB, Chiang MT, Lin JH, Lii CK, et al. Effects of chitosan oligosaccharides on drug-metabolizing enzymes in rat liver and kidneys. Food Chem Toxicol 2012; 50: 1171–7.
17. Charles AL, Chang CK, Wu ML, Huang TC. Studies on the expression of liver detoxifying enzymes in rats fed seaweed (*Monostroma nitidum*). Food Chem Toxicol 2007; 45: 2390–6.
18. Brand W, Schutte ME, Williamson G, Van Zanden JJ, Cnubben NH, Groten JP, et al. Flavonoid-mediated inhibition of intestinal ABC transporters may affect the oral bioavailability of drugs, food-borne toxic compounds and bioactive ingredients. Biomed Pharmacother 2006; 60: 508–19.
19. Zhang L, Zheng Y, Chow MS, Zuo Z. Investigation of intestinal absorption and disposition of green tea catechins by Caco-2 monolayer model. Int J Pharm 2004; 287: 1–12.
20. Vaidyanathan JB, Walle T. Cellular uptake and efflux of the tea flavonoid (-)-epicatechin-3-gallate in the human intestinal cell line Caco-2. J Pharmacol Exp Ther 2003; 307: 745–52.
21. Hong J, Lambert JD, Lee SH, Sinko PJ, Yang CS. Involvement of multidrug resistance-associated proteins in regulating cellular levels of (-)-epigallocatechin-3-gallate and its methyl metabolites. Biochem Biophys Res Commun 2003; 310: 222–7.
22. Cordo Russo RI, García MG, Alaniz L, Blanco G, Alvarez E, Hajos SE. Hyaluronan oligosaccharides sensitize lymphoma

resistant cell lines to vincristine by modulating P-glycoprotein activity and PI3K/Akt pathway. Int J Cancer 2008; 122: 1012–8.
23. Tian QE, Li HD, Yan M, Cai HL, Tan QY, Zhang WY. Astragalus polysaccharides can regulate cytokine and P-glycoprotein expression in H22 tumor-bearing mice. World J Gastroenterol 2012; 18: 7079–86.
24. Van de Schans MG, Bovee TF, Stoopen GM, Lorist M, Gruppen H, Vincken JP. Prenylation and backbone structure of flavonoids and isoflavonoids from licorice and hop influence their phase I and II metabolism. J Agric Food Chem 2015; 63: 10628–40.
25. Chen CJ, Chin JE, Ueda K, Clark DP, Pastan I, Gottesman MM, et al. Internal duplication and homology with bacterial transport proteins in the mdr1 (P-glycoprotein) gene from multidrug-resistant human cells. Cell 1986; 47: 381–9.
26. Zhao M, Lei C, Yang Y, Bu X, Ma H, Gong H, et al. Abraxane, the nanoparticle formulation of paclitaxel can induce drug resistance by up-regulation of P-gp. PLoS One 2015; 10: E0131429.
27. Santos-Buelga C, González-Manzano S, Dueñas M, González-Paramás M. Analysis and characterisation of flavonoid phase II metabolites. Recent Adv Polyphenol Res 2012; 3: 249–86.
28. Matsukawa N, Matsumoto M, Shinoki A, Hagio M, Inoue R, Hara H. Nodigestible saccharides suppress the bacterial degradation of quercetin aglycone in the large intestine and enhance the bioavailability of quercetin glucoside in rats. J Agric Food Chem 2009; 57: 9462–8.
29. Fan YJ, Rong Y, Li PF, Dong WL, Zhang DY, Zhang L, et al. Genistein protection against acetaminophen-induced liver injury via its potential impact on the activation of UDP-glucuronosyltransferase and antioxidant enzymes. Food Chem Toxicol 2013; 55: 172–81.
30. Vaidyanathan JB, Walle T. Transport and metabolism of the tea flavonoid (-)-epicatechin by the human intestinal cell line Caco-2. Pharm Res 2001; 18: 1420–5.
31. Xu X, Harris KS, Wang HJ, Murphy PA, Hendrich S. Bioavailability of soybean isoflavones depends upon gut microflora in women. J Nutr 1995; 125: 2307–15.
32. Yang CS, Pan E. The effects of green tea polyphenols on drug metabolism. Expert Opin Drug Metab Toxicol 2012; 8: 677–89.
33. Csáky I, Fekete S. Soybean: feed quality and safety. Part 1: biologically active components. A review. Acta Vet Hung 2004; 52: 299–313.

---

*Xingbin Yang
Shaanxi Engineering Laboratory for Food Green Processing and Safety Control
College of Food Engineering and Nutritional Science
Shaanxi Normal University
Xi'an 710062
China
Email: xbyang@snnu.edu.cn

14

Development of a Mediterranean diet score adapted to Japan and its relation to obesity risk

Masao Kanauchi[1]* and Kimiko Kanauchi[2]

[1]Department of Health and Nutrition, Faculty of Health Science, Kio University, Koryo-cho, Japan; [2]Department of Internal Medicine, Narahigashi Hospital, Tenri, Japan

Abstract

Background: The Mediterranean diet (MD) is well known as a healthy diet that protects against several chronic diseases. However, there is no appropriate and easy index to assess adherence to the MD pattern in Japan.
Objective: The aim of this study was to develop a novel instrument to measure MD adherence adapted to a Japanese diet and to examine its association with overweight/obesity risk.
Methods: A cross-sectional nutritional survey provided the data for construction of a novel MD score. In total, 1,048 subjects who were employees and university students, aged 18–68 years (645 men and 403 women), completed a 58-item brief-type self-administered dietary history questionnaire. We constructed a Japanese-adapted MD score (jMD score) focusing on 13 components. Adherence to the jMD was categorized as low (score 0–4), moderate (5–7), or high (8–13).
Results: Men had higher jMD scores than women, and adherence to the jMD score increased with age. Only 11.6% of subjects showed high adherence to the jMD, whereas 29.6% showed low adherence. A higher jMD adherence was associated with a higher intake of favorable nutrients with the exception of salt. The jMD adherence was significantly associated with a reduced likelihood of having overweight/obesity for the highest category compared with lowest category (odds ratio [OR] 0.50, 95% confidence interval [CI] 0.30–0.85, $p\text{-}trend = 0.017$) after adjusting for age, sex, smoking, physical activity, alcohol intake, and hypertension. A two-point increment in jMD score was related to a reduced likelihood of having overweight/obesity with an odds ratio of 0.76 (95% CI 0.65–0.90, $p = 0.002$).
Conclusions: Our novel jMD score confirmed reasonable associations with nutrient intakes, and higher MD adherence was associated with a lower prevalence of overweight/obesity.

Keywords: *Mediterranean diet*; *Japanese*; *diet quality*; *obesity*

Responsible Editor: Per Ole Iversen, University of Oslo, Norway.

In the last few decades, the Mediterranean diet (MD) has been recognized as a healthy diet that protects against several chronic diseases (1–4). The traditional MD is characterized by a high consumption of cereals (mostly whole grains), vegetables, legumes, fruits and nuts, and olive oil; a moderate intake of fish; a low-to-moderate intake of dairy products; a low consumption of red and processed meat; and a moderate alcohol intake from red wine (5, 6). Although adherence to the MD has been studied in relation to a lower rate of all-cause mortality and a reduced risk of cancer, metabolic diseases, and cardiovascular disease (7, 8), little is known about the efficacy in a non-Mediterranean population.

The vegetable dietary pattern in Asian populations may also reduce cardiovascular risks (9, 10). A traditional Japanese diet, characterized by whole grains, colorful vegetables, soy products (e.g. tofu), fish, and konbu seaweed, has also been recognized as healthy (11, 12). Some components of this dietary pattern are similar to that of the MD. To date, the prevalence of obesity is increasing rapidly in Japan as well as in Western countries. Over the past few decades, the change from a traditional diet to a westernized dietary pattern had led to an increase in the rate of diabetes and cardiovascular disease in Japan (13). Therefore, switching from a modern dietary pattern to a healthy MD-like pattern may play an important role in the reduction of obesity (14).

Various indexes to assess the adherence to the MD have been proposed and used in nutritional epidemiologic studies (15, 16). However, there are cultural food differences between Mediterranean/European countries and Japan, making these indexes less applicable for Japan. A valid and easy assessment tool should be constructed that can capture the MD pattern in Japan. The aim of this study was to develop a novel instrument to measure MD adherence and compare it to previously reported MD scores. We also examined the relationship of scores on this instrument with overweight/obesity risk.

Methods

Subjects

In total, 1,002 employees at eight workplace settings and 62 university students were invited to participate in this study. Most employees were industrial workers, office workers, formal caregivers, or nursing staff. Of these, we excluded one subject who was older than 70 years, two subjects who did not complete the diet history questionnaire, 11 subjects who had implausibly low or high estimated caloric intake (<700 or >4,500 kcal per day for men and <600 or >3,500 kcal per day for women), and two subjects who had missing information for factors needed for statistical adjustment. Finally, 1,048 participants aged 18–68 years (645 men and 403 women) were included in this analysis. Study protocols were approved by the Institutional Review Board of Kio University, and written informed consent was obtained from each participant.

Dietary assessment

Habitual food consumption and nutrient intake were assessed using the brief-type self-administered diet history questionnaire (BDHQ) (17, 18). The BDHQ is a four-page fixed-portion questionnaire, and food and beverage items contained in the BDHQ were selected from foods commonly consumed in Japan, mainly from a food list used in the National Health and Nutritional Survey of Japan (19). The questionnaire asks about the consumption frequency of 58 food and beverage items and requires that participants recall their dietary habits over the previous 1-month period. Participants were asked to choose from seven possible answers to indicate how often they had consumed specific foods during the past month (never, <one time per week, once per week, two to three times per week, four to six times per week, once per day, and more than twice per day). Combined with standard serving sizes, the intake frequencies were converted into the average daily intake for each food item. Values for the intake of nutrients and energy were estimated based on the food items asked about on the questionnaire and the corresponding food composition list in the Standard Tables of Food Composition in Japan (20).

Mediterranean diet score

We developed a Japanese-adapted MD score (jMD score) by adapting the updated MD pyramid (21) to Japanese eating behaviors; we selected only some components of the MD pyramid and modified some cutoff values to more accurately reflect the standard Japanese diet. This score is based on 13 components: grains (including rice, bread, Japanese wheat noodles, buckwheat noodles, spaghetti, macaroni); vegetables (e.g. green-yellow vegetables, leafy vegetables, root vegetables, cruciferous vegetables, vegetable pickles); fruits (citrus, persimmons, strawberries, kiwifruit, other fruit); legumes (tofu, fermented soybeans, miso); fish (oily fish, non-oily fish, canned tuna, dried fish, fish paste products, shellfish); dairy products (milk, low-fat milk, yogurt); potatoes (all types); eggs; poultry; red meat and processed meat (beef, pork, ham, sausage, bacon); sweets (Japanese confectionaries, Western-type confectionaries, ice creams); alcohol (beer, sake, shochu, wine, whiskey); and the ratio of monounsaturated fatty acids to saturated fatty acids. One point was given to subjects who met criteria for 1) consumption of three to seven servings of grains per day, 2) consumption of five or more servings of vegetables per day, 3) consumption of two or more servings of fruits per day, 4) consumption of 30 g or more of legumes per day, 5) consumption of 84 g or more of fish per day for men and 66 g or more of fish per day for women, 6) consumption of 1.5–2.5 servings of dairy products per day, 7) consumption of potatoes one to three times per week, 8) consumption of poultry two to three times per week, 9) consumption of eggs two to three times per week, 10) consumption of meat or meat products less than three times per week, 11) consumption of sweets less than two times per week, 12) consumption of 10–30 g of alcohol per day for men and 5–15 g of alcohol per day for women, and 13) a ratio of 1.5 or more of monounsaturated fatty acids to saturated fatty acids. Otherwise, a score of zero was assigned. This resulted in scores ranging from 0 to 13, with a higher score indicating better adherence to the jMD. Adherence to the jMD was categorized as low (score 0–4), moderate (score 5–7), or high (score 8–13).

To compare with previously reported MD scores, three MD scores were calculated: the Mediterranean diet scale (T-MDS) proposed by Trichopoulou et al. (22), the Mediterranean Dietary Quality Index (MedDQI) proposed by Gerber (23), and the Mediterranean diet score (S-MDS) proposed by Sofi et al. (24).

Other variables

Body mass index (BMI) was calculated as weight in kilograms divided by the square of height in meters. Overweight/obesity was defined as BMI $\geq$25 kg/m^2, because the percentage of persons with BMI $\geq$30 kg/m^2 is rare in Japan (25). A self-reported questionnaire was used to assess current smoking status (yes, no), physical activity (active, sedentary), and hypertension (yes, no). Alcohol consumption (frequency and daily consumption) was evaluated by BDHQ information and was categorized as low (men, <10 g per day; women, <5 g per day), moderate (men, 10–30 g per day; women, 5–15 g per day), or high (men, >30 g per day; women, >15 g per day).

Statistical analysis

Data are presented as means ± SD or as percentages. Differences between two groups were compared using the Student's *t*-test for continuous variables or the chi-squared test for categorical variables. Differences of food or nutritional parameters across the MD adherence categories were assessed by one-way analysis of variance. Logistic regression analysis was used to evaluate the risk of having obesity. Linear trends were calculated using the median score of the categories of MD adherence. *P*-values <0.05 were considered statistically significant. All statistical analyses were performed using the SPSS statistical version 21.0 (IBM Corp., Armonk, NY).

Results

The mean age of subjects was 42.6 ± 11.4 years (range, 18–68 years), and the prevalence of overweight/obesity (BMI ≥25.0 kg/m^2) was 27.8%. The mean jMD score was 5.45 ± 1.77 (range, 0–11), and scores were symmetrical and normally distributed (data not shown). Men had higher jMD scores than women, and a greater adherence to the jMD was shown in older subjects than in younger subjects (Table 1).

When subjects were classified by jMD adherence categories, only 11.6% of subjects showed high adherence to the jMD, whereas 29.6% showed low adherence. A higher jMD adherence was associated with a higher intake of protein, polyunsaturated fatty acids, dietary fiber, salt, potassium, calcium, magnesium, iron, vitamin D, folate, and vitamin C and a lower intake of saturated fats and sucrose (Table 2).

With respect to the correlations among the four MD indexes, the highest correlations were observed between the jMD score and T-MDS, followed by the T-MDS and S-MDS, and the T-MDS and MedDQI. Lower correlations were seen between the jMD score and MedDQI, and the jMD score and S-MDS (Table 3).

The jMD adherence was significantly associated with a reduced likelihood of having overweight/obesity for the highest category compared with lowest category (odds ratio [OR] 0.50, 95% confidence interval [CI] 0.30–0.85, *p-trend* = 0.017) after adjusting for age, sex, smoking, physical activity, alcohol intake, and hypertension (Table 4). A two-point increment in jMD score was related to a reduced likelihood for having overweight/obesity with an odds ratio of 0.76 (95% CI 0.65–0.90, $p = 0.002$).

Table 1. Association of personal characteristics of study subjects with mean Mediterranean diet score adapted to Japan (jMD)

	Number	jMD score	*P*
Sex			<0.001
Men	645	5.66 ± 1.83	
Women	403	5.11 ± 1.62	
Age group (years)			<0.001
18–29	151	4.92 ± 1.66	
30–39	215	5.42 ± 1.71	
40–49	392	5.38 ± 1.81	
50–59	241	5.80 ± 1.76	
60 +	49	6.00 ± 1.58	
Overweight/obesity[a]			0.150
Yes	291	5.32 ± 1.78	
No	757	5.50 ± 1.76	
Smoking status[b]			0.398
Yes	252	5.54 ± 1.81	
No	732	5.43 ± 1.75	
Physically active[b]			0.314
Yes	445	5.40 ± 1.77	
No	539	5.51 ± 1.77	
Alcohol intake[c]			0.823
No or low	670	5.24 ± 1.69	
Moderate	148	6.63 ± 1.83	
High	230	5.27 ± 1.65	
Hypertension			0.052
Yes	241	5.65 ± 1.90	
No	807	5.39 ± 1.72	

Data are means ± SD.
[a]Overweight/obesity was defined as BMI ≥25 kg/m^2.
[b]Data on smoking status and physical activity status were missing for 64 subjects.
[c]Alcohol consumption was categorized as low (men, <10 g per day; women, <5 g per day), moderate (men, 10–30 g per day; women, 5–15 g per day), or high (men, >30 g per day; women, >15 g per day).

Discussion

This is the first study to develop a novel 13-item MD score adapted to Japan dietary habits and to investigate its association with overweight/obesity. The impact of poor dietary habits on health is an important focus of contemporary health promotion strategies. The MD is now widely promoted for the prevention of cardiometabolic diseases (1–4). Adherence to the MD has been shown to be inversely associated with all-cause mortality, cardiovascular disease mortality, and cancer incidence (7, 8), but evidence of MD adherence in a non-Mediterranean population, especially East Asians, is limited (26–28). A study conducted in Korean adults (26) reported that adherence to the MD evaluated using an alternative MD score was related to lower oxidative stress biomarkers. A study conducted in Chinese elderly (27) reported that adherence to the MD was associated

Table 2. Food and nutrient intake by the adherence levels to the Mediterranean diet adapted to Japan (jMD)

Food/nutrients	jMD score 0–4 ($n = 310$)	jMD score 5–7 ($n = 616$)	jMD score 8–13 ($n = 122$)	p
Grains (g/day)	552±235	548±176	570±145	0.515
Potatoes (g/day)	40±40	55±41	71±44	<0.001
Legumes (g/day)	42±37	65±42	84±56	<0.001
Vegetables (g/day)	214±123	303±139	365±158	<0.001
Fruits (g/day)	92±93	119±125	158±141	<0.001
Fish (g/day)	67±43	94±47	127±63	<0.001
Meat (g/day)	89±54	95±43	95±37	0.194
Dairy (g/day)	166±154	143±119	132±124	0.013
Eggs (g/day)	48±31	51±32	46±27	0.179
Energy (kcal/day)	2,318±305	2,366±296	2,456±247	<0.001
Protein (%E)	13.3±2.8	14.5±2.5	15.6±2.5	<0.001
Fat (%E)	25.7±6.7	25.8±5.4	26.2±4.4	0.780
Carbohydrate (%E)	55.3±8.9	53.7±7.6	53.0±6.0	0.006
SFA (%E)	7.4±2.4	6.7±1.8	6.3±1.4	<0.001
MUFA (%E)	9.3±2.6	9.4±2.2	9.5±1.8	0.740
PUFA (%E)	5.8±1.4	6.4±1.3	6.9±1.3	<0.001
M/S ratio	1.30±0.23	1.42±0.24	1.55±0.25	<0.001
Dietary fiber (g/day)	11.3±3.6	13.9±4.1	16.2±4.2	<0.001
Sucrose (g/day)	20.6±12.2	17.7±10.4	15.6±10.9	<0.001
Salt (g/day)	12.4±3.2	13.7±3.2	15.9±3.9	<0.001
Potassium (mg/day)	2,509±732	2,997±805	3,502±824	<0.001
Calcium (mg/day)	545±230	608±197	689±215	<0.001
Magnesium (mg/day)	259±61	303±62	353±75	<0.001
Iron (mg/day)	7.9±2.1	9.3 ±2.2	10.5±2.3	<0.001
Vitamin D (μg/day)	11.5±8.0	15.3±7.9	20.3±9.8	<0.001
Folate (μg/day)	327±119	402±133	472±140	<0.001
Vitamin C (mg/day)	100±48	130±58	159±63	<0.001

Data are means ± SD.
SFA, saturated fatty acids; MUFA, monounsaturated fatty acids; PUFA, polyunsaturated fatty acids; S, saturated; M, monounsaturated.

with a lower risk for hip fractures. A study conducted in Hong Kong (28) reported that no association was observed between the MD score and 4-year incident frailty in community-dwelling older people. However, adherence to the MD in Japanese people has not been precisely explored. One of the reasons is thought to be the lack of an appropriate assessment tool for this population. In the Mediterranean and European countries, several indexes for assessing MD adherence have been reported (7). The T-MDS, created by Trichopoulou et al. in 1995 (5) and updated thereafter (6, 22), is widely known and is based on consumption of nine items. Other examples are the MedDQI (23), the S-MDS (24), the alternate MD score (29), and the MedDietScore (30) that include 7 components, 9 components, 9 components, and 11 components, respectively. It is interesting to note that the components of these scores and their scoring systems differ across studies (5, 6, 22–24, 29, 30). In addition, there is

Table 3. Correlation among indexes of adherence to the Mediterranean diet

	jMD score (correlation p coefficient)	T-MDS (correlation p coefficient)	MedDQI (correlation p coefficient)	S-MDS (correlation p coefficient)
jMD score	1	–	–	–
T-MDS	0.490 (<0.001)	1	–	–
MedDQI	0.287 (<0.001)	0.457 (<0.001)	1	–
S-MDS	0.184 (<0.001)	0.460 (<0.001)	0.405 (<0.001)	1

jMD, Mediterranean diet score adapted to Japan; T-MDS, Mediterranean diet scale proposed by Trichopoulou et al. (22); MedDQI, Mediterranean Dietary Quality Index proposed by Gerber (23); S-MDS, Mediterranean diet score proposed by Sofi et al. (24).

Table 4. Association of jMD score with the likelihood (odds ratios and 95% CIs) of having overweight/obesity

	Total, *n* (%)	Overweight/obesity, *n* (%)	Crude	Model 1: OR (95% CI)	Model 2: OR (95% CI)	Model 3: OR (95% CI)
jMDS score adherence						
Low (score 0–4)	310 (29.6)	87 (28.1)	1	1	1	1
Moderate (score 5–7)	616 (58.8)	175 (28.4)	1.02 (0.75–1.38)	0.96 (0.71–1.16)	0.89 (0.65–1.22)	0.87 (0.63–1.20)
High (score 8–13)	122 (11.6)	29 (23.8)	0.80 (0.49–1.30)	0.71 (0.43–1.16)	0.56 (0.34–0.92)	0.50 (0.30–0.85)
p-trend			*0.504*	*0.236*	*0.037*	*0.017*

Data are odds ratio (95% CI).
Model 1 is adjusted for age. Model 2 is adjusted for age and sex. Model 3 is adjusted for age, sex, smoking status, physical activity, alcohol intake, and hypertension (yes/no).
jMD, Mediterranean diet score adapted to Japan.

no consensus in the definition of the MD as represented by country-specific features (31).

We created the jMD score based on the updated MD pyramid (21). We incorporated white meat (in Japan, this consists mainly of poultry), potatoes, eggs, and sweets into our score, because the updated MD pyramid recommends that the first three foods should be limited to weekly consumption, and sweets should be consumed occasionally in small amounts. Conversely, we did not incorporate olive oil and nuts into our score, because the BDHQ used in the present study could not calculate the amount of these foods. In addition, consumption of olive oil and nuts are low in Japan. We alternately used an indirect parameter of the monounsaturated fatty acids to saturated fatty acids ratio in the present jMD score, which has been used in several previous studies (5, 6, 22, 29).

When creating the jMD score, we modified some cutoff values to consider Japanese eating habits. First, the MD pyramid today represents a weekly consumption of two or more servings of fish and shellfish (21). However, in general, Japanese people eat a lot of fish and shellfish (32). Almost all of participants might exceed this cutoff level of fish intake. We amended the cutoffs for fish intake with an upward adjustment based on the mean consumption levels of the Japanese population ($\geq$84 g per day for men and $\geq$66 g per day for women) (33). Second, most of the previously reported MD scores consider alcohol intake, especially wine. Japanese people commonly consume several kinds of alcoholic beverages such as sake (Japanese rice wine), beer, or shochu (Japanese distilled alcohol beverage), but the proportion of wine drinkers is relatively low. For this reason, we assessed moderate consumption of all amount of alcohol beverages.

One of the strengths in the present study is that we chose predefined absolute cutoffs of consumption of each food to estimate jMD adherence. In most previous reported MD scores (5, 6, 22, 26–29), the cutoff points are based on the sex-specific medians among the sample population. Under these considerations, their scores are highly dependent on the sample characteristics. Because of the heterogeneity of their cutoff points in each MD score, a result of one study could not be comparable with another study performed in a different cohort even in the same country. This could result in misleading data regarding the association between MD adherence and health outcomes. Indeed, our jMD scores were fairly correlated to T-MDS, but remaining correlations were poor. This is in line with a previous report (16) that compared data from 10 different MD scores in which only three correlations were high but the remaining correlations were fair or poor. This finding implies that the previous proposed MD scores are widely different. As mentioned above, the cutoff point used in the T-MDS reflects their specific sample population, so it is difficult to use in Japanese people, especially in a clinical setting. In contrary, it is noteworthy that our jMD score assigns a value of 0 or 1 to each item according to a predefined absolute cutoff. It seems to be a simple scoring method and to have an advantage of being feasible for assessing or comparing different cohorts studied. Second, we demonstrated an association between jMD adherence and a lower prevalence of overweight/obesity. Two-point increments of jMD score were related to a 24% reduction of having overweight/obesity. Our results indicate that the jMD may help promote healthier eating habits in Japanese people.

On the other hand, we found some unintended results in the present study. The jMD score was shown to be lower among women compared with men, as well as in younger compared with older people. A possible explanation may be that younger women tend to have increased exposure to unhealthy eating habits or unbalanced diets, such as low intakes of grains, legumes, and fish or excess intakes of sweets, resulting in lower jMD scores. In the present study, higher salt intake was observed in the highest jMD category. It is attributable to habitual consumption of higher salt Japanese foods, such as dried fish, canned tuna, and fish paste products (34). In a recent epidemiologic study (35), it is also reported that Japanese adults with higher urinary sodium excretion consumed a significantly greater amount of salty Japanese foods, such as salted fish, miso soup, and Japanese pickles. These salty foods are included in the jMD scores as the fish component, legume component, and vegetable component, respectively. Surprisingly, the MD represents a moderate-to-high salt diet because many of the MD foods such as cheese, bread, some of pastries, anchovies, and salted nuts are pretty salty (36, 37). These foods are recommended to be consumed on a daily basis according to the MD scheme. Nevertheless, the inverse relation of MD adherence and hypertension risk has been shown in epidemiologic studies (38), despite the hidden salt intake supplied from the MD. It may be possible, though not conclusive, that adherence to the MD could be influenced by the impact of salt intake. In this context, based on the updated MD pyramid recommendation (21), use of spices, herbs, and garlic is a good way to contribute to reducing the addition of salt to food. Yet, in Japan, these spices are rarely used despite a frequent use of soy sauce.

This study has several limitations. First, as a cross-sectional study, the present analysis cannot prove a causal relationship between the jMD adherence and the prevalence of overweight/obesity. Second, we assessed the combined risk of overweight and obesity in this study. One reason that we chose the criteria of BMI ≥ 25 kg/m^2 is that the percentage of persons with BMI ≥ 30 kg/m^2 is rare in Japan. In the National Health and Nutrition Survey in Japan, the percentage of persons with BMI ≥ 30 kg/m^2 was only 4.0% in men and 3.3% in women (25); thus, we did not analyze separately the obesity risk of BMI ≥ 30 kg/m^2. Third, evaluation of salt intakes was conducted by dietary assessment questionnaires. It can be measured directly with 24-h urine collection, but this is impractical. Our data were estimated from the BDHQ questionnaire and corresponding food composition list in the Standard Tables of Food Composition in Japan (20). In addition, the questionnaire includes a useful information source that asks about the usual cooking methods for fish, meat, and vegetables, preferable use of soy sauce as a seasoning, and consumption of miso soup or soup for noodles. The validity of this BDHQ questionnaire was reported for several nutrient intakes (17, 18). Fourth, MD cuisine is characterized by pasta tossed with vegetables, herbs, and olive oil, dressing salads with olive oil or vinegar, vegetable soups with added olive oil, and chopped or stewed tomatoes and other carotenoid vegetables. Cooking processes might strongly influence antioxidant or anti-inflammatory compounds, including the MD foods (39). For example, fish that is pan-fried in virgin olive oil is frequently eaten in Mediterranean countries, whereas raw fish or grilled fish is preferred in Japan. However, the present study did not take into consideration the difference in cooking procedures between Mediterranean countries and Japan. Fifth, validation analysis between jMD score and plasma biomarkers was not determined because we did not measure plasma biomarkers such as lipids or vitamin levels. Finally, this study was conducted only among adult employees and university students. Although the geographic characteristics of our study sample are similar to the general Japanese population living in an urban or suburban area setting, we did not include subjects in rural communities, such as farm workers or fisherman. Further investigations including subjects with a wider range of occupations is needed.

In conclusion, the present study showed a novel MD score adapted to Japan by confirming reasonable associations with nutrient intakes. The jMD score is also an easy and useful tool to assess jMD adherence. In addition, jMD adherence was associated with a lower prevalence of overweight/obesity. The MD has been recognized as a healthy diet worldwide. It may be useful to encourage the Japanese population to adapt the jMD to prevent chronic diseases. The use of this score in clinical practice or research may contribute to the promotion of a healthier lifestyle.

Authors' contributions

MK designed the study, researched the data, and wrote the manuscript. KK contributed to the data collection and the discussions.

Conflict of interest and funding

The authors declare that they have no competing interests.

References

1. Estruch R, Ros E, Salas-Salvadó J, Covas MI, Corella D, Arós F, et al. Primary prevention of cardiovascular disease with a Mediterranean diet. N Engl J Med 2013; 368: 1279–90.
2. Esposito K, Kastorini CM, Panagiotakos DB, Giugliano D. Mediterranean diet and metabolic syndrome: an updated systematic review. Rev Endoc Metab Disord 2013; 14: 255–63.
3. Grosso G, Mistretta A, Frigiola A, Gruttadauria S, Biondi A, Basile F, et al. Mediterranean diet and cardiovascular risk factors: a systematic review. Crit Rev Food Sci Nutr 2014; 54: 593–610.
4. Koloverou E, Esposito K, Giugliano D, Panagiotakos D. The effect of Mediterranean diet on the development of type 2 diabetes mellitus: a meta-analysis of 10 prospective studies and 136,846 participants. Metabolism 2014; 63: 903–11.
5. Trichopoulou A, Kouris-Blazos A, Wahlqvist ML, Gnardellis C, Lagiou P, Polychronopoulos E, et al. Diet and overall survival in elderly people. BMJ 1995; 311(7018): 1457–60.
6. Trichopoulou A, Costacou T, Bamia C, Trichopoulos D. Adherence to a Mediterranean diet and survival in a Greek population. N Engl J Med 2003; 348: 2599–608.
7. Sofi F, Macchi C, Abbate R, Gensini GF, Casini A. Mediterranean diet and health status: an updated meta-analysis and a proposal for a literature-based adherence score. Public Health Nutr 2014; 17: 2769–82.
8. D'Alessandro A, DePergola G. Mediterranean diet and cardiovascular disease. Nutrients 2015; 7: 7863–88.

9. Shimazu T, Kuriyama S, Hozawa A, Ohmori K, Sato Y, Nakaya N, et al. Dietary pattern and cardiovascular disease mortality in Japan. Int J Epidemiol 2007; 36: 600–9.
10. Li P, Zhang M, Zhu Y, Liu W, Zhang Y, Gao Y, et al. Dietary patterns and changes in cardiovascular risk factors in apparently healthy Chinese women. J Clin Biochem Nutr 2016; 58: 232–9.
11. Niu K, Momma H, Kobayashi Y, Guan L, Chujo M, Otomo A, et al. The traditional Japanese dietary pattern and longitudinal changes in cardiovascular disease risk factors in apparently healthy Japanese adults. Eur J Nutr 2016; 55: 267–79.
12. Yamamoto K, Shuang E, Hatakeyama Y, Sakamoto Y, Honma T, Jibu Y, et al. The Japanese diet from 1975 delays senescence and prolongs life span in SAMP8 mice. Nutrition 2016; 32: 122–8.
13. Ministry of Health, Labour, and Welfare of Japan (2012). The National Health and Nutrition Survey in Japan. Tokyo, Japan: Ministry of Health, Labour, and Welfare. (in Japanese)
14. Shai I, Schwarzfuchs D, Henkin Y, Shahar DR, Witkow S, Greenberg I, et al. Weight loss with a low-carbohydrate, Mediterranean, or low-fat diet. N Engl J Med 2008; 359: 229–41.
15. Bach A, Serra-Majem L, Carrasco JL, Roman B, Ngo J, Bertomeu I, et al. The use of indexes evaluating the adherence to the Mediterranean diet in epidemiological studies: a review. Public Health Nutr 2006; 9: 132–46.
16. Milà-Villarroel R, Bach-Faig A, Puig J, Puchal A, Farran A, Serra-Majem L, et al. Comparison and evaluation of the reliability of indexes of adherence to the Mediterranean diet. Public Health Nutr 2011; 14: 2338–45.
17. Kobayashi S, Murakami K, Sasaki S, Okubo H, Hirota N, Notsu A, et al. Comparison of relative validity of food group intakes estimated by comprehensive and brief-type self-administered diet history questionnaires against 16 d dietary records in Japanese adults. Public Health Nutr 2011; 11: 1–12.
18. Kobayashi S, Honda S, Murakami K, Sasaki S, Okubo H, Hirota N, et al. Both comprehensive and brief self-administered diet history questionnaires satisfactorily rank nutrient intakes in Japanese adults. J Epidemiol 2012; 22: 151–9.
19. Ministry of Health, Labour, and Welfare of Japan (2008). The National Health and Nutrition Survey in Japan. Tokyo, Japan: Ministry of Health, Labour, and Welfare. (in Japanese)
20. Council for Science and Technology (2010). Standard Tables of Food Composition in Japan, 2010. Tokyo, Japan: Ministry of Education, Culture, Sports, Science and Technology. (in Japanese)
21. Bach-Faig A, Berry EM, Lairon D, Reguant J, Trichopoulou A, Dernini S, et al. Mediterranean diet pyramid today. Public Health Nutr 2011; 14: 2274–84.
22. Trichopoulou A, Orfanos P, Norat T, Bueno-de-Mesquita B, Ocké MC, Peeters PH, et al. Modified Mediterranean diet and survival: EPIC-elderly prospective cohort study. BMJ 2005; 330(7498): 991.
23. Gerber M. Qualitative methods to evaluate Mediterranean diet in adults. Public Health Nutr 2006; 9: 147–51.
24. Sofi F, Abbate R, Gensini GF, Casini A, Trichopoulou A, Bamia C. Identification of change-points in the relationship between food groups in the Mediterranean diet and overall mortality. Eur J Nutr 2012; 51: 167–72.
25. Ministry of Health, Labour, and Welfare of Japan (2015). The National Health and Nutrition Survey in Japan. Tokyo, Japan: Ministry of Health, Labour, and Welfare. (in Japanese)
26. Kim JY, Yang YJ, Yang YK, Oh SY, Hong YC, Lee EK, et al. Diet quality scores and oxidative stress in Korean adults. Eur J Clin Nutr 2011; 65: 1271–8.
27. Zeng FF, Xue WQ, Cao WT, Wu BH, Xie HL, Fan F, et al. Diet-quality scores and risk of hip fractures in elderly urban Chinese in Guangdong, China. Osteoporos Int 2014; 25: 2131–41.
28. Chan R, Leung J, Woo J. Dietary pattern and risk of frailty in Chinese community-dwelling older people in Hong Kong. Nutrients 2015; 7: 7070–84.
29. Fung TT, Rexrode KM, Mantzoros CS, Manson JE, Willett WC, Hu FB. Mediterranean diet and incidence of and mortality from coronary heart disease and stroke in women. Circulation 2009; 119: 1093–100.
30. Panagiotakos DB, Pitsavos C, Stefanadis C. Dietary patterns: a Mediterranean diet score and its relation to clinical and biological markers of cardiovascular disease risk. Nutr Metab Cardiovasc Dis 2006; 16: 559–68.
31. Davis C, Bryan J, Hodgson J, Murphy K. Definition of the Mediterranean diet. Nutrients 2015; 7: 9139–53.
32. Nanri A, Mizoue T, Noda M, Takahashi Y, Matsushita Y, Poudel-Tandukar K, et al. Fish intake and type 2 diabetes in Japanese men and women. Am J Clin Nutr 2011; 94: 884–9.
33. Ministry of Health, Labour, and Welfare of Japan (2016). The National Health and Nutrition Survey in Japan. Tokyo, Japan: Ministry of Health, Labour, and Welfare. (in Japanese)
34. Fujiwara A, Asakura K, Uechi K, Masayasu S, Sasaki S. Dietary patterns extracted from the current Japanese diet and their associations with sodium and potassium intakes estimated by repeated 24 h urine collection. Public Health Nutr 2016; 19: 2580–91.
35. Okuda N, Okayama A, Miura K, Yoshida K, Saito S, Kakagawa H, et al. Food source of dietary sodium in the Japanese adult population: the international study of macro-micronutrients and blood pressure (INTERMAP). Eur J Nutr 2016. doi: http://dx.doi.org/10.1007/s00394-016-1177-1. [Epub ahead of print]
36. Farajian P, Zampelas A. Mediterranean diet and dietary sodium intake. Diet quality. In: Preedy VR, et al., eds., Nutrition and health. New York: Springer Science; 2013, pp. 235–45.
37. Magriplis E, Farajian P, Pounis GD, Risvas G, Panagiotakos DB, Zampelas A. High sodium intake of children through hidden food sources and its association with the Mediterranean diet. J Hypertens 2011; 29: 1069–76.
38. Psaltopoulou T, Naska A, Orfanos P, Trichopoulos D, Mountokalakis T, Trichopoulou A. Olive oil, the Mediterranean diet, and arterial blood pressure. Am J Clin Nutr 2004; 80: 1012–18.
39. Hoffman R, Gerber M. Food processing and the Mediterranean diet. Nutrients 2015; 7: 7925–64.

*Masao Kanauchi
Department of Health and Nutrition
Faculty of Health Science
Kio University
4-2-2 Umami-naka
Koryo-cho Kitakatsuragi-gun
Nara 635-0832, Japan
Email: m.kanauchi@kio.ac.jp

15

Food sources of energy and nutrients in Finnish girls and boys 6–8 years of age – the PANIC study

Aino-Maija Eloranta[1]*†, Taisa Venäläinen[1,2]†, Sonja Soininen[1,3,4], Henna Jalkanen[1], Sanna Kiiskinen[1], Ursula Schwab[2,5], Timo A. Lakka[1,6,7] and Virpi Lindi[1]

[1]Department of Physiology, Institute of Biomedicine, School of Medicine, University of Eastern Finland, Kuopio, Finland; [2]Department of Clinical Nutrition, Institute of Public Health and Clinical Nutrition, School of Medicine, University of Eastern Finland, Kuopio, Finland; [3]Social and Health Center, City of Varkaus, Finland; [4]Institute of Dentistry, School of Medicine, University of Eastern Finland, Kuopio, Finland; [5]Department of Internal Medicine, Institute of Clinical Medicine, Kuopio University Hospital, Kuopio, Finland; [6]Kuopio Research Institute of Exercise Medicine, Kuopio, Finland; [7]Department of Clinical Physiology and Nuclear Medicine, Kuopio University Hospital, Kuopio, Finland

Abstract

Background: Data on food sources of nutrients are needed to improve strategies to enhance nutrient intake among girls and boys in Western countries.
Objective: To identify major food sources of energy, energy nutrients, dietary fibre, and micronutrients, and to study gender differences in these food sources among children.
Design: We assessed food consumption and nutrient intake using 4-day food records in a population sample of Finnish girls ($n = 213$) and boys ($n = 217$) aged 6–8 years from the Physical Activity and Nutrition in Children Study. We calculated the percentual contribution of 55 food groups for energy and nutrient intake using the population proportion method.
Results: Low-fibre grain products, skimmed milk, and high-fibre bread provided almost 23% of total energy intake. Skimmed milk was the top source of protein (18% of total intake), vitamin D (32%), potassium (20%), calcium (39%), magnesium (17%), and zinc (16%). Vegetable oils (15%) and high-fat vegetable oil–based spreads (14%) were the top sources of polyunsaturated fat. High-fibre bread was the top source of fibre (27%) and iron (12%). Non-root vegetables were the top source of folate (14%) and vitamin C (22%). Sugar-sweetened beverages provided 21% of sucrose intake. Pork was a more important source of protein and sausage was a more important source of total fat and monounsaturated fat in boys than in girls. Vegetable oils provided a higher proportion of unsaturated fat and vitamin E among boys, whereas high-fat vegetable oil–based spreads provided a higher proportion of these nutrients among girls.
Conclusion: Commonly recommended foods, such as skimmed milk, high-fibre grain products, vegetables, vegetable oil, and vegetable oil–based spreads, were important sources of several nutrients, whereas sugar-sweetened beverages provided the majority of sucrose intake among children. This knowledge can be used in improving health among children by dietary interventions, nutrition education, and health policy decision making.

Keywords: *food sources; energy; nutrients; vitamins; minerals; children; gender differences*

Children in Western countries fail to meet recommendations for many nutrients that are important for their health, growth, and development (1). For example, the intakes of saturated fat (SFA), sucrose, and salt are higher and the intakes of vitamin D, iron, and dietary fibre as well as unsaturated-to-saturated fatty acid ratio are lower than recommended among children in many Western countries, including Finland (2, 3).

Health promotion messages and nutrition counselling can be made more concrete and easier to adopt if they are based on food consumption rather than nutrient intake. Therefore, recent dietary guidelines, for example in Nordic countries, emphasise healthy dietary choices at food rather than nutrient level (4, 5). Consequently, it is important to have precise data on food sources of nutrients to better design strategies to enhance diet quality in different age groups.

†These authors contributed equally to this work.

There are few studies on the food sources of nutrients in children and most of them have reported the sources of only one or few nutrients (6–9). Milk products have been found to be among the main sources of energy, protein, and SFA among children in Europe (6, 8, 10) and the USA (11–13). Sugar-sweetened beverages have also been observed to be a major source of energy and refined carbohydrates among US children (13, 14). In a Swedish study, girls obtained more sucrose from sweets and chocolate, whereas boys received more sucrose from sugar-sweetened beverages (8). With the exception of the Swedish study (8), there are limited data on differences in the food sources of nutrients among girls and boys (11).

To provide detailed information on food sources of nutrients for health promotion and dietary counselling to correct the observed shortcomings in nutrient intake among children, we investigated the main food sources of energy, energy nutrients, dietary fibre, vitamins, and minerals among Finnish children 6–8 years of age. We also studied the gender differences in food sources of energy and these nutrients.

Methods

Study population

The present analyses are based on the baseline data of the Physical Activity and Nutrition in Children (PANIC) study, which is an ongoing physical activity and dietary intervention study in a population sample of primary school children from the city of Kuopio, Finland. We invited 736 children 6–8 years of age who were registered for the first grade in 16 primary schools, selected out of all 26 primary schools of Kuopio, in 2007–2009. We received the contact information of the children's principal custodians from the city of Kuopio and sent them the invitation letters by mail. Of 736 invited children, 512 (70%) participated in the baseline examinations that were conducted in 2007–2009. The participants did not differ in sex distribution, age, or body mass index standard deviation score (BMI-SDS) from all children who started first grade in primary schools of Kuopio in 2007–2009 based on available school health examination data. Complete dietary data were available for 430 children (213 girls and 217 boys) who were included in the analyses. These children did not differ in sex distribution, age, or BMI-SDS from those 82 children who had incomplete data and were excluded. The PANIC study protocol was approved by the research ethics committee of the Hospital District of Northern Savo. All participating children and their parents gave informed written consent.

Assessments

We assessed food consumption and nutrient intake by food records administered by the parents on 4 predefined consecutive days that included either consecutive 2 weekdays and 2 weekend days (99.5%) or consecutive 3 weekdays and 1 weekend day (0.5%). A clinical nutritionist instructed the parents to record all food and drinks consumed by their child at home, at school, in afternoon care, and elsewhere outside home using household or other measures, such as tablespoons, decilitres, and centimetres, in person at the first study visit. The parents were instructed to report the recipes of mixed dishes and the brands and the contents of food products. A clinical nutritionist reviewed the food records with the parents at the second study visit and completed the records using a picture booklet of portion sizes (15). Moreover, a clinical nutritionist asked the catering company about the details of food and drinks, such as menus, cooking fat, and spread on bread, served at schools and in afternoon care. All prepared foods and mixed dishes were disaggregated into ingredients according to the recipes used. We analysed food consumption and nutrient intake using The Micro Nutrica® dietary analysis software, version 2.5 (The Social Insurance Institution of Finland), that uses Finnish and international data on the nutrient compositions of foods (16). A clinical nutritionist also updated the software by adding new food items and products with their precise nutrient content received from the producers. Vitamin and mineral supplements were not included in these analyses. Food records that contained <4 days, contained inconsecutive days, did not include weekdays and weekend days, or lacked essential information for dietary analysis even after the review were excluded from the analyses. We estimate that 26% of girls and 24% of boys may have underreported their total energy intake in the food records when comparing it with energy expenditure estimated by basal metabolic rate and using the cut-offs for underreporting suggested by Torun et al. (17).

Foods consumed were divided into 55 food groups each of which included foods of similar nutrient composition and type of consumption (Table 1). We divided bread, breakfast cereals, and grain products into six food groups based on their fibre content. Bread, breakfast cereals, and grain products with at least 5% of fibre were considered high-fibre products. Meat products were divided into seven groups and fish was separated from shellfish and fish products. Fats and fat products were divided into five groups based on the amount and the quality of fat. Milk, sour milk products, and cheese were divided into six groups based on their fat content. Milk and sour milk products with <1% of fat were considered low-fat products. Cheese was defined low-fat cheese if it contained no more than 17% of fat. Ice creams and puddings were included in the same group. Sweetened beverages were divided into artificially sweetened and sugar-sweetened beverages. Energy drinks formed one group.

Table 1. Contents and median intakes (interquartile range) of the food groups in girls and boys

Food groups	Contents	All children ($n=430$), median (interquartile range)	Girls ($n=213$), median (interquartile range)	Boys ($n=217$), median (interquartile range)
High-fibre bread	Rye bread, crisp bread, wholegrain bread (fibre $\geq 5\%$)	37.5 (22.5, 59.0)	36.5 (21.1, 58.9)	37.5 (22.5, 59.0)
Low-fibre bread	White bread, white rolls (fibre $<5\%$)	22.0 (7.5, 40.1)	22.3 (7.5, 37.5)	21.7 (7.5, 45.0)
High-fibre breakfast cereals	Mueslis, breakfast cereals (fibre $\geq 5\%$)	0.0 (0.0, 3.8)	0.0 (0.0, 3.8)	0.0 (0.0, 4.1)
Low-fibre breakfast cereals	Breakfast cereals (fibre $<5\%$)	0.0 (0.0, 7.5)	0.0 (0.0, 7.5)	0.0 (0.0, 6.6)
High-fibre grain products	Wholegrain pasta, rice, oatmeal (fibre $\geq 5\%$)	9.6 (0.0, 24.1)	9.4 (0.0, 23.5)	10.5 (0.0, 24.9)
Low-fibre grain products	White pasta, rice, flours (fibre $<5\%$)	70.7 (45.0, 104.7)	71.8 (46.2, 100.4)	69.1 (42.6, 108.5)
Sweet pastry	Biscuits, cookies, cakes, pastries	0.0 (0.0, 6.8)	0.0 (0.0, 6.6)	0.0 (0.0, 7.1)
Potato	Potatoes	70.7 (44.7, 101.2)	68.3 (43.6, 100.4)	75.0 (48.3, 101.9)
Root vegetables	Carrot, beetroot, turnip	14.9 (3.8, 30.2)	16.9 (5.3, 31.6)	12.5 (1.7, 28.2)
Non-root vegetables	Green leafy vegetables, cabbages, cucumber, peppers, tomatoes, onions	68.3 (40.0, 103.9)	68.3 (43.1, 103.9)	68.3 (39.0, 104.8)
Legume and nut	Peas, beans, nuts, almonds, seeds	0.0 (0.0, 2.4)	0.0 (0.0, 2.2)	0.0 (0.0, 2.5)
Mushroom	Mushrooms	0.0 (0.0, 0.0)	0.0 (0.0, 0.0)	0.0 (0.0, 0.0)
Vegetable products	Ready-made vegetable products	0.0 (0.0, 0.0)	0.0 (0.0, 0.0)	0.0 (0.0, 0.0)
Fruit	Fruit and fruit purées	73.8 (33.6, 121.1)	75.8 (40.5, 126.8)	70.0 (27.5, 117.7)
Berry	Berries and berry purées	9.0 (0.0, 25.4)	9.9 (0.0, 28.2)	8.3 (0.0, 23.4)
Jam	Jams, marmalades	0.9 (0.0, 7.7)	1.6 (0.0, 8.0)	0.0 (0.0, 7.4)
Pork	Pork	29.5 (15.7, 46.8)	27.8 (13.8, 42.6)	32.6 (16.7, 56.5)**
Beef	Beef	13.5 (0.0, 29.0)	12.0 (0.0, 27.9)	14.5 (0.0, 30.5)
Sausage	Frankfurter, balkan, salami, ham sausage	15.0 (3.5, 31.8)	11.8 (0.0, 25.3)	18.0 (6.9, 34.6)**
Poultry	Chicken, turkey	10.3 (0.0, 24.5)	10.3 (0.0, 22.9)	10.0 (0.0, 27.2)
Game	Hare, moose, willow grouse	0.0 (0.0, 0.0)	0.0 (0.0, 0.0)	0.0 (0.0, 0.0)
Lamb and other meat	Lamb, horse, reindeer	0.0 (0.0, 0.0)	0.0 (0.0, 0.0)	0.0 (0.0, 0.0)
Organ meats	Liver, kidney, tongue	0.0 (0.0, 0.0)	0.0 (0.0, 0.0)	0.0 (0.0, 0.0)
Fish	Fresh fish	0.0 (0.0, 18.5)	0.0 (0.0, 17.1)	0.0 (0.0, 23.9)
Shellfish	Shellfish	0.0 (0.0, 0.0)	0.0 (0.0, 0.0)	0.0 (0.0, 0.0)
Fish products	Salted fish, smoked fish, canned fish, roe paste	0.0 (0.0, 0.0)	0.0 (0.0, 0.0)	0.0 (0.0, 0.0)
Egg	Eggs	10.0 (5.7, 19.1)	9.8 (5.8, 18.6)	10.9 (5.6, 19.6)
High-fat vegetable oil–based spreads	Vegetable oil–based spreads (fat 60–80%)[a]	5.0 (1.3, 10.3)	5.0 (1.5, 10.6)	4.5 (1.3, 9.9)
Low-fat vegetable oil–based spreads	Low-fat vegetable oil–based spreads (fat $<60\%$)[a]	0.0 (0.0, 5.3)	0.0 (0.0, 5.0)	0.0 (0.0, 6.1)
Vegetable oil	Vegetable oils, vegetable oil–based salad dressings	2.9 (1.2, 5.5)	2.5 (1.1, 5.0)	3.1 (1.2, 6.3)
Butter and butter-based spreads	Butter, butter-based spreads	3.0 (0.9, 7.9)	2.9 (1.0, 6.9)	3.1 (0.8, 10.1)
Shortenings and other added fats	Shortenings, lard, coconut fat	5.1 (2.7, 8.5)	5.1 (2.7, 8.6)	5.2 (2.7, 8.6)
Skimmed milk	Milk,[a] organic milk (fat $<1\%$)	371.7 (88.8, 602.8)	356.4 (91.4, 587.5)	421.2 (87.5, 633.8)
Fat-containing milk	Milk,[a] organic milk, farm milk (fat $\geq 1\%$)	95.8 (33.1, 264.4)	93.4 (31.2, 253.7)	102.6 (36.6, 301.7)
Low-fat sour milk products	Yoghurts, sour milk (fat $<1\%$)	0.0 (0.0, 9.9)	0.0 (0.0, 13.3)	0.0 (0.0, 8.9)
Sour milk products	Yoghurts, sour milk (fat $\geq 1\%$)	66.9 (25.0, 125.0)	65.0 (25.0, 114.4)	75.0 (25.0, 142.6)
Low-fat cheese	Cheese, cottage cheese, processed cheese, fromage frais (fat $\leq 17\%$)	2.5 (0.0, 10.0)	4.2 (0.0, 12.0)	0.6 (0.0, 9.0)*
Cheese	Cheese, processed cheese, blue cheese, fromage frais (fat $>17\%$)	4.2 (0.0, 10.1)	3.8 (0.0, 9.3)	5.0 (0.0, 11.2)
Ice cream and pudding	Ice creams, puddings	17.5 (0.0, 37.9)	16.3 (0.0, 40.9)	18.8 (0.0, 37.5)
Cream and other dairy products	Cream, sour cream, double cream, soya-, rice-, and oat-based milks and creams	10.6 (2.9, 20.0)	11.2 (3.8, 19.9)	10.4 (1.6, 20.2)

Table 1. (Continued)

Food groups	Contents	All children ($n = 430$), median (interquartile range)	Girls ($n = 213$), median (interquartile range)	Boys ($n = 217$), median (interquartile range)
Coffee	Coffee	0.0 (0.0, 0.0)	0.0 (0.0, 0.0)	0.0 (0.0, 0.0)
Tea	Tea	0.0 (0.0, 0.0)	0.0 (0.0, 0.0)	0.0 (0.0, 0.0)
Artificially sweetened beverage	Carbonated and non-carbonated artificially sweetened beverages	0.0 (0.0, 50.0)	0.0 (0.0, 0.0)	0.0 (0.0, 56.7)
Sugar-sweetened beverage	Carbonated and non-carbonated sugar-sweetened beverages	100.0 (43.4, 200.3)	87.5 (42.5, 200.0)	125.0 (50.0, 225.0)
Fruit juice	Natural fruit juices	1.4 (0.0, 50.0)	1.5 (0.0, 50.0)	0.8 (0.0, 50.0)
Energy drink	Energy drinks	0.0 (0.0, 0.0)	0.0 (0.0, 0.0)	0.0 (0.0, 0.0)
Water and other drinks	Water, mineral water, sport drink, mulled wine, berry fool	187.2 (108.2, 319.8)	163.4 (90.1, 277.8)	206.0 (121.6, 350.0)**
Sugar and honey	Table sugar, baking sugar, honey, syrup	7.7 (4.2, 13.3)	7.7 (4.1, 13.3)	7.4 (4.4, 13.3)
Candy	Sweets, chewing gums	12.5 (2.0, 31.1)	12.0 (2.0, 26.8)	15.0 (0.0, 37.5)
Chocolate and hot chocolate powder	Chocolate, hot chocolate powder	5.3 (0.2, 14.1)	5.0 (0.5, 12.5)	6.0 (0.0, 16.2)
Ready meal	Hamburgers, pizzas, nuggets	0.0 (0.0, 10.0)	0.0 (0.0, 5.6)	0.0 (0.0, 15.0)
Salt	Recipe and table salt	2.2 (1.8, 2.8)	2.1 (1.7, 2.6)	2.4 (1.9, 3.0)***
Condiments and sauces	Ketchup, mustard, soy sauce, chilli sauce, barbeque sauce	3.9 (0.4, 12.0)	4.0 (0.5, 13.0)	3.8 (0.3, 11.1)
Salty snacks	Popcorn, potato crisps, nachos, crackers, tacos	0.0 (0.0, 3.8)	0.0 (0.0, 3.8)	0.0 (0.0, 3.9)

[a]Fortified with vitamin D.
*$p < 0.05$ for difference between girls and boys. **$p < 0.01$ for difference between girls and boys. ***$p < 0.001$ for difference between girls and boys.

Statistical methods

Data were analysed using the SPSS for Windows software, Version 21.0 (IBM Corp. IBM SPSS Statistics for Windows, Armonk, NY). We compared differences in food consumption between genders by the Mann–Whitney U-test. The differences between genders with p-value < 0.05 were considered statistically significant. We calculated the contribution of each food group to the intakes of total energy, energy nutrients, dietary fibre, and selected vitamins and minerals using the population proportion method as defined by Krebs-Smith et al. (18). The percentage contribution of each food group to the intakes of total energy, energy nutrients, dietary fibre, and selected vitamins and minerals was estimated by summing the amount of a particular nutrient from the particular food group for all children and dividing this value by the sum of the nutrient from all foods for all children. The food sources of nutrients were ranked and top 10 sources were reported for all children, and for girls and boys separately.

Results

The medians (interquartile ranges) of the consumption of food groups in girls and boys are presented in Table 1. Boys consumed more pork, sausage, water and other drinks, and salt and less low-fat cheese than girls.

Food sources of energy, energy nutrients, and dietary fibre

Several food groups contributed almost similarly to the intake of energy, the two main sources being low-fibre grain products and skimmed milk in girls and boys (Table 2). Skimmed milk was the main source of protein in girls and boys, followed by fat-containing milk in girls and pork in boys. The main source of total fat was high-fat vegetable oil–based spreads, followed by shortenings and other added fats among girls and sausage among boys. The top two sources of SFA were cream and other dairy products and fat-containing milk in girls and fat-containing milk and butter and butter-based spreads in boys. The main source of monounsaturated fatty acids (MUFA) was high-fat vegetable oil–based spreads in girls and boys, followed by shortenings and other added fats among girls and by sausage among boys. The main source of polyunsaturated fatty acids (PUFA) was high-fat vegetable oil–based spreads followed by vegetable oil in girls and vegetable oil followed by high-fat vegetable oil–based spreads in boys. Low-fibre grain products were the major source of carbohydrates, followed by skimmed milk in girls and boys. Sugar-sweetened beverages and sugar and honey were the major sources of sucrose in both girls and boys. High-fibre bread was the major source of dietary fibre, followed by fruit and low-fibre grain products in girls and boys.

Table 2. Dietary sources of energy, energy nutrients, and dietary fibre in all children, girls, and boys

		All ($n = 430$)	Girls ($n = 213$)	Boys ($n = 217$)
Rank[a]	Food group	% of intake	% of intake	% of intake
Energy				
1	Low-fibre grain products	9.4	9.5	9.4
2	Skimmed milk	7.6	7.5	7.7
3	High-fibre bread	5.5	5.7	5.4
4	Fat-containing milk	5.4	5.4	5.3
5	Sour milk products	4.5	4.3	4.6
6	Candy	4.4	4.3	4.6
7	Low-fibre bread	4.0	4.0	4.0
8	Pork	3.7	3.4	3.9
9	Sugar-sweetened beverage	3.3	3.2	3.4
10	Potato	3.3	3.3	3.2
Protein				
1	Skimmed milk	18.3	18.2	18.4
2	Pork	9.2	8.7	9.7
3	Fat-containing milk	9.2	9.4	9.0
4	Low-fibre grain products	6.5	6.6	6.4
5	Beef	5.8	5.9	5.7
6	High-fibre bread	5.0	5.1	4.8
7	Poultry	4.6	4.8	4.4
8	Sour milk products	4.3	4.2	4.3
9	Sausage	3.7	3.1	4.2
10	Low-fibre bread	3.6	3.6	3.6
Total fat				
1	High-fat vegetable oil–based spreads	9.1	10.0	8.4
2	Shortenings and other added fats	8.1	8.6	7.7
3	Sausage	7.2	6.2	8.0
4	Pork	6.9	6.5	7.2
5	Butter and butter-based spreads	6.6	6.3	6.8
6	Vegetable oil	6.5	6.2	6.8
7	Fat-containing milk	5.4	5.3	5.4
8	Cream and other dairy products	5.3	5.8	4.8
9	Chocolate and hot chocolate powder	5.0	4.6	5.3
10	Ice cream and pudding	4.8	5.3	4.4
Saturated fatty acids				
1	Fat-containing milk	8.8	8.7	8.9
2	Cream and other dairy products	8.3	9.2	7.5
3	Butter and butter-based spreads	7.9	7.7	8.1
4	Shortenings and other added fats	7.9	8.3	7.5
5	Ice cream and pudding	7.2	7.9	6.6
6	Chocolate and hot chocolate powder	7.0	6.5	7.4
7	Sausage	6.8	5.8	7.6
8	High-fat vegetable oil–based spreads	6.6	7.3	6.0
9	Pork	6.2	5.9	6.5
10	Cheese	6.2	5.5	6.8
Monounsaturated fatty acids				
1	Vegetable oil–based spreads	12.2	13.4	11.2
2	Sausage	9.6	8.3	10.7
3	Vegetable oil	9.3	8.9	9.6
4	Pork	9.0	8.4	9.4
5	Shortenings and other added fats	8.5	9.0	8.1

Table 2. (Continued)

		All ($n = 430$)	Girls ($n = 213$)	Boys ($n = 217$)
Rank[a]	Food group	% of intake	% of intake	% of intake
6	Butter and butter-based spreads	5.3	5.0	5.7
7	Chocolate and hot chocolate powder	4.8	4.4	5.0
8	Cream and other dairy products	4.0	4.3	3.8
9	Ice cream and pudding	3.5	3.8	3.2
10	Fat-containing milk	3.2	3.2	3.3
Polyunsaturated fatty acids				
1	Vegetable oil	15.0	14.1	15.8
2	High-fat vegetable oil–based spreads	13.8	14.8	12.9
3	Shortenings and other added fats	11.0	11.9	10.2
4	Sausage	5.9	5.1	6.6
5	Pork	5.9	5.5	6.2
6	Low-fat vegetable oil–based spreads	5.5	4.9	6.0
7	Salty snacks	5.5	5.7	5.2
8	Low-fibre grain products	4.2	4.2	4.1
9	High-fibre bread	3.4	3.5	3.3
10	Butter and butter-based spreads	3.2	2.8	3.5
Carbohydrates				
1	Low-fibre grain products	14.8	14.8	14.8
2	Skimmed milk	8.5	8.3	8.7
3	Candy	8.3	7.9	8.7
4	High-fibre bread	8.0	8.2	7.9
5	Sugar-sweetened beverage	6.1	5.9	6.2
6	Low-fibre bread	5.7	5.6	5.7
7	Potato	5.5	5.6	5.4
8	Sour milk products	5.2	4.9	5.4
9	Fruit	5.0	5.5	4.5
10	Sugar and honey	4.5	4.7	4.3
Sucrose				
1	Sugar-sweetened beverage	21.2	20.5	21.7
2	Sugar and honey	17.5	18.4	16.6
3	Sour milk products	14.5	13.6	15.3
4	Candy	9.7	9.2	10.1
5	Chocolate and hot chocolate powder	8.0	7.4	8.5
6	Ice cream and pudding	6.4	6.8	6.0
7	Fruit	6.2	6.8	5.6
8	Sweet pastry	2.4	2.2	2.6
9	Fruit juice	2.4	2.1	2.6
10	Low-fibre breakfast cereals	2.0	2.2	1.9
Dietary fibre				
1	High-fibre bread	27.1	27.1	27.2
2	Fruit	11.7	12.4	11.0
3	Low-fibre grain products	10.9	10.7	11.0
4	High-fibre grain products	8.3	7.7	8.7
5	Potato	8.1	8.1	8.1
6	Low-fibre bread	7.5	7.1	7.8
7	Non-root vegetables	6.0	6.3	5.6
8	Berry	3.6	3.7	3.5
9	Root vegetables	3.3	3.7	3.0
10	High-fibre breakfast cereals	2.0	1.8	2.2

[a]Rank for all children.

Food sources of vitamins

Skimmed milk and fat-containing milk were the most important sources of vitamin D, followed by high-fat vegetable oil–based spreads among girls and by fish among boys (Table 3). The main source of vitamin E was high-fat vegetable oil–based spreads followed by vegetable oil in girls and vegetable oil followed by high-fat vegetable oil–based spreads in boys. The main sources of folate were non-root vegetables and potato in girls and boys. Non-root vegetables were the main source of vitamin C, followed by sugar-sweetened beverages among girls and boys.

Food sources of minerals

Sodium was mainly obtained from salt among girls and boys (Table 4). The main source of potassium was skimmed milk, followed by potato in girls and fat-containing milk in boys. Skimmed milk and fat-containing milk provided the majority of calcium intake in girls and boys. High-fibre bread was the main source of iron, followed by low-fibre grain products in girls and boys. The main sources of magnesium were skimmed milk and high-fibre bread in girls and boys. Similarly, skimmed milk was the main source of zinc, followed by high-fibre bread among girls and boys.

Discussion

Our study in a population sample of girls and boys 6–8 years of age provides new information on the top food sources of energy, energy nutrients, dietary fibre, and several vitamins and minerals among primary school children. Previous studies have mainly focused on the sources of one or few nutrients (9, 19–21), and only few studies have compared the food sources of nutrients among girls and boys (8, 11).

Milk products have been observed to be among the main sources of energy, protein, and SFA among children in Western countries (6, 8, 10–13). However, most of the previous studies have not analysed the contribution of milk products of different fat contents to the intake of nutrients. We found that skimmed milk was among the top sources of energy, protein, carbohydrates, vitamin D, folate, potassium, calcium, magnesium, and zinc. Fat-containing milk provided a lower proportion of all these nutrients than skimmed milk. This finding is due to the higher consumption of skimmed milk than fat-containing milk in the present study sample that is in line with the results of previous studies in Finnish children (1, 22). However, we observed that fat-containing milk was the highest source of SFA among children. Since milk is commonly consumed in large quantities among children, the consumption of fat-containing milk easily leads to an excessive intake of SFA. Because milk is an important source of several nutrients among children, sufficient intake of these nutrients from other sources should be assured among children who do not drink milk regularly.

Bread has been reported to provide 20–45% of the intake of dietary fibre among Finnish children (6) and European adolescents (23). We found that high-fibre bread was among the top sources not only for dietary fibre but also for iron, magnesium, and zinc. However, low-fibre grain products were the top source of energy and carbohydrates among children. These findings are explained by a higher density of dietary fibre and minerals but a lower consumption of high-fibre grain products than those of low-fibre grain products. Enhancing the use of high-fibre grain products at the expense of low-fibre grain products could be effective in improving the intake of several nutrients among children.

Previous studies have reported that sugar-sweetened beverages provide a considerable amount of energy and refined carbohydrates among children (8, 13, 14). In line with those findings, sugar-sweetened beverages were the top source of sucrose in children in this study, providing one-fifth of total sucrose intake. They were also the ninth most common source of energy and the fifth most common source of carbohydrates. The reduction in the consumption of sugar-sweetened beverages among children would markedly decrease their total intake of sucrose, which is currently higher than recommended (1, 24). Moreover, we found that sugar and honey provided almost 18% of the total sucrose intake in children. In this study, the food group of sugar and honey included all sugar used at home in baking, cooking, and as table sugar, and the dietary analysis software was unable to analyse sugar from recipes and sugar as such separately. This led to overestimation of sugar and honey as a source of sucrose at the expense of other food groups and needs to be acknowledged when comparing the dietary sources of sucrose in this study with those of other studies.

Previous studies have shown that the daily intake of vitamin D from food is around 6 μg in Finland (24–26) and even lower in the most Western countries (2, 3, 27). Products fortified with vitamin D have been reported to be major food sources of vitamin D in children across Europe and USA (10, 26–28). Whereas products fortified with vitamin D are available to a lesser extent in many other countries, in Finland most of the liquid dairy products and vegetable oil-based spreads have been fortified with vitamin D since 2003. In line with this, we found that the top sources of vitamin D among children were skimmed milk, fat-containing milk, and high-fat vegetable oil–based spreads that together contributed more than a half of the total intake of vitamin D. The level of fortification was increased in 2010, after the data collection of this study, in both liquid dairy products and fat spreads. Therefore, we suggest that the fortified products are even more abundant sources of vitamin D in Finnish children at the moment. Moreover, because

Table 3. Dietary sources of selected vitamins in all children, girls, and boys

		All ($n = 430$)	Girls ($n = 213$)	Boys ($n = 217$)
Rank[a]	Food group	% of intake	% of intake	% of intake
Vitamin D				
1	Skimmed milk[b]	31.9	32.0	31.8
2	Fat-containing milk[b]	16.1	16.7	15.6
3	High-fat vegetable oil–based spreads[b]	11.1	12.2	10.1
4	Fish	9.7	8.4	10.8
5	Low-fat vegetable oil–based spreads[b]	6.5	6.0	6.9
6	Shortenings and other added fats	6.3	6.7	6.0
7	Fish products	3.0	2.8	3.1
8	Egg	2.9	3.1	2.7
9	Pork	2.5	2.4	2.6
10	Butter and butter-based spreads	1.5	1.3	1.7
Vitamin E				
1	Vegetable oil	14.1	13.1	15.1
2	High-fat vegetable oil-based spreads	12.8	13.5	12.2
3	Non-root vegetables	5.4	5.8	5.0
4	High-fibre bread	5.2	5.4	5.1
5	Low-fat vegetable oil–based spreads	5.1	4.4	5.6
6	Shortenings and other added fats	4.4	4.4	4.4
7	Fruit	4.1	4.6	3.7
8	Low-fibre bread	3.9	4.0	3.8
9	Egg	3.8	3.9	3.6
10	Butter and butter-based spreads	3.1	2.7	3.4
Folate				
1	Non-root vegetables	13.5	14.4	12.7
2	Potato	11.5	11.5	11.5
3	Skimmed milk	9.3	8.9	9.7
4	Sour milk products	6.5	6.2	6.8
5	High-fibre bread	6.0	6.2	5.8
6	Fruit	5.8	6.3	5.3
7	Fat-containing milk	4.5	4.4	4.6
8	Low-fibre grain products	3.9	3.7	4.0
9	Low-fibre bread	3.8	3.6	4.0
10	Egg	3.3	3.3	3.3
Vitamin C				
1	Non-root vegetables	22.3	23.1	21.4
2	Sugar-sweetened beverage	18.4	17.3	19.5
3	Fruit	14.4	15.9	12.9
4	Fruit juice	13.6	12.6	14.5
5	Berry	10.5	10.3	10.7
6	Potato	7.2	7.0	7.3
7	Skimmed milk	4.9	4.6	5.2
8	Fat-containing milk	2.4	2.3	2.5
9	Root vegetables	2.0	2.1	2.0
10	Sour milk products	0.9	0.8	1.0

[a]Rank for all children. [b]Fortified with vitamin D.

skimmed milk was among the top sources of several vitamins and minerals, and high-fat vegetable oil–based spreads were among the top sources of MUFA, PUFA, and vitamin E, these products are not only good sources of vitamin D but also important sources of other nutrients among children.

Table 4. Dietary sources of selected minerals in all children, girls, and boys

		All ($n = 430$)	Girls ($n = 213$)	Boys ($n = 217$)
Rank[a]	Food group	% of intake	% of intake	% of intake
Sodium				
1	Salt	37.8	37.9	37.7
2	High-fibre bread	8.2	8.6	7.9
3	Skimmed milk	6.9	6.9	6.9
4	Sausage	6.6	5.8	7.3
5	Low-fibre bread	4.8	4.8	4.8
6	Pork	4.1	3.7	4.4
7	Fat-containing milk	3.2	3.3	3.1
8	Condiments and sauces	3.2	3.4	3.0
9	Ready meal	2.1	1.9	2.2
10	Low-fibre breakfast cereals	1.8	1.9	1.7
Potassium				
1	Skimmed milk	20.4	19.9	20.9
2	Potato	9.7	9.9	9.5
3	Fat-containing milk	9.7	9.7	9.6
4	Non-root vegetables	6.9	7.3	6.6
5	Fruit	6.3	6.8	5.8
6	Sour milk products	5.4	5.1	5.6
7	High-fibre bread	5.0	5.0	5.0
8	Sugar-sweetened beverages	2.9	2.8	3.0
9	Low-fibre grain products	2.8	2.8	2.8
10	Pork	2.8	2.6	3.0
Calcium				
1	Skimmed milk	38.9	38.6	39.2
2	Fat-containing milk	19.5	19.9	19.2
3	Sour milk products	8.6	8.3	8.8
4	Cheese	5.3	4.6	5.9
5	Low-fat cheese	4.8	5.3	4.4
6	Ice cream and pudding	2.5	2.7	2.4
7	Chocolate and hot chocolate powder	1.9	1.7	2.0
8	Low-fat sour milk products	1.9	1.9	1.8
9	Candy	1.6	1.5	1.6
10	Non-root vegetables	1.5	1.6	1.4
Iron				
1	High-fibre bread	12.4	12.7	12.0
2	Low-fibre grain products	9.3	9.4	9.2
3	Potato	6.2	6.3	6.0
4	Low-fibre bread	5.9	5.8	6.0
5	High-fibre grain products	5.9	5.7	6.1
6	Pork	5.4	5.1	5.6
7	Beef	4.2	4.3	4.2
8	Egg	3.7	3.9	3.6
9	Candy	3.7	3.5	3.9
10	Non-root vegetables	3.6	3.9	3.4
Magnesium				
1	Skimmed milk	16.7	16.4	17.1
2	High-fibre bread	11.7	11.9	11.6
3	Fat-containing milk	7.7	7.8	7.7
4	Potato	6.6	6.6	6.5
5	Fruit	5.0	5.4	4.6

Table 4. (*Continued*)

Rank[a]	Food group	All ($n = 430$) % of intake	Girls ($n = 213$) % of intake	Boys ($n = 217$) % of intake
6	Low-fibre grain products	4.8	4.9	4.7
7	High-fibre grain products	4.6	4.4	4.7
8	Low-fibre bread	4.3	4.2	4.4
9	Non-root vegetables	4.2	4.5	4.0
10	Sour milk products	3.9	3.7	4.1
Zinc				
1	Skimmed milk	16.2	16.1	16.3
2	High-fibre bread	9.8	10.1	9.5
3	Pork	9.0	8.6	9.4
4	Fat-containing milk	7.8	8.0	7.7
5	Beef	7.4	7.6	7.3
6	Low-fibre grain products	4.9	5.0	4.7
7	Low-fibre bread	4.0	3.9	4.0
8	Sour milk products	3.8	3.7	3.9
9	High-fibre grain products	3.8	3.7	4.0
10	Sausage	3.4	2.9	3.9

[a]Rank for all children.

Potato was among the top 10 sources of energy, carbohydrates, dietary fibre, folate, vitamin C, potassium, iron, and magnesium in our study sample. Although potato is not particularly rich in these nutrients (16, 29), high consumption of potato in Finland makes it as a good source of several nutrients. On the contrary, although the consumption of vegetables and fruit was relatively low among children in this study, they contributed markedly to the intakes of dietary fibre, vitamin E, folate, and vitamin C and to a lesser extent to the intakes of several minerals. This is due to the high density of these nutrients in vegetables and fruit (29).

Fish and fish products were among the top 10 sources of vitamin D in our study. However, fish did not markedly contribute to the intakes of any other nutrients, although it is high in protein and several minerals, such as calcium and potassium, and some fish species provide a considerable amount of PUFA (29). This finding is explained by the low consumption of fish among children in our study, which is in line with a previous report among Finnish children (1, 24).

In one previous study, meat provided more total and SFA in boys than in girls among 15-year-old adolescents, but the differences between genders were smaller among 9-year-old children (8). We also found that meat and sausages covered a slightly higher proportion of the intake of protein, fat, and sodium in boys than in girls. Moreover, vegetable oils provided a higher proportion of PUFA and vitamin E among boys, whereas high-fat vegetable oil–based spreads provided a higher proportion of these nutrients among girls. However, the rankings of most sources of nutrients did not differ between girls and boys. One explanation for the minor differences between girls and boys can be that our study sample consisted of primary school children who are provided a free-of-charge school meal every school day which may equalise food consumption between genders at this age. In addition, most of the gender differences in the sources of nutrients may not appear before adulthood (30).

A major strength of this study is the large population-based sample of Finnish primary school children. Another strength is that food consumption and nutrient intake were assessed by 4-day food records that were reviewed by a clinical nutritionist together with the family at return and analysed using a carefully updated nutrition database. A limitation of this study is that the grouping of food items was based on the judgement of a clinical nutritionist which could have had an influence on the rankings. If no detailed information was available, standard recipes were used for foods prepared at home, which could have led to either underestimation or overestimation of the intake of certain nutrients at an individual level. However, at group level this might have a minor effect only.

This study provides comprehensive data on the main food sources of nutrients among primary school girls and boys. Foods that are commonly recommended to be included in a healthy diet, such as skimmed milk, high-fibre grain products, vegetables, vegetable oil, and vegetable oil-based spreads, had a major contribution to the intake of several health-promoting nutrients, whereas sugar-sweetened beverages provided the majority of sucrose intake. This knowledge can be used in improving health among children by dietary interventions, nutrition education, and health policy decision making.

Acknowledgements

We are grateful to all voluntary subjects and their families participating in the PANIC study. We are also gratefully indebted to the research team for the skilful contribution in performing the study. The PANIC study was financially supported by grants from the Ministry of Social Affairs and Health of Finland, the Ministry of Education and Culture of Finland, the Finnish Innovation Fund Sitra, the Social Insurance Institution of Finland, the Finnish Cultural Foundation, the Juho Vainio Foundation, the Foundation for Paediatric Research, the Paavo Nurmi Foundation, the Paulo Foundation, the Diabetes Research Foundation, state research funding from the Research Committee of the Kuopio University Hospital Catchment Area, Kuopio University Hospital EVO funding, and the city of Kuopio.

Conflict of interest and funding

The authors declare that there is no conflict of interest.

References

1. Eloranta A, Lindi V, Schwab U, Kiiskinen S, Kalinkin M, Lakka HM, et al. Dietary factors and their associations with socioeconomic background in Finnish girls and boys 6–8 years of age: the PANIC study. Eur J Clin Nutr 2011; 65: 1211–18.
2. Lambert J, Agostoni C, Elmadfa I, Hulshof K, Krause E, Livingstone B, et al. Dietary intake and nutritional status of children and adolescents in Europe. Br J Nutr 2004; 92: S147–211.
3. Elmadfa I, Meyer AL, Nowak V, Hasenegger V, Putz P, Verstraeten R, et al. European Nutrition and Health Report 2009. Ann Nutr Metab 2009; 55: 1–40.
4. Nordic Council of Ministers (2014). Nordic nutrition recommendations, integrating nutrition and physical activity. Copenhagen, Denmark: Nordic Council of Ministers.
5. National Nutrition Council (2014). Finnish nutrition recommendations. Helsinki, Finland: National Nutrition Council. (in Finnish)
6. Kyttälä P, Ovaskainen M, Kronberg-Kippilä C, Erkkola M, Tapanainen H, Tuokkola J, et al. The diet of Finnish preschoolers. Helsinki, Finland: Publications of the National Public Health Institute; 2008. (in Finnish)
7. Erkkola M, Kronberg-Kippilä C, Kyttälä P, Lehtisalo J, Reinivuo H, Tapanainen H, et al. Sucrose in the diet of 3-year-old Finnish children: sources, determinants and impact on food and nutrient intake. Br J Nutr 2009; 28: 1209–17.
8. Patterson E, Wärnberg J, Kearney J, Sjöström M. Sources of saturated fat and sucrose in the diets of Swedish children and adolescents in the European Youth Heart Study: strategies for improving intakes. Public Health Nutr 2010; 13: 1955–64.
9. Cribb VL, Northstone K, Hopkins D, Emmett PM. Sources of vitamin A in the diets of pre-school children in the Avon longitudinal study of parents and children (ALSPAC). Nutrients 2013; 13: 1609–21.
10. Royo-Bordonada MA, Gorgojo L, de Oya M, Garcés C, Rodríguez-Artalejo F, Rubio R, et al. Food sources of nutrients in the diet of Spanish children: the four provinces study. Br J Nutr 2003; 89: 105–14.
11. Subar AF, Krebs-Smith SM, Cook A, Kahle LL. Dietary sources of nutrients among US children, 1989–1991. Pediatrics 1998; 102: 913–23.
12. Stroehla BC, Malcoe LH, Velie EM. Dietary sources of nutrients among rural native Americans and white children. J Am Diet Assoc 2005; 105: 1908–16.
13. Keast DR, Fulgoni VL, Nicklas TA, O'Neil CE. Food sources of energy and nutrients among children in the United States: National health and nutrition examination survey 2003–2006. Nutrients 2013; 5: 283–301.
14. Reedy J, Krebs-Smith SM. Dietary sources of energy, solid fats, and added sugars among children and adolescents in the United States. J Am Diet Assoc 2010; 110: 1477–84.
15. Paturi M, Nieminen R, Reinivuo H, Ovaskainen ML, editors. Picture book of food portion sizes. Helsinki, Finland: Publications of the National Public Health Institute; 2006.
16. Rastas M, Seppänen R, Knuts LR, Hakala P, Karttila V. Nutrient composition of foods. Helsinki, Finland: Publications of the Social Insurance Institution; 1997.
17. Torun B, Davies PS, Livingstone MB, Paolisso M, Sackett R, Spurr GB. Energy requirements and dietary energy recommendations for children and adolescents 1 to 18 years old. Eur J Clin Nutr 1996; 50: S37–81.
18. Krebs-Smith SM, Kott PS, Guenther PM. Mean proportion and population proportion: two answers to the same question? J Am Diet Assoc 1989; 89: 671–6.
19. Slining MM, Mathias KC, Popkin BM. Trends in food and beverage sources among US children and adolescents: 1989–2010. J Acad Nutr Diet 2013; 113: 1683–94.
20. Vandevijvere S, Michels N, Verstraete S, Ferrari M, Leclercq C, Cuenca-García M, et al. Intake and dietary sources of haem and non-haem iron among European adolescents and their association with iron status and different lifestyle and socio-economic factors. Eur J Clin Nutr 2013; 67: 765–72.
21. Campbell KJ, Hendrie G, Nowson C, Grimes CA, Riley M, Lioret S, et al. Sources and correlates of sodium consumption in the first 2 years of life. J Acad Nutr Diet 2014; 114: 1525–32.
22. Mäki P, Hakulinen-Viitanen T, Kaikkonen R, Koponen P, Ovaskainen ML, Sippola R, et al. Child health – results of the LATE-study of growth, development, health, health behavior and growth environment. Helsinki, Finland: National Institute for Health and Welfare; 2010.
23. Lin Y, Huybrechts I, Vereecken C, Mouratidou T, Valtueña J, Kersting M, et al. Dietary fiber intake and its association with indicators of adiposity and serum biomarkers in European adolescents: the HELENA study. Eur J Nutr 2015; 54: 771–82.
24. Kyttälä P, Erkkola M, Kronberg-Kippilä, Tapanainen H, Veijola R, Simell O, et al. Food consumption and nutrient intake in Finnish 1–6-year-old children. Public Health Nutr 2010; 13: 947–56.
25. Hoppu U, Lehtisalo J, Tapanainen H, Pietinen P. Dietary habits and nutrient intake of Finnish adolescents. Public Health Nutr 2010; 13: 965–72.
26. Soininen S, Eloranta AM, Lindi V, Venäläinen T, Zaproudina N, Mahonen A, et al. Determinants of serum 25-hydroxyvitamin D concentration in Finnish children: the Physical Activity and Nutrition in Children (PANIC) study. Br J Nutr 2016; 115(6): 1080–92.
27. Black LJ, Walton J, Flynn A, Kiely M. Adequacy of vitamin D intakes in children and teenagers from the base diet, fortified foods and supplements. Public Health Nutr 2014; 17: 721–31.

28. Berner LA, Keast DR, Bailey RL, Dwyer JT. Fortified foods are major contributors to nutrient intakes in diets of US children and adolescents. J Acad Nutr Diet 2014; 114: 1009–22.
29. Fineli, Finnish food composition database. Helsinki, Finland: National Institute for Health and Welfare, Nutrition Unit. Release 16. Available from: http://www.fineli.fi [cited 18 May 2015].
30. Helldán A, Raulio S, Kosola M, Tapanainen H, Ovaskainen ML, Virtanen S. The National FINDIET 2012 Survey. Helsinki, Finland: National Institute for Health and Welfare; 2013. (in Finnish)

*Aino-Maija Eloranta
Department of Physiology
Institute of Biomedicine
University of Eastern Finland
PO Box 1627
FI-70211 Kuopio, Finland
Email: aino-maija.eloranta@uef.fi

Dietary apigenin potentiates the inhibitory effect of interferon-α on cancer cell viability through inhibition of 26S proteasome-mediated interferon receptor degradation

Sheng Li[1†], Li-juan Yang[1†], Ping Wang[2], Yu-jiao He[1], Jun-mei Huang[1,2], Han-wei Liu[3], Xiao-fei Shen[1] and Fei Wang[1,4*]

[1]Chengdu Institute of Biology, Chinese Academy of Sciences, Chengdu, China; [2]School of Chinese Pharmacy, Chengdu University of Traditional Chinese Medicine, Chengdu, China; [3]Ningbo Entry-Exit Inspection and Quarantine Bureau Technical Center, Ningbo, China; [4]Sichuan Translational Medicine Research Hospital, Chinese Academy of Sciences, Chengdu, China

Abstract

Background: Type I interferons (IFN-α/β) have broad and potent immunoregulatory and antiproliferative activities. However, it is still known whether the dietary flavonoids exhibit their antiviral and anticancer properties by modulating the function of type I IFNs.
Objective: This study aimed at determining the role of apigenin, a dietary plant flavonoid abundant in common fruits and vegetables, on the type I IFN-mediated inhibition of cancer cell viability.
Design: Inhibitory effect of apigenin on human 26S proteasome, a known negative regulator of type I IFN signaling, was evaluated *in vitro*. Molecular docking was conducted to know the interaction between apigenin and subunits of 26S proteasome. Effects of apigenin on JAK/STAT pathway, 26S proteasome-mediated interferon receptor stability, and cancer cells viability were also investigated.
Results: Apigenin was identified to be a potent inhibitor of human 26S proteasome in a cell-based assay. Apigenin inhibited the chymotrypsin-like, caspase-like, and trypsin-like activities of the human 26S proteasome and increased the ubiquitination of endogenous proteins in cells. Results from computational modeling of the potential interactions of apigenin with the chymotrypsin site (β5 subunit), caspase site (β1 subunit), and trypsin site (β2 subunit) of the proteasome were consistent with the observed proteasome inhibitory activity. Apigenin enhanced the phosphorylation of signal transducer and activator of transcription proteins (STAT1 and STAT2) and promoted the endogenous IFN-α-regulated gene expression. Apigenin inhibited the IFN-α-stimulated ubiquitination and degradation of type I interferon receptor 1 (IFNAR1). Apigenin also sensitized the inhibitory effect of IFN-α on viability of cervical carcinoma HeLa cells.
Conclusion: These results suggest that apigenin potentiates the inhibitory effect of IFN-α on cancer cell viability by activating JAK/STAT signaling pathway through inhibition of 26S proteasome-mediated IFNAR1 degradation. This may provide a novel mechanism for increasing the efficacy of IFN-α/β.

Keywords: *apigenin*; *interferon*; *proteasome*; *STAT*; *ubiquitination*

Considerable attention has been devoted to identifying plant-derived dietary agents that could be developed as chemopreventives. One such agent is apigenin, a naturally occurring plant flavonoid (4′, 5, 7-trihydroxyflavone) abundant in common fruits and vegetables, including parsley, onions, oranges, tea, chamomile, wheat sprouts, and some seasonings. Apigenin exerts anti-inflammatory, antioxidant, and anticarcinogenic effects by targeting multiple cellular factors (1). Previously, apigenin has been reported to potently inhibit

[†]These authors contributed equally to this work.

the chymotrypsin-like activity of 26S proteasome and induce apoptosis in human leukemia cells, breast cancer cells, and other cancer cell lines (2–4). The inhibitory effect of apigenin and other natural flavonoids, such as (-)-epigallocatechin-3-gallate (EGCG), quercetin, chrysin, and resveratrol, on 26S proteasome may partly explain their beneficial effects in cancer prevention (5). However, the differential effects of apigenin on the three peptidase-like activities of the human 26S proteasome are unknown. These include caspase-like activity (β1 subunit), trypsin-like activity (β2 subunit), and chymotrypsin-like activity (β5 subunit), each of which has a distinct role in protein breakdown. These differential effects may influence the development of antineoplastic drugs (6, 7).

Type I interferons (IFN-α/β) are pleiotropic cytokines with broad and potent immunoregulatory and antiproliferative activities. IFNs mediate their effects by binding to cell-surface IFN receptors (IFNAR1/2), activating Janus kinases (Jak1, Tyk2), and subsequently phosphorylating signal transducer and activator of transcription proteins (STAT1, STAT2), which translocate into the nucleus and recognize a specific interferon α-stimulated response element (ISRE) motif in the promoter region of certain transcription genes (8). Type I IFNs have been clinically used for the treatment of various viral or cancerous diseases, such as hepatitis B/C, multiple sclerosis, leukemia, and melanoma. However, the side effects, such as neuropsychiatric and hematologic toxicities, which appear to be directly related to the dose and duration of IFN therapy, and drug tolerance severely limit their clinical use (9). Thus, chemical compounds that can mimic or enhance the effect of type I IFNs on the JAK/STAT signaling pathway have potential to be developed as next-generation antiviral and anticancer drugs. Some compounds have been identified through cell-based ISRE reporter screening to activate JAK/STAT signaling and exhibit antiviral or antiproliferative effects through different mechanisms, including suppression of the cyclic AMP-protein kinase A (PKA) – Src homology phosphatase 2 domain containing phosphatase (SHP2) pathway, inhibition of pyrimidine biosynthesis, or activation of type I IFN receptors (10–12). Thus, it is of interest to further investigate whether dietary compounds can exert beneficial effect on JAK/STAT signaling, the major system in humans for the prevention of infection and carcinogenesis.

The ubiquitin/26S proteasome pathway plays an important role in the negative regulation of IFN signaling. The binding of IFN to IFNAR1 induces the phosphorylation and ubiquitination of IFNAR1, which leads to the subsequent lysosomal degradation of ligand–IFNAR1 complex (13, 14). Phosphorylated Jak2 is polyubiquitinated and degraded by the 26S proteasome, which is regulated by the suppressor of cytokine signaling 1 (SOCS-1) (15). Phosphorylated STAT1 is also recognized by the F-box E3 ligase $SCF^{\beta TRCP}$ for ubquitination and 26S proteasomal degradation (16). Thus, inhibition of 26S proteasome may be a new therapeutic means to enhance the efficacy of IFNs and reduce their side effects.

Apigenin was identified as an activator of the JAK/STAT pathway and was found to increase the endogenous antiviral gene expression regulated by the type I IFNs (17). However, the mechanism by which apigenin acts on the JAK/STAT pathway is still unknown. In this study, we investigated the inhibition of proteasome and potentiation of type I IFN-induced JAK/STAT signaling by apigenin in detail.

Materials and methods

Reagents and plasmids

Apigenin (purity ≥99%, HPLC) was purchased from Must Biotechnology Co., Ltd. (Chengdu, China). IFN-α (recombinant human IFN-α2a) and IFN-β (recombinant human IFN-β1b) were purchased from ProSpec-Tany Techno Gene, Ltd. (Shanghai, China). Bortezomib, anti-ubiquitin antibody, and protein A/G agarose were purchased from Santa Cruz Biotechnology (Santa Cruz, CA). MG132 was purchased from Sigma-Aldrich (Shanghai, China). The purified human 26S proteasome, Ac-Arg-Leu-Arg-AMC, and Suc-Leu-Leu-Val-Tyr-AMC were purchased from Enzo Life Sciences (Farmingdale, NY). Z-Nle-Pro-Nle-Asp-aminoluciferin was purchased from Promega (Beijing, China). Anti-phospho-STAT1, anti-STAT1, anti-phospho-STAT2, anti-STAT2, and anti-GAPDH antibodies were purchased from Abcam (Cambridge, MA). Anti-IFNAR1 and anti-Ki67 antibodies were purchased from Proteintech (Chicago, IL). The 37-amino-acid long C-terminus of mouse ornithine decarboxylase (cODC) was amplified through a plasmid containing full-length mouse ODC (kindly provided by Prof. Philip Coffino, University of California San Francisco). The pCIneo-luciferase-cODC plasmid was obtained by subcloning the cODC fragment into a pCIneo-luciferase plasmid. This plasmid was constructed by cloning the luciferase gene from a pGL4.26 vector (Promega) into the pCI-neo mammalian expression vector (Promega). pCMV-ubiquitin plasmid was constructed by cloning the full-length coding sequence of human ubiquitin cDNA into pCMV 7.1 expression vector (Sigma). TUNEL apoptosis assay kit, Alexa Fluor 555-labeled anti-rabbit IgG and 4′, 6-diamidino-2-phenylindole (DAPI) were obtained from Beyotime (Haimen, China).

Cell culture

Human embryonic kidney 293A (HEK293A) cells (Qbiogene, Carlsbad, CA) and human cervical cancer HeLa cells (American Type Culture Collection, Manassas, VA) were maintained in Dulbecco's Modified Eagle Medium (DMEM; Invitrogen, Carlsbad, CA) containing 10% fetal calf serum (Invitrogen), and 1% penicillin/

streptomycin at 37°C in a 5% CO_2 atmosphere. The HEK293A-luciferase-cODC cell line and HepG2-ISRE-Luc2 cell line were established and maintained as previously reported (17, 18).

Measurement of peptidase activity

The purified human 26S proteasome (0.1 μg) was incubated with or without different concentrations of apigenin in 100 μL assay buffer (50 mM Tris-HCl, pH 7.5) and 40 μM fluorogenic peptide substrate Suc-Leu-Leu-Val-Tyr-AMC (for the proteasomal chymotrypsin-like activity), Ac-Arg-Leu-Arg-AMC (for the proteasomal trypsin-like activity), or Z-Nle-Pro-Nle-Asp-aminoluciferin (for the proteasomal caspase-like activity) for 2 h at 37°C. After incubation, the fluorescence was measured with a Thermo Scientific Varioskan Flash multimode reader.

Computational binding simulation

Molecular docking was carried out as previously reported with minor modifications (2). The crystal structure of eukaryotic yeast 20S proteasome was obtained from the Protein Database (Ref. number 1JD2) and used for all the docking studies presented here. The molecular docking simulation was performed and analyzed using AutoDock 4.2 and AutoDock Vina (19). AutoDock 4.2, a Lamarckian genetic algorithm method implemented in the program suite, was employed to identify appropriate binding modes and conformation of the ligand molecules. Docking pose was chosen based on two criteria. First, the proximity to the N-terminal threonine should lie in 3–4Å (a distance suitable for nucleophilic attack). Second, placement of the A–C ring system of the molecule should be within the S1 hydrophobic pocket. Of the orientations/conformations that fit these two criteria, the docked structure of lowest docked free energy was chosen. The output from AutoDock and all modeling studies as well as images was rendered with PyMOL, which was used to calculate the distances of hydrogen bonds as measured between the hydrogen and its assumed binding partner (20).

Western blotting

Cells were lysed in RIPA buffer and the lysates were subjected to sodium dodecyl sulfate-polyacrylamide gel electrophoresis. The proteins were blotted onto nitrocellulose membranes, probed with each specific antibody and an appropriate peroxidase-conjugated secondary antibody, and detected by enhanced chemiluminescence (Amersham Biosciences, Piscataway, NJ). Protein concentration was measured with a BCA protein assay kit (Bestbio, Shanghai, China).

Real-time quantitative reverse transcription-polymerase chain reaction

Total cellular RNA was isolated by TRIzol reagent, which was then reverse-transcribed using SuperScript III Reverse Transcriptase with oligo dT_{18} primer (Invitrogen). Equal amounts of complementary DNA were subjected to real-time quantitative PCR with the fluorescent dye SYBR Green I. The primer pairs used in the assay for IFN-induced double-stranded RNA-activated protein kinase (PKR), 2′,5′-oligoadenylate synthetase 1 (2′,5′-OAS1), and GAPDH were the following: 5′-GTTTGCTTCT CTGGCGGTCTT-3′/5′-GCCATTTCTTCTTCCCGTAT CC-3′ (PKR), 5′-AGGTGGTAAAGGGTGGCTCC-3′/5′-ACAACCAGGTCAGCGTCAGAT-3′ (2′,5′-OAS1), 5′-TGCACCACCAACTGCTTAGC-3′/5′-GGCATGGACT GTGGTCATGAG-3′ (GAPDH). The quantity of PKR and 2′,5′-OAS1 mRNA was normalized to the endogenous reference (GAPDH) mRNA in the same samples.

Immunoprecipitation

Cell lysates were prepared in ice-cold immunoprecipitation buffer (20 mM Tris-HCl, 200 mM NaCl, 1 mM EDTA, 0.5% Nonidet P-40, pH 8.0) with PMSF and protease cocktail inhibitors (Sigma). The mixture was centrifuged at 13,000 × g for 15 min, cleared with normal immunoglobulin G coupled to agarose beads (protein A/G) for 1 h, incubated overnight at 4°C with IFNAR1 antibody, and then incubated with protein A/G agarose beads for 4 h. The precipitates were washed thrice in PBS buffer, centrifuged at 3,000 × g for 3 min, resuspended in 5 × loading buffer, and boiled for 5 min. The supernatants were loaded onto sodium dodecyl sulfate-polyacrylamide gel electrophoresis and immunoblotted with anti-ubiquitin antibody.

Cell viability assay

HeLa cells were seeded in 96-well plates at a density of 5×10^3 cells/well in 100 μL of media. Cultured cells were treated with apigenin or a combination of apigenin with IFN-α at the indicated concentrations. After 72 h, 10 μL of Alamar Blue reagent was added to the media and incubated for another 2–4 h until the development of pink color. The relative fluorescence intensity was measured using a Thermo Scientific Varioskan Flash multimode reader.

Colony formation assay

The HeLa cells, at the logarithmic phase, were plated in 6-well plates at the density of 600 cells/well. Cells were treated with emodin in combination with IFN-α and allowed to grow for 12 days to form colonies. A colony was defined as a cluster of more than 50 cells. Then, cells were fixed with methanol and stained with 0.1% crystal violet solution for 20 min, and the colonies (>50 cells) were counted under microscope.

Statistical analysis

Statistical analyses were performed with GraphPad Prism 5.0 software (GraphPad, La Jolla, CA). All experiments were repeated at least thrice. Representative results are presented. Data were compared by one-way ANOVA followed by Dunnett's post hoc test. The differences were considered statistically significant when $p \leq 0.05$.

Results

Identification of apigenin as an inhibitor of 26S proteasome

To identify inhibitors of 26S proteasome, we established a HEK293A cell line stably transfected with pCIneo-luciferase-cODC plasmid (HEK293A-luciferase-cODC). The native ODC is recognized by 26S proteasome for degradation through a small conserved degradation tag (37 amino acids in mouse and human) at its C-terminus (cODC) without the need of ubiquitin modification (21). Using this ubiquitin-independent, 26S proteasome-specific cell-based assay, we screened our chemical library consisting of 1,431 natural products and synthetic analogues (17). After hit reconfirmation, apigenin was identified as potently increasing luciferase expression. The chemical structure of apigenin is illustrated in Fig. 1a. Bortezomib, a specific 26S proteasome inhibitor used in clinic for the treatment of multiple myeloma, also increased luciferase expression, confirming that HEK293A-luiferase-cODC cells specifically respond to inhibition of 26S proteasome (Fig. 1b). Apigenin at 1 and 10 μM increased luciferase activity 1.3- and 2.3-fold, respectively, over that of DMSO-treated control cells (Fig. 1b). The EC_{50} value for apigenin to inhibit luciferase-cODC degradation was 4.08 μM (Fig. 1c). Apigenin did not exhibit cytotoxicity at the concentrations examined (Supplementary Fig. 1). Promotion of luciferase-cODC expression by apigenin at 10 μM was first evident at 2 h and was sustained until 12 h, at which time luciferase-cODC expression increased by approximately 1.8-fold compared to that in the control (Fig. 1d). Similarly, a proteasomal inhibitor MG132 at 1 μM also promoted luciferase-cODC expression in a time-dependent manner (Supplementary Fig. 2). These results suggest that apigenin inhibits 26S proteasome to stabilize luciferase-cODC.

Inhibitory effect of apigenin on 26S proteasome activity

Purified human 26S proteasome was used to examine whether apigenin directly inhibits 26S proteasome. As shown in Fig. 2a, apigenin inhibited the chymotrypsin-like activity of purified 26S proteasome, with an IC_{50} value of 11.5 μM. Apigenin inhibited the trypsin-like activity of 26S proteasome with an IC_{50} value of 20 μM (Fig. 2b). Apigenin also potently inhibited the caspase-like activity of 26S proteasome, with an IC_{50} value of 1.5 μM (Fig. 2c).

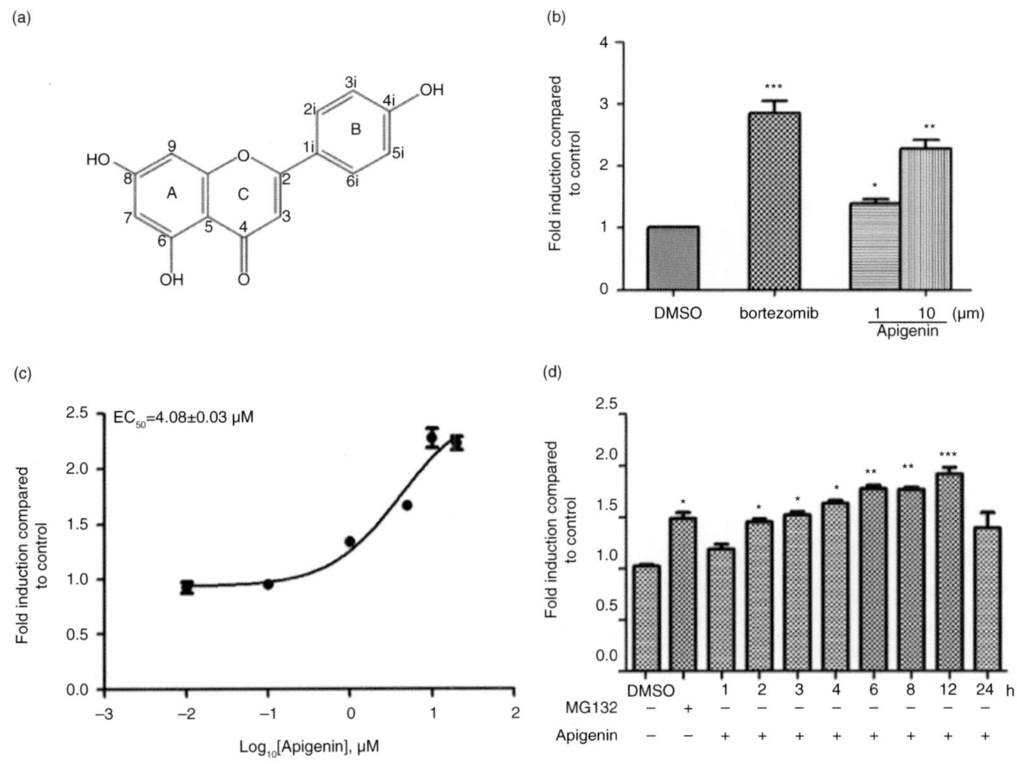

Fig. 1. Identification of apigenin as an inhibitor of 26S proteasome in HEK293A-luciferase-cODC cells. (a) Chemical structure of apigenin. (b) HEK293A-luciferase-cODC cells were seeded in 96-well plates and treated in the presence of indicated concentrations of apigenin or bortezomib for 3 h. (c) Concentration–response curve for apigenin. The calculated EC_{50} value was 4.08 μM. (d) HEK293A-luciferase-cODC cells were seeded in 96-well plates and treated with 10 μM apigenin for the indicated time, or treated with 1 μM MG132 for 4 h. Results are representative of three separate experiments. The error bars represent the standard deviation of the measurements. (*) $p < 0.05$, (**) $p < 0.01$, (***) $p < 0.001$ compared to the DMSO control.

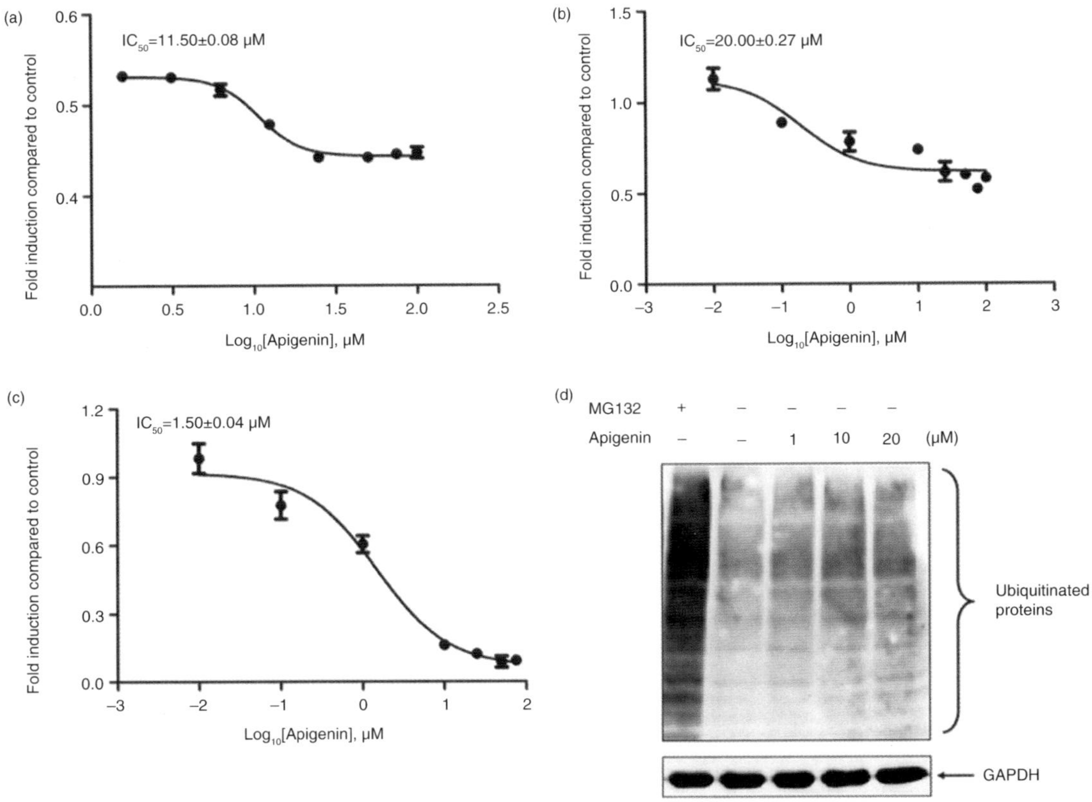

Fig. 2. Inhibitory effect of apigenin on 26S proteasome activity. The purified human 26S proteasome (0.1 μg) was treated with different concentrations of apigenin and (a) 40 μM Suc-Leu-Leu-Val-Tyr-AMC (for the chymotrypsin-like activity), (b) 40 μM Ac-Arg-Leu-Arg-AMC (for the trypsin-like activity), (c) 40 μM Z-Nle-Pro-Nle-Asp-aminoluciferin (for the caspase-like activity) for 2 h at 37°C. (d) HeLa cells were treated with the indicated concentrations of apigenin or 10 μM MG132 for 3 h, and the cell lysates were probed with anti-ubiquitin antibody. GAPDH was used as an internal control.

To examine the effect of apigenin on endogenous protein ubiquitination, we treated cells with apigenin (1–20 μM) and the total cell lysates were probed with ubiquitin antibody. As shown in Fig. 2d, inhibition of 26S proteasome by MG132 treatment significantly increased the endogenous protein ubiquitination level. Apigenin also increased endogenous protein ubiquitination levels. These results indicate that apigenin inhibits the activity of 26S proteasome, which can lead to the accumulation of protein ubiquitination in cells.

Molecular docking of apigenin on the proteasome subunits

To investigate the nature of the interactions through which apigenin inhibits the activity of the proteasome, the compound was docked to the active site of the proteasome β1, β2, and β5 subunits, which are responsible for the caspase-like, trypsin-like, and chymotrypsin-like activity, respectively. AutoDock arranges its results by energy and clusters of solutions that adopt the same conformation (see Materials and Methods for details). As shown in Fig. 3a, apigenin adopted a conformation favorable for nucleophilic attack at the active site of the β5 subunit with an energy of −5.97 kcal/mol. To further investigate the favorable binding mode of apigenin to the proteasomal chymotrypsin active site, we analyzed hydrogen-bond (H-bond) formation and hydrophobic interactions between apigenin and the β5 subunit. There are three polar hydrogens and two carbonyl-oxygens on apigenin that are available for H-bonding (see Fig. 1a). It appears that two hydrogens and one carbonyl-oxygen are capable of actively participating in H-bonding with the side chains of Thr1, Arg19, Lys33, and Ala49 (Fig. 3b). The A–C ring system of apigenin was favorably oriented in the middle of the S1 hydrophobic pocket of the β5 subunit driven by hydrophobic interactions (Fig. 3c). Similarly, apigenin adopted a conformation favorable for nucleophilic attack at the active site of the β2 subunit with an energy of −7.19 kcal/mol (Fig. 3d). Two hydrogens in the A ring and two oxygens in the C ring of apigenin were capable of participating in H-bonding with the side chains of Thr21, Ser20, Thr52, Gly45, and Gly47 (Fig. 3e). The A–C ring of apigenin was favorably inserted within the S1 pocket of the β2 subunit by hydrophobic interactions (Fig. 3f). Apigenin also adopted a conformation favorable for nucleophilic attack at the active site of the β1 subunit with an energy of −5.32 kcal/mol (Fig. 3g). Two hydrogens in the A ring and two oxygens in the C ring of apigenin were capable of participating in H-bonding with the side chains of Thr1, Arg19, and Ser68 (Fig. 3h). The A–C ring of apigenin was

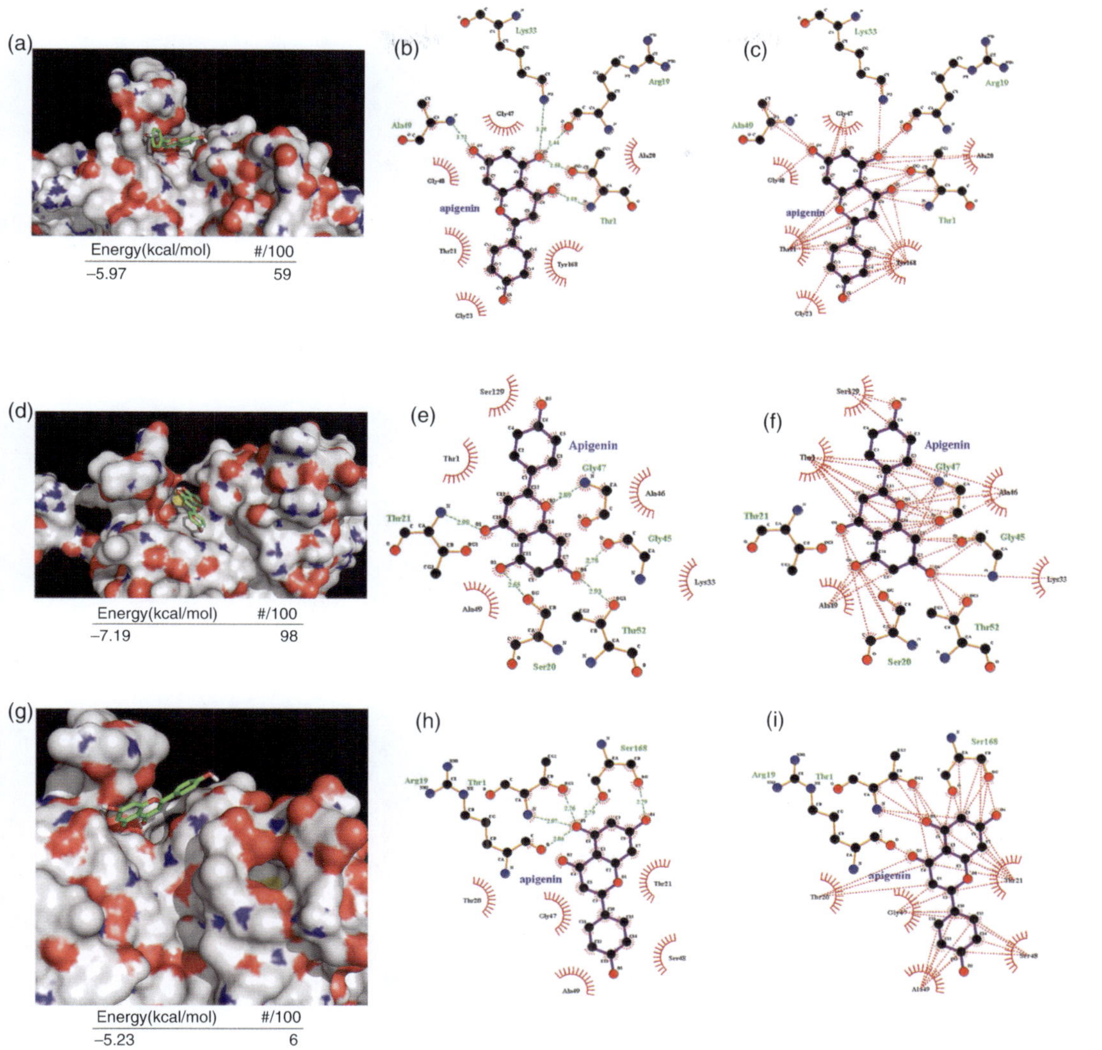

Fig. 3. Molecular docking of apigenin on the proteasome subunits. (a–c) Apigenin was docked to β5 subunit of the proteasome. The energy of the inhibitory pose and the number of runs (out of 100) that adopted the inhibitory pose was shown below (a). The threonine catalytic residue and all amino acids in the S1 pocket of β5 subunit involved in the formation of H-bonds (b) and hydrophobic interactions (c) with apigenin are highlighted. (d–f) Apigenin was docked to β2 subunit of the proteasome. The energy of the inhibitory pose and the number of runs (out of 100) that adopted the inhibitory pose was shown below (d). The threonine catalytic residue and all amino acids in the S1 pocket of β2 subunit involved in the formation of H-bonds (e) and hydrophobic interactions (f) with apigenin are highlighted. (g–i) Apigenin was docked to β1 subunit of the proteasome. The energy of the inhibitory pose and the number of runs (out of 100) that adopted the inhibitory pose was shown below (g). The threonine catalytic residue and all amino acids in the S1 pocket of β1 subunit involved in the formation of H-bonds (h) and hydrophobic interactions (i) with apigenin are highlighted.

also favorably inserted within the S1 pocket of the β1 subunit by hydrophobic interactions (Fig. 3i). These results suggest that apigenin can exhibit an orientation/conformation in the proximity to the N-terminal Thr1 of β1, β2, and β5 catalytic subunits making them subject to nucleophilic attack.

Apigenin enhances the IFN-α/β-induced activation of the JAK/STAT pathway

Considering the important role of 26S proteasome in the attenuation of JAK/STAT pathway signaling, we hypothesize that apigenin may enhance the activation of JAK/STAT pathway by inhibiting 26S proteasome. To test this, we first examined the effect of apigenin on IFNα/β-induced JAK/STAT signaling. As shown in Fig. 4a, apigenin potently increased ISRE luciferase reporter expression induced by IFN-α or IFN-β in a concentration-dependent manner. Apigenin at 10 μM alone significantly increased ISRE reporter expression, as previously reported (17). We then examined the effect of apigenin alone on tyrosine phosphorylation of STAT1, the key factor mediating ISRE gene transcription. However, no obvious tyrosine phosphorylation of STAT1 was observed, possibly owing to the limitation of detection using

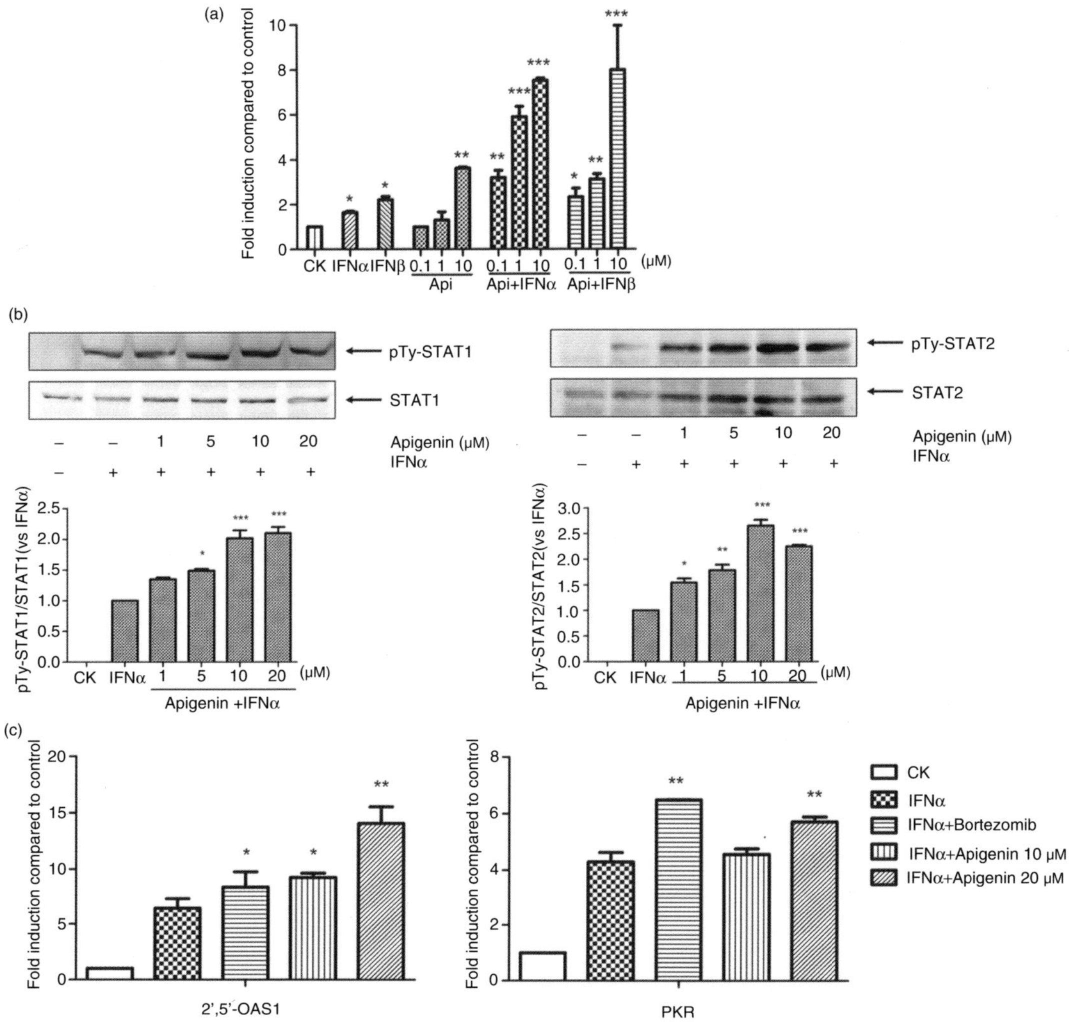

Fig. 4. Apigenin enhances IFN-α/β-induced JAK/STAT activation. (a) HepG2-ISRE-Luc2 cells were seeded in 96-well plates (1×10^4/well) and treated with the various concentrations of apigenin for 2 h, then with 200 U/mL IFN-α or IFN-β for 24 h. (b) HEK293A cells were incubated with indicated concentrations of apigenin for 2 h, then with 2000 U/mL IFN-α for another 1 h. The cell lysates were immunoblotted with phospho-STAT1 (Tyr701), STAT1, phospho-STAT2 (Tyr690), or STAT2 antibodies. The quantitative results are shown. (c) HEK293A cells were treated 200 U/mL IFN-α with or without 10 μM bortezomib or the indicated concentrations of apigenin for 24 h. Real-time quantitative reverse transcription-PCR was used to determine the mRNA expression of PKR or 2′,5′-OAS1. The result is presented as induction (n-fold) relative to basal levels in untreated cells. GAPDH was used as an internal control. (*) $p < 0.05$, (**) $p < 0.01$, (***) $p < 0.001$ versus control ($n = 3$).

anti-phospho-STAT1 antibody (data not shown). To further determine the effect of apigenin on type I IFNs, we examined the phosphorylation state of STATs in response to IFN-α. Apigenin increased the tyrosine phosphorylation of STAT1 and STAT2 in a concentration-dependent manner over that observed with IFN-α alone (Fig. 4b). The tyrosine phosphorylation of STAT1 was also increased in combination with luteolin and various concentrations of IFN-α (Supplementary Fig. 3). PKR and 2′,5′-OAS1 are IFN-α-responsive genes that contain an ISRE consensus sequence in their promoter regions. We examined the effect of apigenin on the mRNA expression of these two genes in combination with IFN-α. As shown in Fig. 4c, the mRNA expression of both IFN-regulated genes significantly increased after treatment with a combination of apigenin and IFN-α over that accompanying IFN-α treatment alone. These results indicate that apigenin enhances the activation of type I IFNs-induced JAK/STAT signaling.

Apigenin inhibits the ubiquitination and degradation of IFNAR1

Ligand-induced degradation of IFNAR1 is a key step in the negative regulation of IFN signaling. As an inhibitor of 26S proteasome, apigenin may activate the JAK/STAT pathway by inhibiting IFNAR1 degradation. To test this hypothesis, we examined the effect of apigenin on IFNAR1 degradation. As shown in Fig. 5a, in the presence of

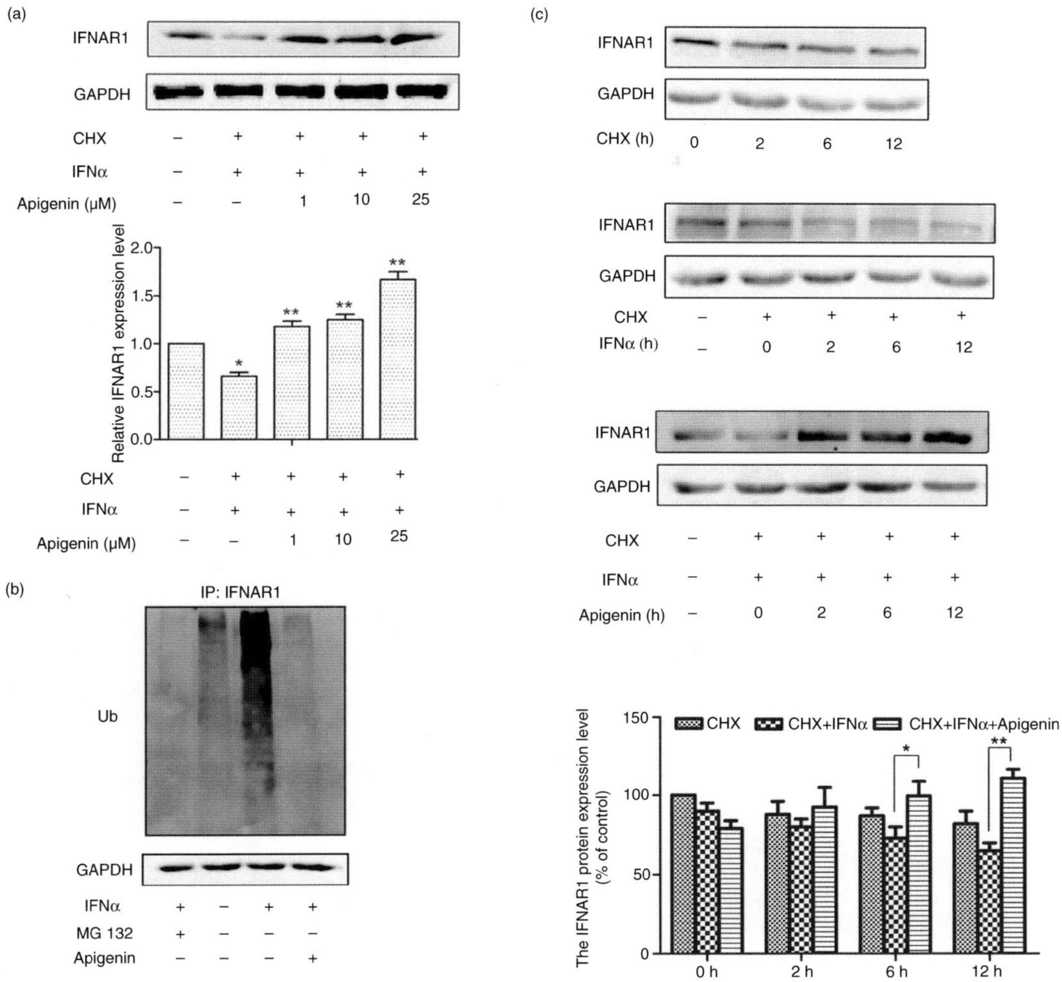

Fig. 5. Apigenin inhibits IFN-α-induced degradation of IFNAR1. (a) HEK293A cells were treated with 20 μM cycloheximde (CHX) for 2 h, and then with apigenin (1 μM, 10 μM, 25 μM) for 12 h before the treatment with IFN-α (1×10^4 U/mL) for an additional 2 h. The cell lysates were immunoblotted with anti-IFNAR1 antibody. GAPDH staining is shown as a loading control. (b) HeLa cells were transfected with pCMV-ubiquitin plasmid for 48 h and incubated with MG132 (20 μM) or apigenin (20 μM) for 12 h before treatment with IFN-α (1×10^4 U/mL) for another 2 h. Cell lysates were immunoprecipitated with the IFNAR1 antibody. Immunoblotting was performed using ubiquitin antibody. GAPDH antibody staining represents 5% of the total cell lysates used in immunoprecipitation. (c) HeLa cells were treated with 20 μM CHX, IFN-α (1×10^4 U/mL) or apigenin (20 μM) for the indicated time. The cell lysates were immunoblotted with anti-IFNAR1 antibodies. GAPDH staining is shown as a loading control.

cycloheximde (CHX) to block *de novo* protein synthesis, IFN-α treatment stimulated the degradation of IFNAR1, as previously reported (13). Apigenin significantly inhibited the degradation of IFNAR1 stimulated by IFN-α. IFNAR1 is ubiquitinated for lysosomal degradation, which can be inhibited by 26S proteasome inhibitors (13). We next examined the effect of apigenin on IFNAR1 ubiquitination. We transiently overexpressed ubiquitin in cells and performed a co-immunoprecipitation experiment using the anti-IFNAR1 antibody. As shown in Fig. 5b, IFN-α treatment simulated the ubiquitination level of IFNAR1, which was inhibited by the 26S proteasome inhibitor MG132 and by apigenin. We also examined the effect of apigenin on ubiquitination level of endogenous proteins in the cell lysates transiently overexpressing ubiquitin. IFN-α slightly decreased ubiquitination level of endogenous proteins compared with DMSO control. Compared with that, addition of MG132 or apigenin increased ubiquitination level of endogenous proteins (Supplementary Fig. 4). We then examined the time course of apigenin in the inhibition of IFN-α-induced IFNAR1 degradation. As shown in Fig. 5c, apigenin significantly increased the expression of IFNAR1 in the presence of IFN-α in a time-dependent manner, compared with that in the presence of IFN-α alone. MG132 also inhibited IFN-α-induced IFNAR1 degradation in a time-dependent manner (Supplementary Fig. 5). These results indicate that apigenin protects IFNAR1 from degradation.

Apigenin potentiates the inhibitory effect of IFN-α on cancer cell viability

To examine whether apigenin can potentiate the inhibitory effect on cell viability induced by IFN, we treated human cervical cancer HeLa cells with apigenin and IFN-α. As shown in Fig. 6a, apigenin, in a concentration-dependent manner, significantly enhanced the inhibitory effect of IFN-α on cell viability, whereas apigenin alone at 1–20 μM had no effect on HeLa cell viability (Supplementary Fig. 6). Furthermore, INF-α alone or IFN-α plus apigenin did not exhibit the suppression on the cell viability of non-carcinoma HEK293A cells (Supplementary Fig. 7). We then examined the effect of apigenin on the proliferation and apoptosis of HeLa cells. As shown in Supplementary Fig. 8, the pro-apoptotic effects of INF-α alone or IFN-α plus apigenin were not observed. Moreover, treatment with IFN-α resulted in decreased colony formation in HeLa cells compared with the untreated control cells. The addition of apigenin significantly decreased the number and size of colonies, respectively, compared with cells treated by IFN-α alone (Fig. 6b). These results suggest that apigenin enhances the inhibitory effect of IFN-α on viability but not on proliferation and apoptosis in HeLa cancer cells.

Discussion

By using a cell-based screening assay, apigenin was identified as an inhibitor of 26S proteasome-mediated luciferase-cODC degradation. This result is well supported by previous findings that apigenin inhibits the chymotrypsin-like activity of 20S proteasome and induces apoptosis in tumor cells, thus validating that the assay can be used for the screening and evaluation of 26S proteasome activity (2, 3) Apigenin has been found to inhibit, in a concentration-dependent manner from 1 to 20 μM, skin cancer promotion by directly inhibiting epidermal ODC activity induced by 12-O-tetradecanoyl phorbol-13-acetate (TPA) (22). In this study, apigenin was found to inhibit cODC-induced luciferase degradation at similar concentrations (1–20 μM), indicating that apigenin may not only inhibit ODC activity but also stabilize ODC protein. Apigenin inhibited the chymotrypsin-like activity of purified 26S proteasome with a potency different from that observed in previous studies; this difference was possibly owing to the fact that the proteasome used in these studies was from different species (2, 23). The specificity of apigenin for the three peptidase activities of human 26S proteasome was previously unknown. In this study, apigenin inhibited the three peptidase activities in the following order of potency caspase-like activity > chymotrypsin-like activity > trypsin-like activity. This result is consistent with the previous finding that flavones have strong inhibitory effects on chymotrypsin-like and caspase-like activities (23). Structure–proteasome inhibitory activity relationship studies of dietary flavonoids suggest that dietary flavonoids with OH groups on the B ring and/or the double bond between C2 and C3 of the pyranosyl moiety are natural potent proteasome inhibitors (24). This is further supported by our finding that apigenin could be favorably inserted within the S1 hydrophobic pockets of

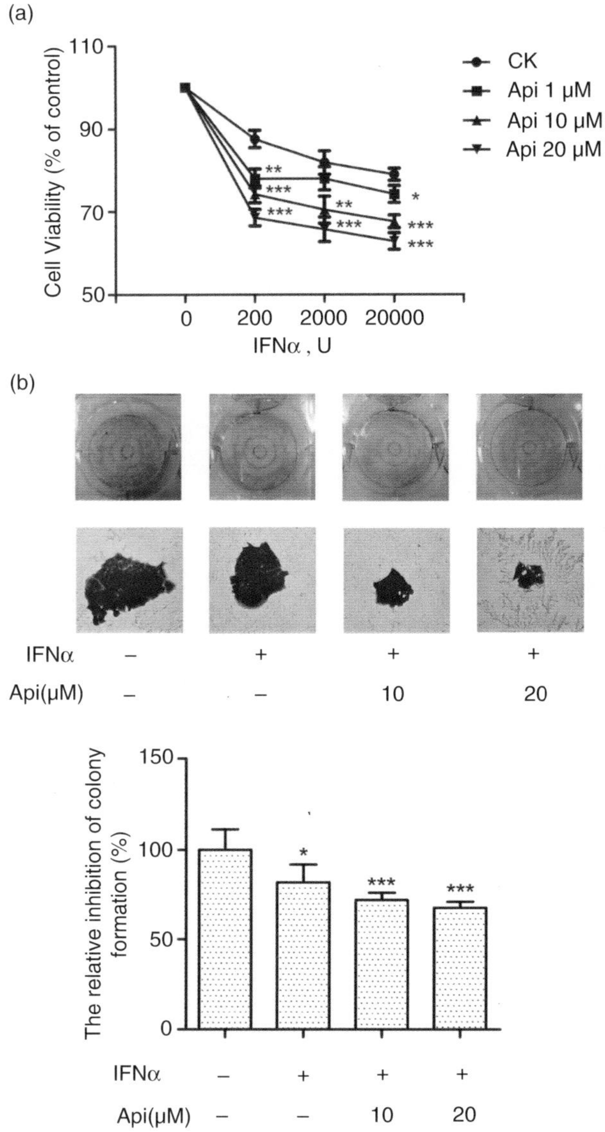

Fig. 6. Apigenin potentiates the inhibitory effect of IFN-α on cancer cell viability. (a) The HeLa cells (5×10^3 cells/well) were seeded in 96-well plates and treated under indicated concentrations of apigenin and IFN-α for 72 h. Cell viability was measured by Alamar Blue assay and the values are expressed as the percentage cell viability relative to the DMSO control. (b) The HeLa cells growing in 6-well plates were treated with the indicated concentrations of apigenin and IFN-α (1×10^4 U/mL) for 12 days, and then colonies were visualized by staining with crystal violet and counted manually. The bar graph was obtained by calculating the percentages of colony numbers from each well relative to the DMSO-treated control. (*) $p < 0.05$, (**) $p < 0.01$, (***) $p < 0.001$ versus control ($n = 3$).

the β1, β2, and β5 subunits through H-bonding and hydrophobic interactions. The two hydroxyl groups on ring A of apigenin play a key role in the formation of H-bonds with residues in the active site of β1, β2, and β5 subunits to inhibit the Thr1 residue-mediated cleavage of peptides. These results also further support the finding that the 6-hydroxy group of the flavones may have an important role in targeting 26S proteasome, and this would help in the development of new 26S proteasome inhibitors (23).

Apigenin at high concentrations (>40 μM) induces apoptosis in leukemia cells and breast cancer cells and sensitizes the malignant tumor cells to tumor necrosis factor-related apoptosis-inducing ligand (TRAIL)-induced apoptosis (2–4). However, the daily dietary intake of apigenin is less likely to increase the concentration of apigenin to such high levels. This is the first study to report that apigenin at physiologically achievable concentrations (1–20 μM) can activate the type I IFN-induced JAK/STAT pathway and increase the endogenous IFN-regulated gene expression, resulting in the sensitization of cancer cells to the anti-cell viability effect of type I IFNs. In this study, we found that apigenin increased IFNAR1 accumulation in a time- and concentration-dependent manner, indicating that it may stabilize IFN-bound IFNAR1 via proteasome inhibition. Ubiquitination of IFNAR1 is required for IFNAR1 endocytosis and lysosomal degradation, similar with other cytokine receptors such as epidermal growth factor receptor and interleukin-2 receptor, which is mediated by 26S proteasome (14, 25, 26). Here, we found that IFN-α treatment could increase IFNAR1 ubiquitination, which was significantly inhibited by MG132 or apigenin. This result indicated that apigenin suppressed IFNAR1 degradation by inhibition of the 26S proteasome, similar to a previous finding that MG132 and lysosomal inhibitors promoted IFNAR1 accumulation (13). The manner in which inhibition of 26S proteasome activity decreases IFNAR1 ubiquitination is unknown. It is possible that inhibition of the 26S proteasome suppresses the activity of E3 ubiquitin ligase $SCF^{\beta Trcp}$, which is responsible for IFNAR1 ubiquitination, or promotes the activity of an unknown deubiquitinase responsible for decreasing IFNAR1 ubiquitination (14, 27). Ligand-induced degradation of IFNAR1 is one of the key steps in the negative regulation of IFN signaling and is associated with the clinical efficacy of IFNs. Thus, protection of IFNAR1 from degradation in the presence of IFNs is proposed to be a new therapeutic means to enhance the efficacy of type I IFNs for the treatment of tumorigenesis, which requires higher doses of type I IFNs than those used for the treatment of viral diseases (28). In addition, apigenin is found to exhibit antiviral effects, but the role of JAK/STAT pathway in its inhibitory effects on viral replication is unknown (29–32). Here, for the first time we found that apigenin can inhibit the ubiquitination and degradation of IFNAR1, suggesting its potential as a new adjuvant for improving the efficacy of type I IFNs in the treatment of viral infections or cancers.

The antiviral and anticancer properties of phytoestrogens such as flavonoids have been widely reported, but their roles in the JAK/STAT pathway have not been studied in detail. Luteolin, another dietary flavonoid, has been found to inhibit 26S proteasome (24) and activate the type I IFNs-induced JAK/STAT pathway by enhancing cAMP-hydrolyzing activity of phosphodiesterases and decreasing intracellular cAMP levels for the suppression of PKA-mediated inhibition of protein tyrosine phosphatase SHP2 in cancer cells (12). This indicates that dietary flavonoids may sensitize the effects of type I IFNs through mechanisms other than the inhibition of 26S proteasome. Low levels of IFN-α/β are produced even in the absence of viral infection so as to maintain a constitutive weak IFN-α/β signal to elicit a rapid and strong cellular response against infection (33). Various flavonoids show additive antiproliferative activity with IFN-α via an unknown mechanism (34). This study provides new insights into how phytoestrogens exert their antiviral effects and their possible roles in potentiating the antiviral and anticancerous JAK/STAT signaling pathway. Apigenin is abundant in common fruits and vegetables, including parsley, onions, oranges, tea, chamomile, wheat sprouts, and some seasonings. In clinical trials, apigenin has shown good safety (35–37). In this study, apigenin was used at concentrations previously reported to translate into well-tolerated and active human serum concentrations (35–37). Thus, to a certain extent, the old saying that 'an apple a day keeps the doctor away' is indeed true because the dietary flavonoids keep the virus at bay through the synergistic action with the type I IFNs (38).

In conclusion, we found that apigenin, distributed widely in fruits and vegetables, potentiates the inhibitory effects of type I IFNs on cancer cell viability by the activation of JAK/STAT pathway through the inhibition of 26S proteasome and stabilization of IFNAR1. Apigenin warrants further investigation as a potential adjuvant for type I IFNs therapy in the treatment of viral or cancerous diseases. Consumption of fruits and vegetables rich in apigenin could prevent viral infection and reduce tumorigenesis.

Acknowledgements

This work was supported by the National Natural Science Foundation of China (No. 21372214, 91413108, 21561142003), Sichuan Youth Science & Technology Foundation (No. 2014JQ0028), the West Light Foundation of the Chinese Academy of Sciences, and Research Foundation of State General Administration of The

People's Republic of China for Quality Supervision and Inspection and Quarantine (No. 2015IK180).

Conflict of interest and funding

The authors have not received any funding or benefits from industry or elsewhere to conduct this study.

References

1. Shukla S, Gupta S. Apigenin: a promising molecule for cancer prevention. Pharm Res 2010; 27: 962–78.
2. Chen D, Daniel KG, Chen MS, Kuhn DJ, Landis-Piwowar KR, Dou QP. Dietary flavonoids as proteasome inhibitors and apoptosis inducers in human leukemia cells. Biochem Pharmacol 2005; 69: 1421–32.
3. Chen D, Landis-Piwowar KR, Chen MS, Dou QP. Inhibition of proteasome activity by the dietary flavonoid apigenin is associated with growth inhibition in cultured breast cancer cells and xenografts. Breast Cancer Res 2007; 9: R80.
4. Horinaka M, Yoshida T, Shiraishi T, Nakata S, Wakada M, Sakai T. The dietary flavonoid apigenin sensitizes malignant tumor cells to tumor necrosis factor-related apoptosis-inducing ligand. Mol Cancer Ther 2006; 5: 945–51.
5. Bonfili L, Cecarini V, Amici M, Cuccioloni M, Angeletti M, Keller JN, et al. Natural polyphenols as proteasome modulators and their role as anti-cancer compounds. FEBS J 2008; 275: 5512–26.
6. Voges D, Zwickl P, Baumeister W. The 26S proteasome: a molecular machine designed for controlled proteolysis. Annu Rev Biochem 1999; 68: 1015–68.
7. Kisselev AF, van der Linden WA, Overkleeft HS. Proteasome inhibitors: an expanding army attacking a unique target. Chem Biol 2012; 19: 99–115.
8. Borden EC, Sen GC, Uze G, Silverman RH, Ransohoff RM, Foster GR, et al. Interferons at age 50: past, current and future impact on biomedicine. Nat Rev Drug Discov 2007; 6: 975–90.
9. Jonasch E, Haluska FG. Interferon in oncological practice: review of interferon biology, clinical applications, and toxicities. Oncologist 2001; 6: 34–55.
10. Konishi H, Okamoto K, Ohmori Y, Yoshino H, Ohmori H, Ashihara M, et al. An orally available, small-molecule interferon inhibits viral replication. Sci Rep 2012; 2: 259.
11. Lucas-Hourani M, Dauzonne D, Jorda P, Cousin G, Lupan A, Helynck O, et al. Inhibition of pyrimidine biosynthesis pathway suppresses viral growth through innate immunity. PLoS Pathog 2013; 9: e1003678.
12. Tai Z, Lin Y, He Y, Huang J, Guo J, Yang L, et al. Luteolin sensitizes the antiproliferative effect of interferon α/β by activation of Janus kinase/signal transducer and activator of transcription pathway signaling through protein kinase A-mediated inhibition of protein tyrosine phosphatase SHP-2 in cancer cells. Cell Signal 2014; 26: 619–28.
13. Ragimbeau J, Dondi E, Alcover A, Eid P, Uze G, Pellegrini S. The tyrosine kinase Tyk2 controls IFNAR1 cell surface expression. EMBO J 2003; 22: 537–47.
14. Kumar KGS, Krolewski JJ, Fuchs SY. Phosphorylation and specific ubiquitin acceptor sites are required for ubiquitination and degradation of the IFNAR1 subunit of type I interferon receptor. J Biol Chem 2004; 279: 46614–20.
15. Ungureanu D, Saharinen P, Junttila I, Hilton DJ, Silvennoinen O. Regulation of Jak2 through the ubiquitin-proteasome pathway involves phosphorylation of Jak2 on Y1007 and interaction with SOCS-1. Mol Cell Biol 2002; 22: 3316–26.
16. Soond SM, Townsend PA, Barry SP, Knight RA, Latchman DS, Stephanou A. ERK and the F-box protein βTRCP target STAT1 for degradation. J Biol Chem 2008; 283: 16077–83.
17. Tai ZF, Zhang GL, Wang F. Identification of small molecule activators of the janus kinase/signal transducer and activator of transcription pathway using a cell-based screen. Biol Pharm Bull 2012; 35: 65–71.
18. He Y, Huang J, Wang P, Shen X, Li S, Yang L, et al. Emodin potentiates the antiproliferative effect of interferon α/β by activation of JAK/STAT pathway signaling through inhibition of the 26S proteasome. Oncotarget 2016; 7: 4664–79.
19. Trott O, Olson AJ. AutoDock Vina: improving the speed and accuracy of docking with a new scoring function, efficient optimization, and multithreading. J Comput Chem 2010; 31: 455–61.
20. Vetrivel U, Pilla K. Open discovery: an integrated live Linux platform of Bioinformatics tools. Bioinformation 2008; 3: 144–6.
21. Erales J, Coffino P. Ubiquitin-independent proteasomal degradation. Biochim Biophys Acta 2014; 1843: 216–21.
22. Wei HC, Tye L, Bresnick E, Birt DF. Inhibitory effect of apigenin, a plant flavonoid, on epidermal ornithine decarboxylase and skin tumor promotion in mice. Cancer Res 1990; 50: 499–502.
23. Chang TL. Inhibitory effect of flavonoids on 26S proteasome activity. J Agric Food Chem 2009; 57: 9706–15.
24. Chen D, Chen MS, Cui QC, Yang H, Dou QP. Structure-proteasome-inhibitory activity relationships of dietary flavonoids in human cancer cells. Front Biosci 2007; 12: 1935–45.
25. Yu A, Malek TR. The Proteasome regulates receptor-mediated endocytosis of interleukin-2. J Biol Chem 2001; 276: 381–5.
26. Longva KE, Blystad FD, Stang E, Larsen AM, Johannessen LE, Madshus IH. Ubiquitination and proteasomal activity is required for transport of the EGF receptor to inner membranes of multivesicular bodies. J Cell Biol 2002; 156: 843–54.
27. Kumar KGS, Tang W, Ravindranath AK, Clark WA, Croze E, Fuchs SY. SCF^{HOS} ubiquitin ligase mediates the ligand-induced down-regulation of the interferon-α receptor. EMBO J 2003; 22: 5480–90.
28. Fuchs SY. Hope and fear for interferon: the receptor-centric outlook on the future of interferon therapy. J Interferon Cytokine Res 2013; 33: 211–25.
29. Chiang LC, Ng LT, Cheng PW, Chiang W, Lin CC. Antiviral activities of extracts and selected pure constituents of *Ocimum basilicum*. Clin Exp Pharmacol Physiol 2005; 32: 811–16.
30. Kanerva A, Raki M, Ranki T, Sarkioja M, Koponen J, Desmond RA, et al. Chlorpromazine and apigenin reduce adenovirus replication and decrease replication associated toxicity. J Gene Med 2007; 9: 3–9.
31. Liu AL, Liu B, Qin HL, Lee SMY, Wang YT, Du GH. Anti-influenza virus activities of flavonoids from the medicinal plant *Elsholtzia rugulosa*. Planta Med 2008; 74: 847–51.
32. Lv X, Qiu M, Chen D, Zheng N, Jin Y, Wu Z. Apigenin inhibits enterovirus 71 replication through suppressing viral IRES activity and modulating cellular JNK pathway. Antivir Res 2014; 109: 30–41.
33. Taniguchi T, Takaoka A. A weak signal for strong responses: interferon-α/β revisited. Nat Rev Mol Cell Biol 2001; 2: 378–86.
34. Blank VC, Poll C, Marder M, Roguin LP. Antiproliferative activity of various flavonoids and related compounds: additive effect of interferon-α2b. Bioorg Med Chem Lett 2004; 14: 133–6.
35. Nielsen SE, Young JF, Daneshvar B, Lauridsen ST, Knuthsen P, Sandström B, et al. Effect of parsley (*Petroselinum crispum*) intake on urinary apigenin excretion, blood antioxidant enzymes

and biomarkers for oxidative stress in human subjects. Br J Nutr 1999; 81: 447–55.

36. Gradolatto A, Basly JP, Berges R, Teyssier C, Chagnon MC, Siess MH, et al. Pharmacokinetics and metabolism of apigenin in female and male rats after a single oral administration. Drug Metab Dispos 2005; 33: 49–54.
37. Chen T, Li LP, Lu XY, Jiang HD, Zeng S. Absorption and excretion of luteolin and apigenin in rats after oral administration of *Chrysanthemum morifolium* extract. J Agric Food Chem 2007; 55: 273–7.
38. Martin JHJ, Crotty S, Warren P, Nelson PN. Does an apple a day keep the doctor away because a phytoestrogen a day kîps the virus at bay? A review of the anti-viral properties of phytoestrogens. Phytochemistry 2007; 68: 266–74.

***Fei Wang**
Chengdu Institute of Biology
Chinese Academy of Sciences. No.9 Section 4
Renmin South Road
Chengdu 610041, China
Email: wangfei@cib.ac.cn

School meal provision, health, and cognitive function in a Nordic setting – the ProMeal-study: description of methodology and the Nordic context

Maria Waling[1]*, Anna S. Olafsdottir[2], Hanna Lagström[3], Hege Wergedahl[4], Bert Jonsson[5], Cecilia Olsson[1], Eldbjørg Fossgard[4], Asle Holthe[4], Sanna Talvia[3], Ingibjorg Gunnarsdottir[6] and Agneta Hörnell[1]

[1]Department of Food and Nutrition, Umeå University, Umeå, Sweden; [2]School of Education, University of Iceland, Reykjavik, Iceland; [3]Turku Institute of Child and Youth Research, University of Turku, Turku, Finland; [4]Faculty of Education, Bergen University College, Bergen, Norway; [5]Department of Psychology, Umeå University, Umeå, Sweden; [6]Unit for Nutrition Research, Landspitali - The National University Hospital of Iceland and Faculty of Food Science and Nutrition, School of Health Sciences, University of Iceland, Reykjavík, Iceland

Abstract

Background: School meals, if both nutritious and attractive, provide a unique opportunity to improve health equality and public health.

Objective: To describe the study rationale, data collection, and background of participants in the study 'Prospects for promoting health and performance by school meals in Nordic countries' (ProMeal). The general aim was to determine whether overall healthiness of the diet and learning conditions in children can be improved by school lunches, and to capture the main concerns regarding school lunches among children in a Nordic context.

Design: A cross-sectional, multidisciplinary study was performed in Finland, Iceland, Norway, and Sweden on pupils ($n = 837$) born in 2003.

Results: In total 3,928 pictures of school lunches were taken to capture pupils' school lunch intake. A mean of 85% of all parents responded to a questionnaire about socioeconomic background, dietary intake, and habitual physical activity at home. Cognitive function was measured on one occasion on 93% of the pupils during optimal conditions with a Stroop and a Child Operation Span test. A mean of 169 pupils also did an Integrated Visual and Auditory Continuous Performance Test after lunch over 3 days. In total, 37,413 10-sec observations of classroom learning behavior were performed. In addition, 753 empathy-based stories were written and 78 focus groups were conducted. The pupils had high socioeconomic status.

Conclusions: This study will give new insights into which future interventions are needed to improve pupils' school lunch intake and learning. The study will provide valuable information for policy making, not least in countries where the history of school meals is shorter than in some of the Nordic countries.

Keywords: *school meals*; *Nordic countries*; *education*; *cognitive function*; *dietary intake*

School meals, if both nutritious and attractive, provide a unique opportunity to improve health equality and public health (1). Despite this, only a few studies have been conducted to evaluate the effect of both school meals and the organization of these meals on total dietary intake (2), classroom learning behavior (3, 4), and cognitive function (5, 6).

The Nordic countries have common dietary recommendations (7), but there are differences in the implementation of guidelines for municipalities and others responsible for organizing school lunches. Furthermore, there are important differences in legislation related to the organization of school lunches in the Nordic countries (8). Finland and Sweden are two of the few countries in the world with a legislation that makes school meals free of charge. In Finland, it is further legislated that school meals should be 'well-balanced', and in Sweden 'nutritious'. The school meal organizations of the other Nordic countries range from giving parents/caregivers total economic and practical responsibility to government subsidizing at varying levels.

The Nordic countries' similar dietary habits but different ways of organizing school lunches give a unique opportunity to study the effect of different ways of school meal organization on pupils' total dietary intake, classroom learning behavior, and cognitive function. The overall aim of the study, 'Prospects for promoting health and performance by school meals in Nordic countries' (ProMeal), was to determine whether the overall healthiness of the diet and learning conditions in children can be improved by school lunches, and to capture the main concerns regarding school lunches among children in a Nordic context. More specific aims were to study the relationship between school lunch intake and overall healthiness of the diet, the effect of school lunches on cognitive function and classroom learning behavior, as well as the school meal environment and pupils' perspectives of school lunches. The present paper describes the study rationale, design, data collection, and participating pupils in the ProMeal-study.

Methods

School meal organization

Among the four Nordic countries included in this study, three different school meal organization systems were represented.

Finland

Dating back to a law from 1943 (9), all Finnish school children in compulsory school (aged 7–15), should be provided with a hot, well-balanced school lunch free of charge (10). In 2008, the National Nutrition Council published the so called Finnish School Lunch Recommendations, based on the Finnish Nutrition Recommendations (11), which in turn are based on the Nordic Nutrition Recommendations (7). The Finnish School Lunch Recommendations describe the requirements of food quality and how often various food items should be served. Education acts and decrees, along with national core curricula, local curricula, and school-level curricula, are central documents governing school lunches. Municipalities and other education providers are responsible for resources and the practical implementation of school meals. A community unit, a public utility, or a private company is responsible for planning, preparing, and serving the meals. These units are responsible for ensuring that nutritious meals are served by self-regulation, but there is no governmental monitoring of the school meals in Finland. A typical Finnish school lunch includes a hot meal, vegetables and/or fruit, bread, a spreadable fat, and a drink (water or milk).

Iceland

In 1995, it was stated in the Icelandic Educational Act that school meals should be provided at school time. It is most common for the cost to be covered partly by the pupils' families and partly by the municipalities. In the revised version of the act published in 2008 (12), it was stated that the nutrient composition of school meals should meet the Icelandic nutrient and food-based recommendations (13). These recommendations are based on the Nordic Nutrition Recommendations (7). There is no official or governmental monitoring of the school meals, but the schools are expected to follow the recommendations. Prior to 1995, all pupils brought a packed lunch, and some pupils still bring their own lunches to school. In some schools, private companies are responsible for the planning, preparing, and serving of school meals, while other schools provide the meals themselves. In both cases, the individual schools are always responsible for the eating environment, including providing an eating space, as well as organizing the pupil flow and eating. A typical Icelandic school lunch includes a warm meal and water as a drink. Fruit and/or vegetables are expected to be a part of each school meal, but serving methods are diverse. By default, fruit and/or vegetables are self-served or provided at a salad bar. Unlike Sweden and Finland, bread is only served occasionally as a part of Icelandic school lunches.

Norway

In Norway, pupils usually bring their own packed lunch to school. There is no national legislation for school meal provision, but in 2003, guidelines were published for healthy school meals in primary and secondary schools (aged 6–18) (14). The guidelines are built on the concept that children bring their own lunch boxes and state that schools should offer sufficient time for eating, supervision during school meals, a pleasant eating environment, and a maximum of 3 to 4 h between meals.

The pupils often eat their lunch in the class room. Schools have been offered a government-subsided milk subscription since the late 1960s, allowing 3 dl of milk to be served daily, and a fruit and vegetable subscription from the 1990s. Beginning in 2009, it was statutory to offer pupils at lower secondary and combined primary/lower secondary schools (aged 6–15) a free piece of fruit or vegetable daily, but this requirement was eliminated by the new government, in 2014. A typical Norwegian lunch box includes sandwiches of bread or crispbread with a spreadable fat, ham, salted meat, cheese, liver paté or a sweet spread with fruit and some vegetables, and milk or water to drink. Since there is no legislation regarding school meals, there is no monitoring of them in Norway.

Sweden

The foundation of the Swedish school meal system was laid during the 1940s, and since the early 1970s, free school meals have been served to all pupils in compulsory school (pupils aged 7 to 15). In 1997, the Swedish Educational Act was instituted with the requirement that school meals should be free of charge in all schools. In 2011, an addition to the act required that the meal should be nutritious, that is, corresponding to the Swedish nutrition recommendations, which were based on Nordic Nutrition Recommendations (7), (15). The meals are government funded, but the responsibility for serving school meals lies with municipalities for municipality schools and company owners for independent schools. A local municipality unit is usually responsible for planning, preparing, and serving the school lunches in the municipality schools, while the school is responsible for the eating environment (pupils usually eat in a special school restaurant within the school), timing, and the teachers' roles during meal time. The Swedish Schools Inspectorate is responsible for ensuring that schools have routines and work systematically to serve nutritious meals. A typical Swedish school lunch includes a hot meal, a choice of four to six different kinds of vegetables or salads (sometimes fruit is served), crispbread, a spreadable fat, and a drink (water or milk).

Study design

ProMeal is a cross-sectional study with a multidisciplinary approach in which data were collected between October 2013 and May 2014.

Recruitment

We aimed to recruit children born in 2003, that is, children in grade 4 in Finland and Sweden, and grade 5 in Iceland and Norway. Some children included in the classes were born 1 year earlier ($n = 11$) or 1 year later than 2003 ($n = 4$). Schools were recruited at each study site with the goal of including schools from areas with diverse socioeconomic and ethnic characteristics. The recruitment started during spring 2013 and continued in parallel to the data collection until spring 2014. In Sweden, school leaders, and after their acceptance teachers, were contacted directly and informed about the study. In Finland, Iceland, and Norway, the municipalities were contacted first for consent to contact school leaders and, once the school leaders accepted, the teachers were contacted. Information letters and informed consent forms were sent home to parents/caregivers and pupils to consider participation.

A power calculation showed that including 200 children in each country would enable detection of differences in cognitive functions and classroom learning behavior related to dietary intake with a power of 80% and significance level of $P < 0.05$.

Data collection

An overview of the data collection methods can be found in Fig. 1. In each class, data were collected during a 3-week period. During the first and the third week, the class was visited on 1 day, and during the second week, the class was visited on 5 days. Data were collected with the same instruments and in the same structured way in all countries to facilitate comparisons. Sometimes protocols were slightly modified to better fit country-specific circumstances. Protocols were tested in a Swedish school during a workshop, before the data collection began. Researchers who were involved in data collection tested and discussed the different methods to form a common view of different aspects of data collection. During the data collection process, regular web-based meetings were held and issues that came up were discussed.

Anthropometric and socioeconomic data

Pupils' body weight and height was measured by a trained researcher in each country. Body weight was weighed to the nearest kilogram (with one decimal) in light clothing and without shoes with an electronic scale (Seca Robusta 813, USA). Height was measured to the nearest millimeter with a portable wall stadiometer (Marsden HM-250P, United Kingdom). Pupils were classified as normal weight, overweight, or obese using the International Obesity Task Force (IOTF) definition (16).

Socioeconomic and background data were collected through a parent/caregiver questionnaire. In Iceland, Norway, and Sweden, the questionnaire was sent to parents/caregivers through an e-mail, which was filled out online. Parents/caregivers who did not respond to the

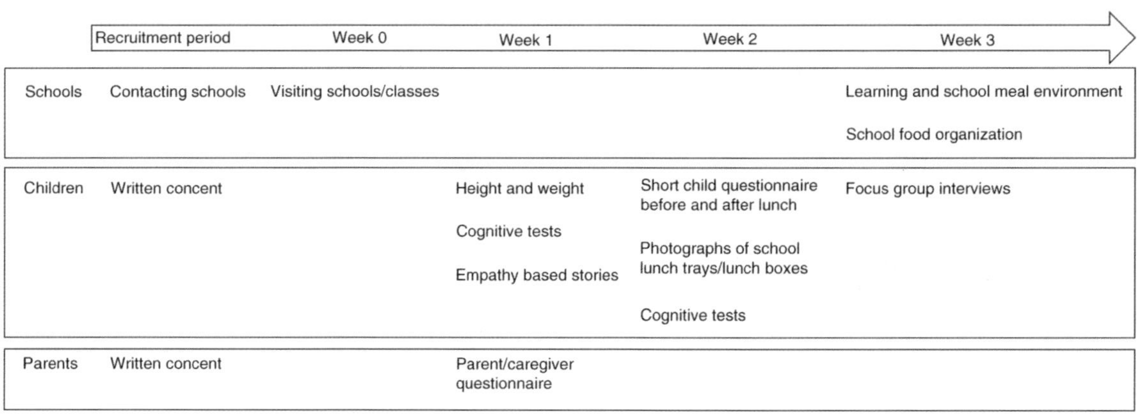

Fig. 1. Study design and measurement overview of the ProMeal-study.

questionnaire inquiry were reminded. In Finland, the questionnaire was only administrated through a telephone interview. The questionnaire covered aspects regarding education and occupation of parents/caregivers, ethnicity, family constellation, rating of the child's health, and the child's diseases/health conditions, if any. In Norway, the questionnaire did not include questions about ethnicity, the education of the parent/caregiver not filling out the questionnaire, the parent's/caregivers' occupations, who the child lived with, or a rating of the child's health. These questions were added to the questionnaire after the application for ethical approval was approved in Norway and there was no time to revise the previously approved application. The total parent/caregiver questionnaire took about 15–20 min to fill out.

Dietary intake and physical activity level outside school

Dietary habits at home were assessed through a quantitative food frequency questionnaire (FFQ), which was developed and validated as part of the Nordic Monitoring project (17, 18). This FFQ was developed to monitor the intake of selected food items and food groups (20 questions), known to contribute to the total healthiness of the diet in the Nordic countries. The questions concerned the frequency of intake of commonly consumed foods that contribute substantially to the total intake of fat, saturated fatty acids, sucrose, and dietary fiber in the Nordic diet. The questions covered usual consumption during the past 12 months and were answered by the parents/caregivers as part of the parent/caregiver questionnaire described above. The questionnaire had already been translated into the different Nordic languages.

Daily dietary intake from school lunch was assessed through a photographic method (19, 20), that was validated as part of the ProMeal-study (unpublished observation). During study week two, all school lunch trays/boxes (including extra helpings and leftovers) were photographed by researchers and trained assistants from two angles; from above and at 45 degrees. A half- and full-weighed reference portion was photographed and used for comparison with amounts taken, any additional helpings, and leftovers in Finland, Iceland, and Sweden. These were then used for estimating the total amount eaten and, most importantly to be used in future analysis to define a very low intake (less than one-half of the meal provided). In Norway, standard portions from a nutritional calculation program were used to assess amounts. On a few occasions, the pupils forgot to photograph extra helpings or leftovers, and if no notes had been taken (e.g. 'missed leftover photograph, but all food eaten'), that day was noted as 'missing'. The following nutritional calculation programs and food databases were used in the participating countries: in Finland, AivoDiet 2.0.2.3 and Fineli® – the Finnish Food Composition Database; in Iceland, Icefood 2.0 and the National Nutrition Database, ISGEM; in Norway, Kostholdsplanleggeren and the Norwegian food composition database from 2014 (both from the Norwegian Directorate of health and the Norwegian Food Safety Authority); and in Sweden, Dietist Net Pro version 15.02.14 and the National Food Agency's Nutrition Database 15.12.13.

The pupils also filled out two short structured questionnaires daily during study week two; one before and one after lunch. In both questionnaires, they were instructed to rate how hungry they were on a visual analogue scale (VAS), which is a method that has been used in earlier studies for similar ratings of satiety and appetite (21, 22). After lunch, they were further instructed to rate both the lunch meal and how they felt on a VAS. If they did not finish their meals, they were asked to give the main reason for the same. Before lunch, they were also asked if and what they had eaten for breakfast, as well as snacks between breakfast and lunch. The questionnaire also included a question about when they went to bed the evening before and when they got up in the morning of the present day.

Physical activity level at home was assessed through four questions as part of the parental/caregiver questionnaire in Finland, Iceland, and Sweden. The aim was not to capture the total physical activity of each individual, but rather to get a general estimate of the pupil's physical activity level outside school for use as a co-variate in future analyses. One question concerned daily sedentary behavior, that is, how many hours per day the pupils spent using a computer, tablet, or smartphone, as well as playing video games and watching television. Two questions were regarding physical activity and were divided into moderate (activities in which one gets slightly out of breath, for example, dancing, horseback riding, or line skating) and strenuous (activities in which one gets out of breath and sweaty, for example, activities like running, ball games, and cross-country skiing). Five predefined frequencies were given (never, 1–2 times per week, 3–4 times per week, 5–6 times per week, or all days of the week). The fourth question was regarding how many times per week the child walked or biked to school and back home.

Children's perspective of school lunches

Empathy-based stories (23) were used to study pupils' experiences and perspectives of school meal situations. Pupils were randomly selected to write short stories based on one of two different frame stories. The frame story helped direct the child to write a story about a school lunch that was either a bad or a good experience. Pupils could write about something that they had experienced themselves, been told, or an imaginary but still possible story.

Further, focus groups were conducted to study children's understandings and way of discussing school lunches (24). The purpose of the focus groups was to investigate and compare experiences and beliefs about the school meals. A structured topic guide was used and the interviews were monitored by one moderator and one assistant. A selection of photos of various dishes, meals, and school lunch contexts were shown in order to stimulate the pupils to talk. The interviews were digitally recorded and transcribed verbatim. In Iceland and Sweden, all groups were separated by gender; in Norway, most groups (16 of 25) were separated by gender; and in Finland, most groups (13 of 19) were mixed gender.

Cognitive function and classroom learning behavior

Measures of cognitive functioning were conducted during study week one and two. Cognitive functioning in the present project is defined as working memory (WM) capacity, the ability to inhibit a prepotent response, speed of information processing, and attention and self-control. In the first study week, a complex WM task (25) and a computerized Stroop test (26) was administered. Operation span (27) is frequently denoted as one of the most reliable and valid instruments of WM (28). In the present study, a child version was used, which in a previous study was found to have high internal consistency with other measures of WM capacity, digit span, and block span (25). There are a number of versions of Stroop task tests available that differ slightly, but the overall picture is that the Stroop effects are a robust phenomenon (29). Analysis of test–re-test reliability have found that computerized Stroop tests have higher reliability than the conventional test (30). These tests were performed with all participating pupils during an early lesson in order to get a reference value of cognitive function in conditions as 'optimal' as possible. In the complex WM task, denoted as the Child Operation span (CO-span), the children were required to solve mathematical tasks while retaining letters in their short-term memory. The number of letters retained was used as measure of WM capacity. In the Stroop task, the participants were shown a sequence of words in the national language and were required to indicate the color of the letters that either was incongruent (the word 'red' printed in 'blue'), congruent (the word 'red' printed in 'red'), or neutral (the word presented in color with no relation to the semantic meaning). Reaction times to incongruent and congruent conditions were used as measures of cognitive inhibition and processing speed, respectively.

The second study week, the Integrated Visual and Auditory Continuous Performance Test (IVA + Plus) (31), which measures a person's ability to concentrate and remain focused, was performed on a random subsample of five pupils in each class during 3 days, 1 to 2 h after lunch. In Sweden, the CO-span and Stroop tests were also performed on an additional five randomized pupils on the same 3 days as the IVA + Plus test was performed. The IVA + Plus test is a standardized instrument with normative data based on 1,700 individuals. The practice effects for IVA + Plus are generally quite small (32).

In addition to the computer tests, structured observations were performed by researchers and trained research assistants to study learning-related classroom behavior in the first lesson after lunch, during study week two. The observation schedule was based on the procedure by Blatchford et al. (33, 34) and comprised categories for time spent in different social settings (child-teacher interaction, child-child interaction, or individual behavior) and in different work settings (individual, group, or whole class). Within the social settings, there were mutually exclusive categories to describe how children behaved (work, social, off-task). The goal was to capture whether or not the child was on-task (concentrated on the task) or off-task (disengaged, disrupted).

School meal and learning environment

The school meal environment was systematically observed in Finland, Iceland, and Sweden with a standardized protocol constructed by the research group. The first area observed was the physical eating environment, for example, size of room, noise-protective materials, temperature, light, art, tables, chairs, material of plates, and cups. Other observations were the number of children eating at the same time, queueing, written rules, staff eating with the pupils, serving practices, commercial messages, and the accessibility of the school menu for pupils and parents. In Norway, an adapted protocol was used since pupils there eat in the classroom.

Physical learning environment was also studied through observations of the class rooms; for example, the size of the classroom, how pupils were seated, the placement of the teacher, teaching-related equipment, extra work stations, art, light, noise-protective materials, and written rules.

School food organization

Different aspects of school food organization were evaluated in all countries with a validated instrument called School Food Sweden (35). The instrument consists of three levels/areas: 1) Variety, nutrition, and food safety; 2) Service, pedagogical thinking, and environmental impact; and 3) Organization and management. The full instrument was only used in Sweden since it was country-specific. Adapted versions of levels 2 and 3 were used in Finland, Iceland, and Norway. In Sweden, the head food service personnel at each school answered the original developed web-based tool. In Finland, the questionnaires were answered by the researchers after observations and conversations with food service personnel. In Iceland, a translated paper questionnaire was answered by food service personnel. In Norway, parts of the questionnaire in level 3 was used, and modified to better fit Norwegian circumstances.

Statistical analysis

In the analysis presented in the present paper, the Chi-square test for independence was used to test potential differences in distribution between categorical variables in the parent/caregiver questionnaire. For variables with cells with an expected count less than five, the Fisher's exact test was used. Descriptive data are presented as mean and standard deviation. For continuous variables, a one-way between-groups analysis of variance was used. If statistically significant differences were seen, a *post-hoc* test (Tukey's HSD) was used to show between which groups the difference occurred. Eta squared was calculated to estimate effect size, and Cohen's classification was used for interpretation of the effect size: 0.01 = small effect; 0.06 = medium effect; and 0.14 = large effect. Results were considered statistically significant if the P-value was <0.05. IBM SPSS Statistics, version 22.0, was used (Armonk, NY: IBM Corp.) for all statistical analysis.

This study was conducted according to the guidelines laid down in the Helsinki Declaration of 1975, as revised in 2008, and all procedures involving human subjects were approved by the Ethical Committee of the University of Turku in Finland, The National Bioethics Committee (56363); The Icelandic Data Protection Authority (VSN-13-088) in Iceland; The Data Protection Official for Research in Norway; and The Regional Research Ethics Review Board, the Faculty of Medicine, Umeå University, in Sweden (2013-212-31Ö). Written informed consent was obtained from all parents/caregivers in the participating countries. In Finland, informed consent was also collected from the pupils. In all countries, the pupils were able to deny participation even if parents/caregivers had consented participation.

Results

In total, 75 schools were invited to participate in the study (variation between countries 7–31) and 30 schools accepted the invitation (variation between countries 6–9). For country-specific numbers, please see Fig. 2. The schools that accepted the invitation had a total of 1,216 pupils in grade 4 (Finland and Sweden) and grade 5 (Iceland and Norway) from 62 different classes. Of these, 842 (69%) parents consented to participate. However, during the study, five pupils dropped out (one each in Iceland and Norway, and three in Sweden), leaving 837 (99% of those who consented to participate) pupils to participate throughout the whole study (Finland $n = 206$, Iceland $n = 224$, Norway $n = 210$, and Sweden $n = 197$). All included schools were run by the municipality and four of the five included towns were university towns with between 118,000 and 275,000 inhabitants at the time of the study.

In total, 85% of the participants' parents/caregivers filled out the parent questionnaire (Table 1). Body weight and height was measured on 97% of the pupils. In total, 3,928 lunches were photographed, and for a majority of the pupils (78%), lunches for all 5 days were photographed. The short questionnaires before and after lunch were answered by 82 and 83% of the pupils, respectively, who had five complete days. The computer tests Stroop and CO-span were conducted for 93% of the pupils during the first study week. During 3 days in study week two, 46 randomly selected pupils from Sweden conducted Stroop and CO-span, and the computer test IVA + Plus was conducted in all countries by a mean of 169 randomly selected pupils per day (mean 25–68 pupils per country). A total of 37,413 observations of classroom learning behavior were performed.

Empathy-based stories were written by 90% of the participating pupils and focus groups were performed in 56 gender-based divided groups and 22 mixed gender groups.

Participants

There was no difference in the gender distribution between the countries ($P = 0.472$) (Table 2). Eighty-five percent of those filling out the parent/caregiver questionnaire were mothers/stepmothers. Pupils had a mean age of 10.5 ± 0.36 years. The Finnish pupils were older than the Norwegian and Swedish pupils (10.7 ± 0.34 years old in Finland versus 10.5 ± 0.35 years old in Norway ($P < 0.001$) and 10.6 ± 0.33 years old in Sweden ($P = 0.002$)). The mean body weight and height of the children was 38.3 ± 7.70 kg and 145 ± 6.80 cm. Mean body mass index (BMI) was 18.1 ± 2.71 kg/m^2. There was a difference in both body weight and BMI between pupils in Finland and Norway

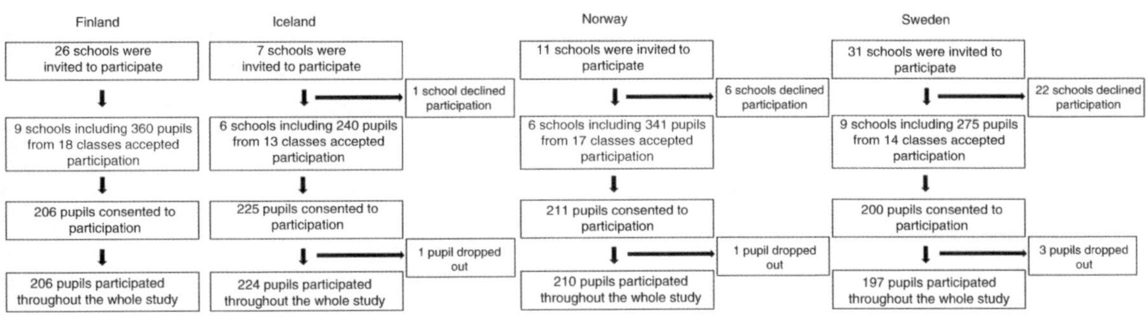

Fig. 2. Flow-cart of participants in Finland, Iceland, Norway, and Sweden in the ProMeal-study.

Table 1. Collected data in the ProMeal-study between October 2013 and May 2014 in Finland, Iceland, Norway, and Sweden

	Finland ($n=206$)	Iceland ($n=224$)	Norway ($n=210$)	Sweden ($n=197$)	Total ($n=837$)
	n (%[a])	*n* (%[a])	*n* (%[a])	*n* (%[a])	*n* (%[a])
Parent questionnaire	187 (91)	221 (99)	144 (69)	161 (82)	713 (85)
Body weight (kg)	200 (97)	224 (100)	209 (99)	179 (91)	812 (97)
Height (cm)	200 (97)	224 (100)	210 (100)	179 (91)	813 (97)
Body mass index (kg/m^2)	200 (97)	224 (100)	209 (99)	179 (91)	812 (97)
School meal lunches					
Total lunches photographed	976 (95)	1,067 (95)	989 (94)	896 (91)	3,928 (94)
Number of pupils with 5 days photographed[b]	171 (83)	186 (83)	164 (78)	135 (69)	656 (78)
Questionnaire before lunch					
Total number of questionnaires filled out	966 (94)	1,072 (96)	1,005 (96)	919 (93)	3,962 (95)
Number of pupils with 5 days of filled out questionnaires	178 (86)	184 (82)	177 (84)	149 (76)	688 (82)
Questionnaire after lunch					
Total number of questionnaires filled out	976 (95)	1,056 (94)	991 (94)	912 (87)	3,935 (94)
Number of pupils with 5 days of filled out questionnaires	193 (94)	183 (82)	168 (80)	150 (76)	694 (83)
Observations in the classroom (number of observations in total)[c]	6,179 (60)	10,844 (97)	11,887 (113[d])	8,503 (86)	37,413 (89)
Child Operation span and Stroop[e]					
Baseline measurement study week one	197 (96)	212 (95)	204 (97)	167 (85)	780 (93)
Measurements during study week 2 (only measured in Sweden)	–	–	–	46 (23)	46 (3)
The Integrated Visual and Auditory Continuous Performance Test (done by a randomized sub-sample of the pupils)[f]					
Test day 1	65 (32)	43 (19)	27 (13)	34 (17)	169 (20)
Test day 2	71 (34)	44 (20)	27 (13)	44 (22)	186 (22)
Test day 3	67 (33)	39 (17)	21 (10)	26 (13)	153 (18)
Empathy-based stories (total number of stories)					
Positive	95 (46)	103 (46)	104 (50)	86 (44)	388 (46)
Negative	95 (46)	100 (45)	85 (40)	85 (43)	365 (44)
Focus groups (number of groups, 5–8 pupils in each group)					
Gender-based divide	6 (3)	18 (8)	16 (8)	16 (8)	56 (7)
Mixed gender	13 (6)	0 (0)	9 (4)	0 (0)	22 (3)
School meal environment (number of schools observed)	9 (100)	6 (100)	6 (100)	9 (100)	30 (100)
Learning environment (number of schools observed)	9 (100)	6 (100)	6 (100)	9 (100)	30 (100)
School food organization[g]					
Level 1 (only measured in Sweden)	–	–	–	6 (100)	6 (100)
Level 2	9 (100)	6 (100)	6 (100)	6 (67)	27 (90)
Level 3	9 (100)	6 (100)	–	5 (56)	20 (67)

[a]The percentage of the total number of possible measurements of the participating pupils.
[b]The reason for less than 5 days were that the pupils either were absent from school one or more days, or that one or more pictures were missing in the series of photographs.
[c]Observations were made according to Blatchford et al. (33, 34).
[d]In Norway, more observations than planned were made on each pupil and, consequently, the percentage exceeds 100%.
[e]Child Operation span (25) and Stroop test (26).
[f]The Integrated Visual and Auditory Continuous Performance Test (31).
[g]School food organization was studied with the e-tool School Food Sweden (35) in Sweden and adapted versions in the other countries.

where the Norwegian pupils had lower body weight (37.2 ± 6.60 kg versus 39.2 ± 8.50 kg, $P=0.033$) and BMI (17.7 ± 2.20 kg/m^2 versus 18.5 ± 3.20 kg/m^2, $P=0.020$) than the Finnish pupils. The effect size for both differences was, however, low. The majority (81%) of the pupils were classified as normal weight, 16% overweight, and 3% as obese. There was a difference in the proportion of pupils classified as normal weight, overweight, and obese between countries. Finland had the highest proportion of pupils with obesity (6.5% versus 3%, 0.5%, and 3% in Iceland, Norway, and Sweden, respectively) ($P=0.010$). Iceland, on the contrary, had the highest proportion of

Table 2. Background information about pupils and parents/caregivers participating in the ProMeal-study between October 2013 and May 2014 in Finland, Iceland, Norway, and Sweden

	Finland ($n = 187$)		Iceland ($n = 221$)		Norway ($n = 144$)		Sweden ($n = 161$)		
	Mean	SD	Mean	SD	Mean	SD	Mean	SD	P^a
Age (years)[a]	10.7	0.3	10.6	0.3	10.5	0.3	10.6	0.3	**<0.001**
Body weight (kg)[b]	39.2	8.5	38.9	8.1	37.2	6.6	37.9	7.2	**0.022**
Height (cm)[c]	145	6.8	146	6.8	145	6.9	145	6.5	0.463
BMI (kg/m^2)[d]	18.5	3.2	18.3	2.8	17.7	2.2	17.9	2.6	**0.016**
	%		%		%		%		
Sex, girls[e]	52.0		49.0		56.0		51.0		0.472
Non-native pupils	2.0		7.0		–		5.0		**0.028**
Child live with both parents all the time	62.0		89.0		–		90.0		**<0.001**
Education parent 1[f]									
≥10–12 y	38.5		32.0		27.0		34.0		
University degree	53.5		58.0		73.0		64.0		**<0.001**
Other/none	8.0		10.0		0.0		1.0		
Employed parent one (or other occupation)[f]	89.0		87.0		–		91.0		0.488
Body mass index classification									
Overweight	16.5		18.0		16.0		12.0		**0.010**
Obesity	6.5		3.0		0.5		3.0		
Child has a diet-related disease	13.0		7.0		11.0		6.0		0.067
Child has other chronic disease	17.0		15.0		11.0		9.0		0.123
Parents who estimate the child's health as good[g]	98.0		94.0		–		89.0		**0.002**

The difference between the groups were compared with a Chi-Square test on categorical variables (the Fishers exact test was used for the variables in which the parents rate the child's health and BMI classification). One-way between-groups ANOVA with *post-hoc* tests was used to compare means of continuous variables. (In the present table, only *P*-values from the ANOVA are presented. *P*-values from *post-hoc* tests are presented in the text.)
[a]Finland $n = 206$, Iceland $n = 224$, Norway $n = 208$, and Sweden $n = 190$.
[b]Finland $n = 200$, Iceland $n = 224$, Norway $n = 209$, and Sweden $n = 179$.
[c]Finland $n = 200$, Iceland $n = 224$, Norway $n = 210$, and Sweden $n = 179$.
[d]Body mass index: Finland $n = 200$, Iceland $n = 224$, Norway $n = 209$, and Sweden $n = 1,879$.
[e]Finland $n = 206$, Iceland $n = 224$, Norway $n = 210$, and Sweden $n = 197$.
[f]Education degree and employment for the parent who filled out the questionnaire.
[g]Parents were asked to rate their child's health on a visual analogue scale, 1–10. In the present paper, 8–10 on the VAS scale is defined as good health.
Bold P-values indicate a statistically significant difference between countries.

children with overweight (18% versus 17%, 16%, and 12% in Finland, Norway, and Sweden, respectively) ($P = 0.010$). A majority of the children from Finland, Iceland, and Sweden were born in the respective country (no data on Norway available). Iceland and Sweden had a higher proportion of non-native children than Finland ($P = 0.028$). A somewhat higher proportion of children lived with parents/caregivers all of the time in Iceland and Sweden compared with Finland ($P < 0.001$). In all countries, it was most common that the parents/caregivers had a university degree ($P < 0.001$). There were no differences between countries in parents/caregivers reporting that their child had a diet-related disease or a chronic disease. A larger proportion of parents/caregivers rated their child's health as good (meaning, 8 to 10 on a VAS with 10 being the best possible condition) in Finland (98%) compared with Iceland (94%) and Sweden (89%) ($P = 0.002$).

Discussion

The present study is unique with its Nordic approach in studying the effect of school lunch on overall healthiness of diet, cognitive function, classroom learning behavior, and pupils' own understandings and experiences of school lunch. The Nordic countries have been proposed as a global health lab (36), given their many similarities in, for example, culture, dietary habits, and diet-related diseases. The present study has used these similarities as a base for studying different aspects of school meals in the Nordic countries.

An overall strength with the present study is the large number of participating children. We aimed to recruit at least 200 pupils in each country and that goal was reached. The drop-out rate was low in all countries. Some of the children said they dropped out because of the strain of photographing the school lunch. The large number of participants made statistical comparisons more reliable and results more representative. Another unique aspect of the study is the multidisciplinary approach, such that different disciplines, in this case, food and nutrition, education, and psychology, met and studied a common research aim. To our knowledge, no other similar size studies have done this.

Cognitive function was tested through objective measures and will be evaluated in relation to dietary intake during the school lunch. Systematic observations of classroom learning behavior were also performed in order to be evaluated in relation to school lunch intake. To date, only a few studies have focused on the relationship between school lunch and cognitive function or classroom learning behavior in relation to lunch intake (5, 6, 33). A study situated in relatively poor areas in England showed substantial improvements in the national Key Stage 2 tests (literacy and science), as well as decreased absenteeism in schools as a result of the Jamie Oliver Campaign to improve the food in English schools (37). Improvement in children's classroom learning behavior has been shown in other intervention studies with an improved school lunch and eating environment (3, 4). One reason so few studies have been done in this area may be the methodological challenges of measuring dietary intake, cognitive function, and learning behavior. There are also many confounders involved that complicate the evaluation of cognitive function. Confounders that may affect a child's cognitive performance are sleep duration, physical activity, previous meals, physical or pedagogical environments, as well as social background, to name a few. In the present study, we tried to take into account as many of these confounders as possible because they may help explain some variations.

For future interventions aiming to improve children's food habits through school lunch, it is vital to know more about pupils' own experiences and understandings of the school meal. This area has been little studied, and the present study will, to our knowledge, be the first to explore this important topic using qualitative methodology among a large sample of Nordic pupils. The two different methods used, focus group discussions and empathy-based stories, are expected to complement each other. In the focus groups, children are constructing understanding within groups (38), whereas empathy-based stories give children space to express their experiences and perspectives individually (23).

The participating pupils had a mean BMI within what is considered as normal weight according to the definition by Cole et al. (16). The proportion of overweight children in ProMeal was somewhat lower in Finland and Iceland and substantially lower in Sweden compared with what earlier studies have shown regarding the prevalence of overweight in these countries (39–41). In Norway, the prevalence of overweight was, in contrast, slightly higher than what earlier studies have reported (42). The proportion of children with obesity was lower in ProMeal than what earlier studies have reported in Iceland, Norway, and Sweden (40–42). In Finland, the obesity rate among the participating pupils was much higher than what has been reported before (39). The differences from earlier studies may be due to the relatively few pupils from each country compared with previous studies. The statistically significant difference of 0.8 kg/m^2 in BMI between Finland and Norway had a low effect size according to Cohen's classification, which means that it is of little practical relevance. The Swedish parents/caregivers rated their children's health as somewhat lower compared to the other countries. Nevertheless, there was no statistically significant difference between countries as to how parents responded regarding whether their child had a diet-related disease or a chronic disease. The meaning parents/caregivers put into the word 'health' may vary within and between countries, which must be kept in mind when questions about health are interpreted.

The participation rate varied in the participating classes while Finland and Norway had the lowest participation rate in the included classes. A low participation rate increases the risk of selection bias, and there is a possibility that those who chose not to participate differ from the ones who chose to participate. A limitation is that it is not possible to study whether the groups differ since we do not have any information about those who declined participation. The participation rates in the parent/caregiver questionnaire were relatively good in Finland, Iceland, and Sweden (99, 91, and 82%) but lower than desired in Norway (69%) in spite of reminders through e-mails and phone calls. The background data for those not filling out the questionnaire are not known, but an analysis showed that the parents who did not answer the questionnaire were fairly evenly distributed among the participating schools. This is positive since the schools were situated in different socioeconomic areas. A further limitation is that some background questions from the parent/caregiver questionnaire were not included in the Norwegian questionnaire. This unfortunately, made comparisons of some background variables between all countries impossible. Missing data in the measurements carried out at school are due to, for example, ill children not present in school or practical difficulties in collecting data if the pupils were not at the same place at the same time. At many measuring occasions, pupils from one class were spread out in the school, for example, in smaller groups or individual pupils left the class for special teaching. Efforts were made to locate children not present in the classroom during measurements but not always successfully.

In spite of the schools being situated in different socioeconomic areas, the study population was homogeneous from a socioeconomic perspective because most of the parents/caregivers were highly educated and employed. A majority of the children lived continuously with parents/caregivers all the time, and a low proportion of children were non-native. Iceland and Sweden had a somewhat higher proportion of non-native pupils, which may add important information to the group as a whole. Efforts were made to recruit pupils from areas with different socioeconomic backgrounds, but not completely successfully. Because of the high inclusion of university towns and, consequently, the high education levels, the variation in socioeconomic status within each town was limited. Schools in areas with lower socioeconomic status were more difficult to recruit because the teachers thought that they already had enough to deal with and did not think they had the time to participate in a study. Because of the high socioeconomic status among the study population, the results must be interpreted with caution in relation to different socioeconomic contexts. From a methodological point of view, the homogenous groups can be an advantage, for example, when measuring the relationship between school lunch intake and cognitive function.

Dietary intake from lunches was assessed by a photographic method, which has been validated on the pupils in ProMeal (unpublished observations). The method worked well for the dietary assessment of pupils in the often time-limited and stressful school meal environment. Furthermore, the method is practical since it does not interfere much with the daily routine of the personnel and children, which is important when performing research involving the school setting. One downside of the method was missing photographs of taken left over food, for example, because pupils forgot to have their plates photographed, showing either what was taken or thrown away. In these instances, it was not possible to assess the child's total dietary intake from that particular lunch.

Conclusion

ProMeal is, to date, the largest study done with the aim of studying Nordic pupils' school lunch intake, total diet, cognitive function, learning behavior, and pupils' own perspectives of school meals. The results of the study will give new insights into what future interventions need to focus on to improve pupils' dietary intake and learning. The study will also provide valuable information for policy making, not least in countries where the history of school meals is shorter than in some of the Nordic countries.

Acknowledgements

The authors are thankful to all pupils, parents/caregivers, and participating schools in the study, as well as Ana Karina Pastrana Polo, Marléne Hedelin, Linda Berggren, Maarit Laurinen, Soile Kotilainen, Elli Heino, Gudrun Kristin Sigurgeirsdottir, Cindy Mary Imai, Bryndis Elva Gunnarsdottir, Ragnheidur Juniusdottir, Kristin Jonsdottir, Unnur Bjork Arnfjord, Steingerdur Olafsdottir, Linda Manner, Tormod Bjørkkjær, Synneve Skei, Cecilie Johansson, and Kristin Skjetne Berg who worked with the data collection in schools. The authors also want to thank Jenni Iirola, the statistical consultant. The ProMeal-study was funded by Nord Forsk (grant number 54761) and the Juho Vainio Foundation.

Conflict of interest and funding

The authors have not received any funding or benefits from industry or elsewhere to conduct this study.

References

1. Mikkelsen BE. School – a multitude of opportunities for promoting healthier eating. Public Health Nutr 2014; 17(6): 1191–4.
2. Andersen R, Biltoft-Jensen A, Christensen T, Andersen EW, Ege M, Thorsen AV, et al. Dietary effects of introducing school meals based on the New Nordic Diet – a randomised controlled trial in Danish children. The OPUS School Meal Study. Br J Nutr 2014; 111(11): 1967–76.
3. Golley R, Baines E, Bassett P, Wood L, Pearce J, Nelson M. School lunch and learning behaviour in primary schools: an intervention study. Eur J Clin Nutr 2010; 64(11): 1280–8.
4. Storey HC, Pearce J, Ashfield-Watt PA, Wood L, Baines E, Nelson M. A randomized controlled trial of the effect of school food and dining room modifications on classroom behaviour in secondary school children. Eur J Clin Nutr 2011; 65(1): 32–8.
5. Muller K, Libuda L, Gawehn N, Drossard C, Bolzenius K, Kunz C, et al. Effects of lunch on children's short-term cognitive functioning: a randomized crossover study. Eur J Clin Nutr 2013; 67(2): 185–9.
6. Schroder M, Muller K, Falkenstein M, Stehle P, Kersting M, Libuda L. Short-term effects of lunch on children's executive cognitive functioning: the randomized crossover cognition intervention study Dortmund PLUS (CogniDo PLUS). Physiol Behav 2015; 152: 307–14.
7. Nordic Council of Ministers Nordic Nutrition Recommendations 2012. Integrating nutrition and physical activity. 5th ed. Nordisk. Copenhagen, Denmark: Nordisk Ministerråd 2014.
8. Kainulainen K, Benn J, Fjellström C, Palojoki P. Nordic adolescents' school lunch patterns and their suggestions for making healthy choices at school easier. Appetite 2012; 59(1): 53–62.
9. Finnish National Board of Education 2014. School meals in Finland. Available from: http://www.edu.fi/yleissivistava_koulutus/hyvinvointi_koulussa/kouluruokailu/verkkomateriaalia_kouluruokailuun [cited 9 June 2016].
10. Finnish Basic Education Act 628/1998, 31§.
11. Valtion ravitsemusneuvottelukunta (2008). Kouluruokailusuositus (in Finnish). Available from: http://www.ravitsemusneuvottelukunta.fi/portal/fi/ravitsemussuositukset/erillisryhmat/koululaiset/ [cited 9 June 2016].
12. Icelandic Educational Act nr. 66/1995 and 91/2008.
13. Icelandic Directorate for Health. Dietary guidelines for adults and children from the age of two. Available from: http://www.landlaeknir.is/servlet/file/store93/item25796/radleggingar-um-mataraedi-2015.pdf [cited 9 June 2016].
14. The Norwegian Directorate for Health and Social Affairs, #1946 (2003).

15. SFS 2010:800 (2010) Education Act. Stockholm: Ministry of Education.
16. Cole TJ, Bellizzi MC, Flegal KM, Dietz WH. Establishing a standard definition for child overweight and obesity worldwide: international survey. BMJ 2000; 320(7244): 1240–3.
17. Fagt S, Andersen L, Anderssen S, Becker W, Borodulin K, Fogelholm M, et al. Nordic monitoring on diet, physical activity and overweight. Part 1. Description of a common Nordic method for collecting representative data. Copenhagen, Denmark: National Food Institute, Technical University of Denmark; 2009.
18. Fagt S, Andersen L, Anderssen S, Becker W, Borodulin K, Fogelholm M, et al. Nordic monitoring of diet, physical activity and overweight. Validation of indicators. TemaNord. Copenhagen, Denmark: Nordic Council of Ministers; 2012.
19. Gemming L, Utter J, Ni Mhurchu C. Image-assisted dietary assessment: a systematic review of the evidence. J Acad Nutr Diet 2015; 115(1): 64–77.
20. Swanson M. Digital photography as a tool to measure school cafeteria consumption. J Sch Health 2008; 78(8): 432–7.
21. Parker BA, Sturm K, MacIntosh CG, Feinle C, Horowitz M, Chapman IM. Relation between food intake and visual analogue scale ratings of appetite and other sensations in healthy older and young subjects. Eur J Clin Nutr 2004; 58(2): 212–18.
22. Olsen A, Ritz C, Hartvig DL, Moller P. Comparison of sensory specific satiety and sensory specific desires to eat in children and adults. Appetite 2011; 57(1): 6–13.
23. Lehtomäki E, Janhonen-Abruquah H, Tuomi MT, Okkolin M-A, Posti-Ahokas H, Palojoki P. Research to engage voices on the ground in educational development. Int J Educ Dev 2014; 35: 37–43.
24. Wilkinson S. Focus groups in health research: exploring the meanings of health and illness. J Health Psychol 1998; 3(3): 329–48.
25. Nyroos M, Jonsson B, Korhonen J, Eklöf H. Children's mathematical achievement and how it relates to working memory, test anxiety and self-regulation: a person-centred approach. Educ Inq 2015; 6(1): 73–97.
26. Stroop JR. Studies of interference in serial verbal reactions. J Exp Psychol 1992; 121(1): 15–23.
27. Turner ML, Engle RW. Is working memory capacity task dependent? J Mem Lang 1989; 28(2): 127–54.
28. Chein JM, Moore AB, Conway AR. Domain-general mechanisms of complex working memory span. Neuroimage 2011; 54(1): 550–9.
29. MacLeod CM. Half a century of research on the Stroop effect: an integrative review. Psychol Bull 1991; 109(2): 163–203.
30. Gualtieri CT, Johnson LG. Reliability and validity of a computerized neurocognitive test battery, CNS Vital Signs. Arch Clin Neuropsychol 2006; 21(7): 623–43.
31. Sandford JA, Turner A. Manual for the integrated visual and auditory continuous performance test. Richmond, VA: Brain Train; 1995.
32. Strauss E, Sherman EMS, Spreen O. A compendium of neuropsychological tests: administration, norms, and commentary. 3rd ed. Oxford: Oxford University Press; 2006.
33. Blatchford P, Bassett P, Brown P. Teachers' and pupils' behavior in large and small classes: a systematic observation study of pupils aged 10 and 11 years. J Educ Psychol 2005; 97(3): 454–67.
34. Blatchford P, Baines E, Rubie-Davis C, Basset P, Chowne A. The effect of a new approach to group work on pupil-pupil and teacher-pupil interactions. J Educ Psychol 2006; 98: 750–65.
35. Patterson E, Quetel AK, Lilja K, Simma M, Olsson L, Elinder LS. Design, testing and validation of an innovative web-based instrument to evaluate school meal quality. Public Health Nutr 2013; 16(6): 1028–36.
36. Monday Morning, Scandinavian 'think-tank' (2008). The Nordic region as a global health lab. NordForsk policy briefs 2008–4. Oslo: Norden, NordForsk.
37. Belot M, James J. Healthy school meals and educational outcomes (Report No. 2009-01). Essex, UK: Institute for Social and Economic Justice; 2009.
38. McLafferty I. Focus group interviews as a data collecting strategy. J Adv Nurs 2004; 48(2): 187–94.
39. Vuorela N, Saha MT, Salo M. Prevalence of overweight and obesity in 5- and 12-year-old Finnish children in 1986 and 2006. Acta Paediatr 2009; 98(3): 507–12.
40. Lager A, Fossum B, Rorvall G, Bremberg S. Children's overweight and obesity: local and national monitoring using electronic health records. Scand J Public Health 2009; 37(2): 201–5.
41. Jonsson SH, Hedinsdottir M, Erlendsson RO, Gudlaugsson JO, Danielsdottir S, Reynisson JA. Body weight of children in the capital area: results from Iskra on childrens' weight measurements 2003/04-2011/12. Reykjavik, Directorate of Health and Primary Health Care of the Capital Area; 2013.
42. Juliusson PB, Eide GE, Roelants M, Waaler PE, Hauspie R, Bjerknes R. Overweight and obesity in Norwegian children: prevalence and socio-demographic risk factors. Acta Paediatr 2010; 99(6): 900–5.

*Maria Waling
Department of Food and Nutrition
Umeå University
SE-901 87 Umeå
Sweden
Email: maria.waling@umu.se

18

Zolfino landrace (*Phaseolus vulgaris* L.) from Pratomagno: general and specific features of a functional food

Francesco Balestri[1,2], Rossella Rotondo[1], Roberta Moschini[1,2], Mario Pellegrino[3], Mario Cappiello[1,2], Vito Barracco[1], Livia Misuri[1], Carlo Sorce[1,2], Andrea Andreucci[1,2], Antonella Del-Corso[1,2]* and Umberto Mura[1,2]

[1]Department of Biology, University of Pisa, Pisa, Italy; [2]Interdepartmental Research Center Nutrafood 'Nutraceuticals and Food for Health', University of Pisa, Pisa, Italy; [3]Department of Translational Research on New Technologies in Medicine and Surgery, University of Pisa, Pisa, Italy

Abstract

Background: The Zolfino bean is a variety of *Phaseolus vulgaris*, which is cultivated in a limited area of Tuscany, Italy, and is widely appreciated for its flavor and culinary uses.
Objectives: A yellow Zolfino landrace cultivated in the Leccio-Reggello area was characterized and compared with three other varieties of *Phaseolus vulgaris* (i.e. the Borlotto, Cannellino, and Corona beans) in terms of its general features and potential as an antioxidant/anti-inflammatory agent.
Design: The length, width, thickness, equatorial section surface, weight, volume, and seed coat section were measured in all the beans. The seed surface area was also estimated by an original empirical method. The ability of the different beans to interfere with the enzymes of the polyol pathway (that is, aldose reductase (AR) and sorbitol dehydrogenase) was tested using the supernatant after soaking the beans at room temperature and after thermal treatment, which simulated the bean-cooking process in a controlled fashion.
Results: Concerning the general features, Zolfino was comparable with other beans, except Corona, in terms of surface–volume ratio, which possesses the lowest tegument thickness. Moreover, Zolfino appears the most effective in inhibiting AR activity. The inhibitory ability is unaffected by thermal treatment and appears to be associated with compound(s) present in the coat of the bean.
Conclusions: The ability of Zolfino to inhibit AR, thus reducing the flux of glucose through the polyol pathway, highlights the features of Zolfino as a functional food, potentially useful in treating the dysfunctions linked to the hyperactivity of AR, such as diabetic complications or inflammatory responses.

Keywords: *Zolfino bean*; *Phaseolus vulgaris*; *aldose reductase*; *sorbitol dehydrogenase*; *polyol pathway*

The Zolfino bean is a variety of *Phaseolus vulgaris*, which is cultivated in the area between Arezzo and Florence in Tuscany, Italy. Zolfino has a thin coat, which means that it does not need to be pre-treated before cooking. In addition, its soft texture, special flavor, sweet taste, as well as digestibility make this bean an excellent food, appreciated for long, and a perfect complement to the traditional Tuscan cuisine (1). The Zolfino is a bush-type bean that is particularly sensitive to temperature, humidity, and soil conditions. The passion and business acumen of a few farmers have saved this variety, as well as other bean landraces, from extinction (2).

The basic nutrition parameters for the Zolfino bean, such as its protein or trypsin inhibitor content, are not complete or adequate characterizations (2). More specifically, although not exclusively, the Zolfino's pattern of secondary metabolites and antioxidant properties (3) may mean that it can be officially categorized as a functional food. The flavonoid content and the characterization of a number of Zolfino phenotypes, defined by the colors of the coat (namely, yellow, tobacco, and black), have been reported (4). Although differently represented in the three landraces, glycosylated kaempferol derivatives have been identified as the major components in alcoholic extracts, while the isoflavones daidzein and genistein have also been reported to a much lesser extent.

Essentially, the same pattern of flavonoid derivatives has been identified in 10 different analyzed ecotypes of *Zolfino del Pratomagno* grown in different areas of Arezzo (5). The variability in the composition of flavonoids observed among these samples, which was also observed among samples from the same area harvested over a 3-year period, highlights how these molecules respond dynamically to environmental and meteorological changes.

In order to extend the ability of the Zolfino bean to interact with biotargets linked to human oxidative stress conditions, the susceptibility to inhibition by components of the bean of the two polyol pathway enzymes, namely aldose reductase (AR) and sorbitol dehydrogenase (SDH), was evaluated. AR, which is the first enzyme of the pathway, catalyzes the NADPH-dependent reduction of glucose and a number of different aldehyde compounds (6). SDH, the second and last enzyme of the polyol pathway, removes the sorbitol generated by AR through an NAD^+ dependent oxidation leading to fructose (7). As it is involved in the etiology of diabetic complications and in the NFkB-linked inflammatory signaling (8), AR is also involved in the detoxification from cytotoxic aldehydes generated from membrane peroxidative processes (9, 10). AR has thus received much attention as a target of inhibitors, capable of counteracting and/or ameliorating the pathological states linked to hyperglycemic conditions (11–13).

We characterized and compared a yellow Zolfino landrace cultivated in the Leccio-Reggello area (Tuscany) with three other varieties of *Phaseolus vulgaris* (i.e. the Borlotto, Cannellino, and Corona beans) in terms of its general features and its inhibitory potential on the polyol pathway enzymes.

Materials and methods

Materials

D,L-Dithiothreitol (DTT), EDTA, β-D($-$) fructose, bovine serum albumin (BSA), NADH, and sheep liver SDH (E.C. 1.1.1.14, 40 U/mg) were obtained from Sigma-Aldrich (Saint Louis, MO, USA). NADPH and L-idose were supplied by Carbosynth (Compton, England); YM10 ultrafiltration membranes were obtained from Merck-Millipore (Darmstadt, Germany). The electrophoretic equipment was from Bio-Rad Laboratories (Hercules, CA, USA). All other chemicals were reagent grade. Molecular-weight markers for SDS-PAGE were obtained from Thermo Fisher Scientific (Waltham, MA, USA).

Dry beans of the yellow Zolfino landrace were obtained from the farm Agostinelli Mario in Leccio-Reggello (Florence, Italy; 43° 42' N, 11° 27' E), and their authenticity was confirmed by comparing their features with those registered in the 'Regione Toscana' germplasm data bank (access VE_027): www.germoplasma.arsia.toscana.it/.

Dry beans of the Borlotto (also referred to as the 'cranberry' bean), the Cannellino (also referred to as the 'alubia' bean), and the Corona (also referred to as the 'sweet white runner' bean) are in the National Register under horticultural varieties access number 307, 301, and 386, respectively (www.sementi.it/articoli/164/registro-nazionale-varieta-specie-ortaggi), and were obtained from the market. The Borlotto and Cannellino beans were from Frantoio Oleario Bartolini Emilio s.r.l., Arrone, Terni, Italy; the Corona beans were from Pedon SpA, Molvena, Vicenza, Italy.

Methods

Bean size evaluation

The length (L), width (g), and thickness (p) of the beans were measured by a vernier caliper with a precision to 0.01 mm. The perimeter and area of the equatorial section of the beans were quantitated on a scanned image of 30 beans by Image Measurement software KLONK (Ringsted, Denmark). The area was also measured by weighing the paper of the bean image carefully cut out after scanner printing. The actual surface was obtained by a surface standard reference scanned with the beans.

Bean weight was determined by weighing 20 independent samples, each composed of 10 randomly chosen beans. The weight of each sample was divided by 10 and the values averaged.

Bean volume was determined by evaluating the water displacement by the addition of 20 independent samples, each composed of 10 randomly chosen beans. The volume of each sample was divided by 10 and the values averaged.

Bean surface estimation

The bean surface was estimated by averaging the values from two different empirical approaches.

A. The beans were first assumed to be represented by a regular geometric solid (i.e. a 'capsule'), composed of a cylinder ending with two hemispheres with the same radius of the cylinder base. The length of the capsule is the measured length of the bean, while its radius comes from the mean between the width and thickness of the bean, divided by two. Thus, the height of the cylinder that makes up the capsule is obtained by subtracting the diameter of the sphere from the measured bean length. The shape and size of this solid is then corrected by subtracting, from the original capsule volume, the volume of a slice cut in the equatorial region of the capsule. The thickness of the slice, approximated to a cylindroid, is calculated as described below.

The difference between the volume of the capsule (V) and the measured volume of the bean (v), was set as:

$$V - v = \Delta V = Ah\frac{g}{p}$$

in which A is the equatorial area of the capsule and $\frac{g}{p}$ is a factor introduced to take into account the effect of the shape of the bean on the evaluation. The virtual height of the cylindroid, that is, the thickness of the slice, h, is then used to evaluate the lateral area of the cylindroid. This value is then subtracted from the surface of the capsule in order to estimate the surface of the bean (see Supplementary Fig. 1, Panel A).

B. The bean is first assumed to be a cylindroid, whose base is shaped as the equatorial section of a capsule as defined above (see method A) in which the length and the width are the length and width of the bean. The height of the cylindroid is the thickness of the bean. The shape and size of this regular solid, which can be assumed to contain the bean, is then corrected as described below.

The difference between the volume of the cylindroid (V) and the measured volume of the bean (v) was set as:

$$\Delta V = V - \nu = p\frac{1}{2}Pk\frac{p}{g}$$

in which P is the perimeter of the cylindroid base. Through this approach, the original cylindroid may be transformed into a new regular solid with the same width and approximately the same length as the original solid but consisting of a smaller cylindroid surrounded by a prism with a triangular base. The base and height of this triangle are p and k, respectively. Also, in this case, the factor $\frac{p}{g}$ was introduced to take into account the effect of the bean shape on the evaluation. The base of the new cylindroid will have a width of $g^* = g - 2k$, a radius of terminal semicircles $r^* = g/2 - k$, and a length of the rectangular component $l^* = L - 2r$. This new solid, whose perimeter and surface of the base are $P^* = 2\pi r^* + 2L^*$ and $A^* = \pi(r^*)^2 + 2r^*L^*$, respectively, is complemented by a triangular base prism, whose exposed lateral surface S* is $S^* = 2P^*\left[k^2 + \left(\frac{p}{2}\right)^2\right]^{\frac{1}{2}}$.

The surface of the emerging solid: $S = 2A^* + S^*$ is then taken as an estimate of the bean surface (see Supplementary Fig. 1, Panel B).

The surface evaluation of the bean is finally obtained from the average of the surfaces measured with both methods A and B. Because of comparable errors in direct measurements (Table 1) on different beans, no error propagation analysis of measured parameters in the calculated parameters was performed.

In order to validate the surface estimate of the beans, the Corona beans were used as a reference, because they are relatively large and their coats are easy to remove. Thus, 25 beans were cut in order to separate the cotyledons, very rapidly wetted (15–20 sec), and the teguments gently removed. In these conditions, the tegument, which comes

Table 1. Size parameters of different beans

	Measured parameters		Zolfino	Borlotto	Cannellino	Corona
1	Weight (g)[a]		0.34 ± 0.01	0.58 ± 0.02	0.72 ± 0.02	2.40 ± 0.12
2	Weight of tegument (g)[b]		0.021 ± 0.002	0.044 ± 0.008	0.050 ± 0.006	0.382 ± 0.03
3	Tegument w/total w (w/w %)		6.18	7.59	6.94	15.91
4	Volume (cm^3)[c]		0.27 ± 0.02	0.47 ± 0.04	0.55 ± 0.02	2.58 ± 0.04
5	Length (cm)		1.04 ± 0.13	1.39 ± 0.08	1.63 ± 0.08	2.77 ± 0.13
6	Minor section (thickness) (cm)		0.64 ± 0.05	0.67 ± 0.05	0.73 ± 0.04	0.98 ± 0.10
7	Major section (width) (cm)		0.71 ± 0.08	0.89 ± 0.06	0.82 ± 0.04	1.70 ± 0.09
8	Equatorial surface by weight (cm^2)		0.65 ± 0.13	0.98 ± 0.13	1.12 ± 0,14	3.48 ± 0.40
9	Equatorial surface by Klonk[d] (cm^2)		0.55 ± 0.08	0.91 ± 0.10	0.97 ± 0.11	3.44 ± 0.45
10	Perimeter by Klonk[d] (cm)		3.35 ± 0.26	4.39 ± 0.30	4.70 ± 0.22	8.60 ± 0.63
11	Tegument thickness	By caliper[e]	79 ± 34	160 ± 49	112 ± 59	270 ± 98
12		By image analysis	93 ± 8	147 ± 14	133 ± 10	312 ± 21
13		Density (g/cm^3)	1.26 ± 0.1	1.23 ± 0.11	1.31 ± 0.06	0.93 ± 0.05
	Calculated parameters					
14	Surface (cm^2)	Method A[d]	2.1	3.2	3.7	10.8
15		Method B[d]	2.0	3.3	3.5	11.7
16		A, B average	2.0	3.2	3.6	11.3
17	Surface/volume (cm^{-1})		7.7	6.9	6.5	4.4
18	Tegument weight/surface (g/cm^2)		0.010	0.013	0.014	0.034
19	Thickness (μm)	Referred to Zolfino	93	121	130	316
20		Referred to Corona	92	120	128	312

[a]20 independent measurements of groups of 30 beans.
[b]3 independent measurements of groups of 10 beans.
[c]10 independent measurements of groups of 10 beans.
[d]See Methods.
[e]At least 15 independent measurements.

out almost as an integer, was transversely cut in order to make it flat, kept for few minutes, gently squeezed between sheets of filter paper, and then scanned. The area was then measured as above.

Seed coat section measurements

In order to evaluate the contribution of the seed coat (i.e. the outer integument plus the inner integument and residual endosperm) to the total weight of the bean, the coat was gently removed. The part of the endosperm that had remained attached to the cotyledons was gently scraped and added to the removed coat. The weight of the material recovered after this approach (i.e. the tegument plus cotyledons) was never less than 99% of the weight of the integer bean.

In order to measure the thickness of the coat, parts of the tegument were gently removed to prevent any endosperm detachment and checked by optical microscopy for the absence of particles, possibly from the cotyledons, taken during the coat removal. The thickness was measured by a Vernier caliper with a 0.01-mm precision. Because of the difficulties in controlling the pressure applied on the caliper in each measurement, thickness determination was also performed by optical microscopy imaging. Tegument transverse sections were mounted on the stage of a Nikon Eclipse E600FN microscope with a 10 × objective. The epi-illumination of the sample was performed with an optical fiber. Images were acquired by a CCD camera (WV-BP514E, Panasonic, Kadoma, Japan) and collected using Axon Imaging Workbench 2.2 software (Molecular Device, Sunnyvale, CA, USA), by averaging 16 frames (time of exposure 528 ms). Acquired images were processed using the open source Image-J software.

Assay, expression, and purification of AR

The activity of AR (E.C. 1.1.1.21) was determined at 37°C, following the decrease in absorbance at 340 nm due to NADPH oxidation ($\varepsilon_{340} = 6.22\ mM^{-1} \cdot cm^{-1}$). Briefly, the standard assay mixture (700 μL) contained 0.25-M sodium phosphate buffer pH 6.8, 0.18-mM NADPH, 0.4-M ammonium sulfate, 0.5-mM EDTA, and 4.7- mM glyceraldehyde. The oxidation rate of NADPH oxidation in the absence of the substrate was subtracted as a blank. One unit of enzyme activity is the amount that catalyzes the conversion of 1 μmol of substrate/min in the above assay conditions. These assay conditions were also adopted to evaluate the effectiveness as inhibitors of the bean extracts when 0.6-mM L-idose was used as a substrate.

The human placental aldose reductase (*h*AR) was expressed and purified as previously described (14, 15). The specific activity of purified *h*AR was 5.3 U/mg of protein. The purified *h*AR was stored at −80°C in a 10-mM sodium phosphate, buffer pH 7.0 containing 2-mM DTT with 30% (w/v) glycerol. Before use, the enzyme was extensively dialyzed against sodium phosphate buffer pH 7.0.

Assay of SDH

The SDH assay was performed at 37°C, essentially as previously described (16), by following the decrease in absorbance at 340 nm in a reaction mixture (700 μL) containing 0.18-mM NADH and 0.4-M D-fructose in 100-mM Tris/HCl, buffer pH 7.4. The rate of NADH oxidation measured in a parallel assay, in which the substrate was omitted, was subtracted as a blank. One unit of enzyme activity is the amount of SDH that catalyzes the oxidation of 1 μmol substrate/min in the above assay conditions.

Other methods

Protein concentration was determined according to Bradford (17), using BSA as a standard protein. The protein pattern of bean extracts was assessed through SDS-PAGE (18); gels were stained with 0.1% Coomassie blue R250, in 10% acetic acid and 20% ethanol. Acquired images of stained gels were processed using the open source Image-J software.

Absorption spectra were acquired through a Biochrom Libra S35PC single beam spectrophotometer (1-nm bandwidth), calibrated with water as a reference. If not otherwise specified, the absorbance data acquired within the instrumental linear dynamic range were then converted into true values by multiplying the absorbance values by the dilution factor.

All the samples of seed extracts and seed-flour extracts analyzed for both absorption spectra and enzyme inhibitory activity were centrifuged at 4°C for 1 h at $9.6 \times 10^4 \times g$ in a Beckman Optima L-90K ultracentrifuge before analysis.

Statistical analysis was performed using standard statistical software (GraphPad Instat version 3.05, San Diego, CA); the results are reported as the mean of the values ± standard deviation and the number of replicates is indicated each time.

Results and discussion

The distinctive size parameters of the Zolfino landrace used in this study, such as length, width, thickness, equatorial section surface, weight, and volume, were measured. The results are summarized in Table 1. The bean surface was also estimated (Table 1) as described in the 'Methods' section. The method was validated using the Corona bean, whose calculated surface was 11.3 cm^2, which compares well with the measured value of 11.1 ± 1.7 cm^2. With this approach, the Zolfino surface was 2.0 cm^2, which is indicative of the highest exposed surface per unit weight (5.9 cm^2/g) and per unit volume (7.4 cm^{-1}) of the tested beans. The ratios of both surface/weight and surface/volume of all the beans were similar, except for the Corona beans, whose surface/volume ratio was significantly lower (approximately 40% of that of the Zolfino bean). To quantify the thinness of the Zolfino coat, portions of the coat

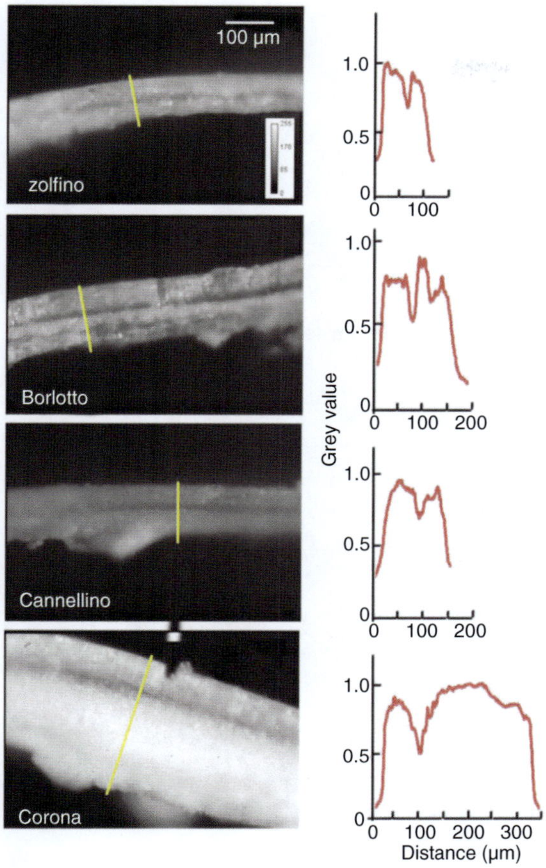

Fig. 1. Epi-illumination micrographs of tegument transverse sections from four varieties of beans. On the right of each image, a two-dimensional graph of the pixel value as a function of the distance along the yellow line is displayed.

were used by measuring the section thickness with a caliper. The variability of the measurements (Table 1, line 11), even in the same sample, was overcome by evaluating the coat section with microscopy imaging. The typical organization of the teguments was analyzed on a digital image, through the distribution of the pixel-grade level along lines crossing the coat sections. The images of the different beans and the relative profile graphs are shown in Fig. 1. As can be seen, the endosperm is mainly responsible for the observed differences, as the inner and the outer integuments are very similar among the beans. The results of the analysis are reported in Table 1, line 12.

Using these measured values, we evaluated the tegument thickness from the weight/surface ratio of the tegument. The calculated thickness was in a good agreement with the measured values, suggesting that the beans were similar in terms of coat density. This is shown in Table 1, in which the measured coat thickness of both the Zolfino and the Corona were used as a reference value (compare lines 19 and 20 with lines 11 and 12).

Despite a lower coat thickness and larger surface contact, conceivably leading to more efficient fluid entry, no correlation between the relative surface exposure and the time course of water absorption could be found. Indeed, the Zolfino bean, closely followed by the Cannellino bean, is more resistant to water entry than the Corona and Borlotto beans (Fig. 2a). This is not surprising, as water and solutes trafficking in and out of the tegument are perhaps governed by the overall structural differences in permeability and composition linked to different bean varieties (19–21).

The extrusion of compounds from the beans undergoing water imbibition was monitored by absorption spectroscopy. The difference between different bean varieties is clearly shown in Fig. 2b, which reports the absorption spectra of the incubation medium of different beans after 1 h of incubation at room temperature (22–25°C). The absorption spectra obtained at different times of incubation are shown in the Supplementary Fig. 2. The difference in the extruded compounds during incubation is highlighted

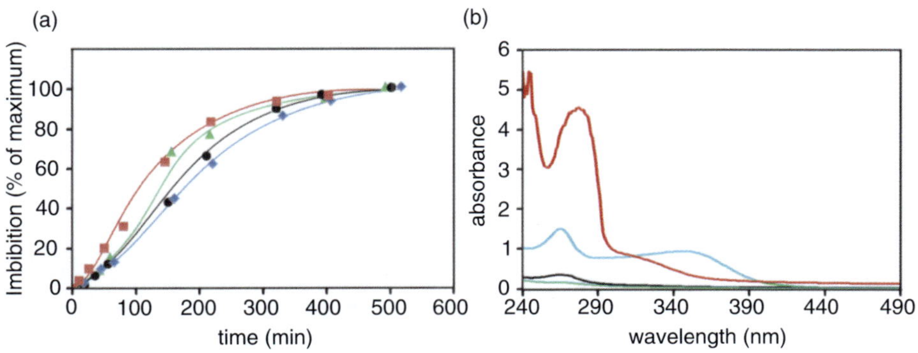

Fig. 2. Water entry and extrusion of molecular species. Beans were suspended (0.4 g/mL) in deionized water and left at room temperature (22–25°C). Panel a: at the indicated times, the incubation medium was carefully removed and the water entry, reported as a percentage of maximal imbibition, was evaluated by the increase in bean weight. Symbols (◆), (■), (●), and (▲) refer to Zolfino, Borlotto, Cannellino, and Corona, respectively. Panel b: the absorption spectra are reported in the UV-visible region of the imbibition medium after 1 h of incubation. The spectra were acquired directly on the incubation media except for Borlotto for which a twofold dilution in water of the medium was required; data are normalized for the dilution. Blue, red, black, and green lines refer to Zolfino, Borlotto, Cannellino, and Corona, respectively.

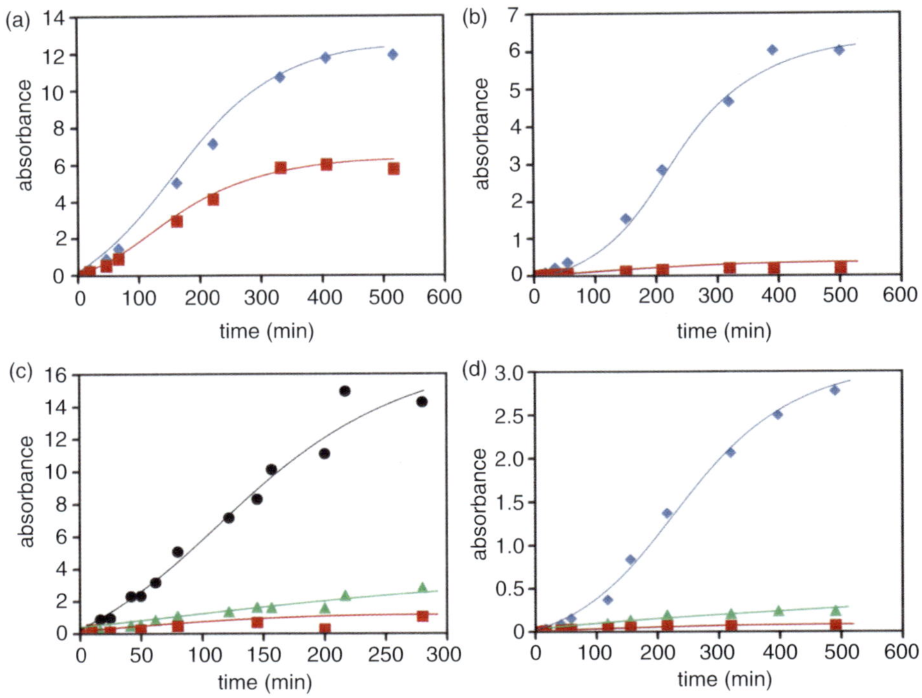

Fig. 3. Time course of chromophores extrusion during beans imbibition. The release of bean components and incubation times are reported for different beans as the absorbance measured at distinctive wavelengths, namely 265 (◆), 273 (●), 310 (▲), and 345 (■) nm. Panels a, b, c, d refer to Zolfino, Cannellino, Borlotto, and Corona, respectively.

in Fig. 3, which reports the absorbance at different wavelengths for the different beans at different times.

Beside an absorption peak in the region 260–280 nm, which is common to all the bean varieties, an absorbance peak is evident in the Zolfino spectrum at approximately 350 nm, with a tail protruding over 400 nm, which is not present in other beans. Although no attempt was performed to specifically identify the yellow-colored component(s), the spectral features are consistent with those of the flavonoid family, previously identified in the Zolfino (4, 22). This is supported by the comparison, reported in Fig. 4a, of the spectra of a methanolic extract of the Zolfino coat and of a solution of authentic kaempferol 3-O-glucoside, which is the most representative flavonol present in the Zolfino bean. Thus, the ratio of the absorbance at 265 and 345 nm, observed in the water extract media, which is too high for a typical kaempferol derivative (Figs. 3 and 4b), may derive from the presence in the incubating medium of other water-soluble chromophores extruded from the cotyledons or/and from the bean coat. As shown in Fig. 4b,

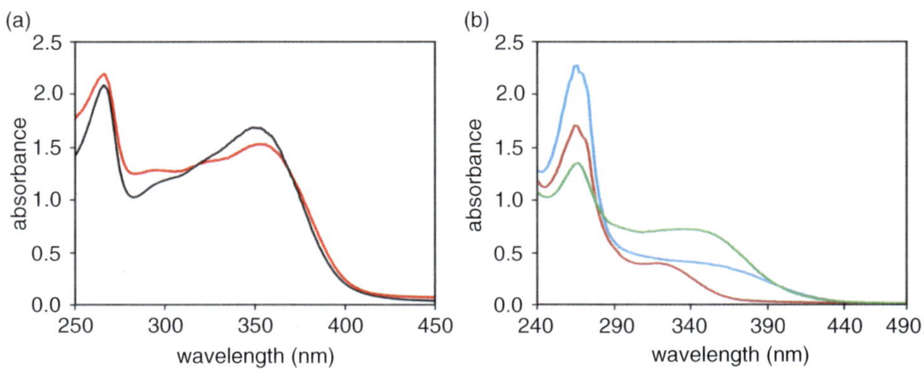

Fig. 4. Yellow chromophores from Zolfino. Panel a: Absorption spectra of methanol extract of Zolfino tegument (the tegument from 1.5 g of seeds soaked in 3 mL methanol for 1 h at room temperature) (red line) and of 20 μM in methanol of authentic kaempferol-3O-glucoside (black line) are reported. Panel b: absorption spectra of water extract from tegument (green line), cotyledons (red line), and whole (blue line) Zolfino bean are reported. Teguments and cotyledons derived from 1.5 g of Zolfino seeds were soaked for 1 h at room temperature in 3 and 6 mL of water, respectively, and the medium analyzed. Whole seeds (1.5 g) were soaked as above in 6 mL of water and the medium analyzed.

Table 2. Some nutritional parameters of different beans

Measured parameters g/100 g dry bean	Zolfino[a]	Borlotto[b]	Cannellino[b]	Corona[b]
Proteins	23.10 ± 1.85	19.4	23.6	23.4
Total carbohydrates	39.16 ± 0.48	47.2	43.1	45.1
Total fat	2.43 ± 0.10	0.8	0.8	0.9
Saturated fat	0.40 ± 0.01	0.1	0.1	0.2
Fibers	19.50 ± 5.85	16.5	17.2	15.2

[a]Values certified by ChelabSilliker Italia, a Mérieux NutriSciences company, Test Report No. 1433658.02 (2014).
[b]Values certified by the producer company; no standard deviation is available.

the absorption spectra of aqueous extracts from the integer bean, coat, and cotyledons indicate that the yellow component(s), which may be responsible for the pale yellow color of the bean, from which the name Zolfino is derived, as expected (2), is essentially from the coat. Conversely, the material that contributes most to the absorption in the 260–280-nm region appears to mainly originate from the inside of the bean embryo.

Protein pattern

Various certified nutritional parameters of the Zolfino bean are reported in Table 2, together with those of other more common varieties of *Phaseolus vulgaris.* Although the reported values suggest that this bean variety is a valuable food, these parameters are limited in their ability to distinguish Zolfino from the other more common bean varieties (2). In this regard, the literature reports a wide

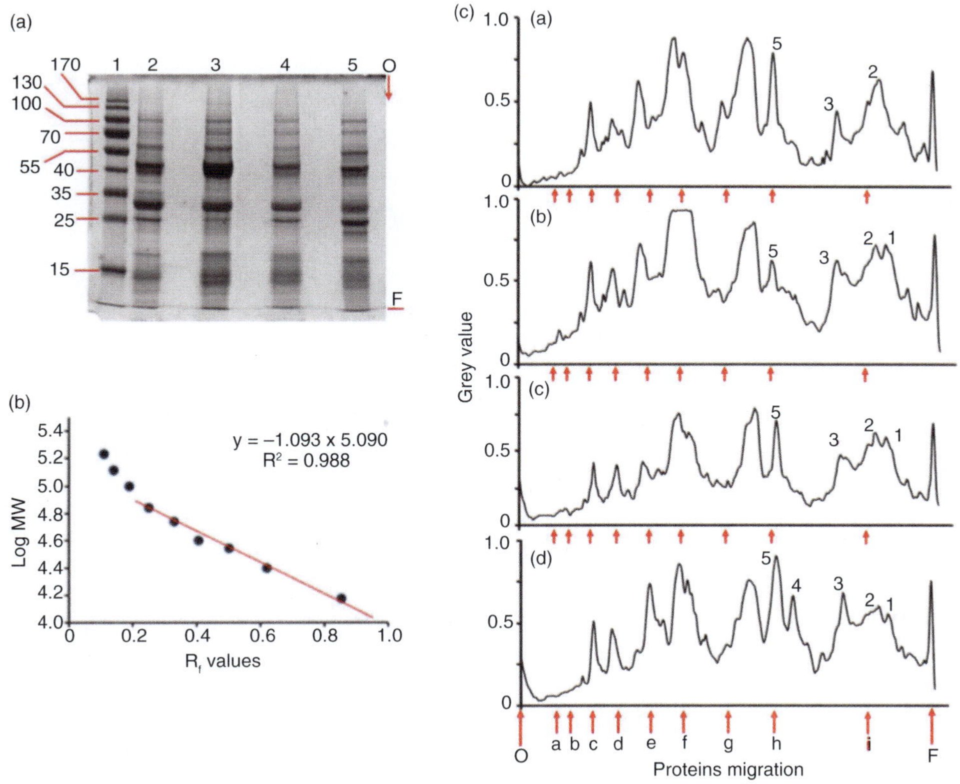

Fig. 5. Electrophoretic pattern of water-soluble proteins from different bean varieties. Water-soluble proteins extracts from bean flours (100 mg/mL) were analyzed by SDS-PAGE on 12% acrylamide gels. 3 μg of proteins were applied to each well. Panel a: Coomassie blue–stained gel of water flour extracts of Zolfino, Cannellino, Borlotto, and Corona beans (lanes 2 to 5, respectively). Lane 1 refers to MW standard proteins. Numbers alongside the gel represent their apparent molecular weights divided by 1,000. Panel b: molecular-weight calibration curve using standard proteins (lane 1 of the stained gel). The equation reported was obtained by linear regression analysis of standards migration Panel c: aligned electropherogram profiles for Zolfino (a), Cannellino (b), Borlotto (c), and Corona (d). Arrows marked with letters *a–h* refer to the migration of MW standards reported in Panel b. Numbers on the profiles refer to specific protein bands characterizing the protein patterns. The letters O and F refer to the origin and to the front of the migration, respectively.

range of values for these parameters (23, 24). Furthermore, a direct comparison of the percentage content (g/100 g dry bean) of water-soluble proteins in the bean flours (4.6±0.3, 3.8±0.3, 3.9±0.4, and 4.4±0.3, for the Zolfino, Cannellino, Borlotto, and Corona beans, respectively) does not reveal significant differences among the beans. When the comparison was extended to the electrophoretic pattern, some specific features emerged (Fig. 5). A much more detailed investigation, which is beyond the scope of this study, would be required for a complete analysis of the protein characterizations (25). However, in terms of the aligned electropherogram profiles of the beans, we found differences in the relative distributions of protein bands in the phaseolin (47,000–50,000 MW) and phytohemagglutinin (29,000–30,000 MW) regions. The triplet of bands (Fig. 5c, bands 1, 2, and 3) present in the MW range of 13,000–18,000, also appears to be a discriminating factor. In fact, these bands appear equally represented in the Cannellino and Borlotto beans, while band 1 is poorly represented or unrepresented in the Zolfino bean, and band 3 appears to prevail in the Corona bean. Other examples of particular protein patterns are the 23,400 MW band (band 4), well represented in the Corona bean, but lacking in the Zolfino, Cannellino, and Borlotto beans; and the 26,000 MW band (band 5), which is poorly represented in the Borlotto bean compared with all other beans.

Bio-interactions

The ability of different beans to interfere with the activity of the enzymes of the polyol pathway (i.e. AR and SDH) was tested by using the supernatant of the suspending medium from the imbibition curves performed at room temperature. The inhibitory potential on *h*AR of different extracts is reported in Fig. 6a. The Zolfino and Borlotto beans were found to extrude the most active inhibitory mixtures; each displayed an IC_{50} of approximately 14.3 mg equivalents of dry bean/mL of assay mixture (DBeq mg/mL). In the same conditions, the Cannellino and Corona beans did not reach 50% inhibition, and at the maximal tested level of 28.6 DBeq mg/mL showed

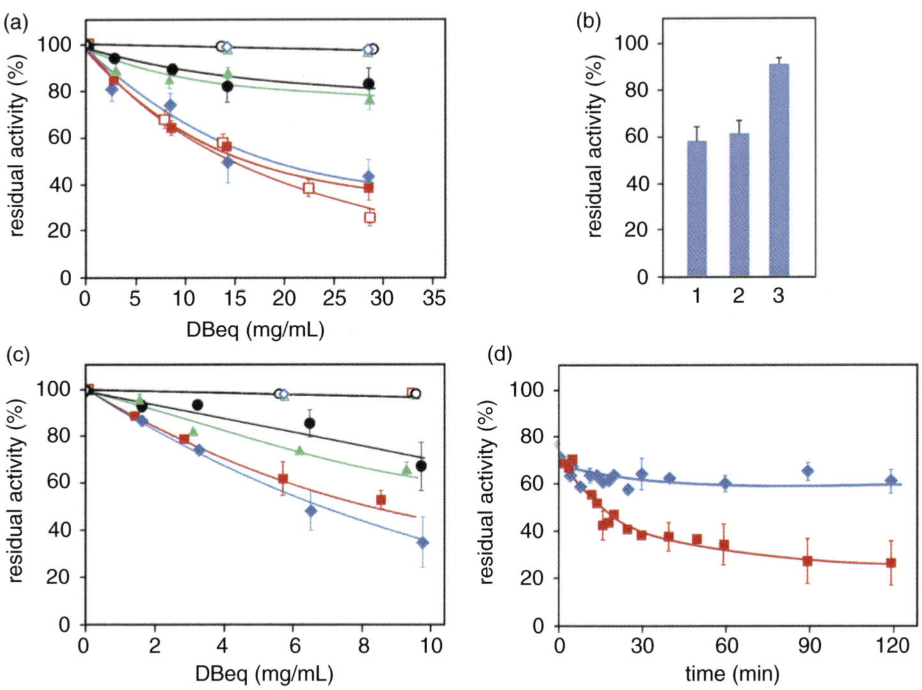

Fig. 6. Polyol pathway enzymes inhibition by bean water extracts. The effect of different extracts from Zolfino (◆, ◇), Borlotto (■, □), Cannellino (●, ○), and Corona (▲, △) was tested on AR (closed symbols) and SDH (open symbols). The residual activity is reported as a% of the activity measured in the absence of the effector, which accounts for 8 and 3.1 mU for AR and SDH, respectively. Error bars (when not visible, these are within the symbol size) represent the standard deviation from three independent measurements. Panel a: The aqueous medium derived from an overnight incubation at room temperature of the bean seeds (400 mg/mL) was centrifuged; various amounts of the supernatants (expressed as DBeq mg/mL, see text) were added to the standard assay mixture of AR and SDH. Panel b: the whole Zolfino bean (bar 1), tegument (bar 2), and cotyledons (bar 3) were incubated overnight at room temperature in water at 200, 12, and 190 mg/mL, respectively. After centrifugation, aliquots of the supernatants (corresponding to 8.6 DBeq mg/mL) were tested for AR inhibition effectiveness. Panel c: Bean seeds were incubated (200 mg/mL) in a boiling water bath for 2 h. After the seeds had been separated, the medium was centrifuged and tested for AR and SDH inhibitory efficiency. Panel d: The aqueous medium from an overnight incubation at room temperature (400 mg/mL) was centrifuged and the supernatant incubated in a boiling water bath. At the times indicated, aliquots were withdrawn and tested (4.3 DBeq mg/mL) for AR inhibition effectiveness.

17 and 23% AR inhibition, respectively. As happens with the yellow chromophores of beans (Fig. 4b), the inhibitory potential on AR activity of the extract resulting from the imbibition process also appears to be confined to the coat. This is highlighted in Fig. 6b, which reports a comparable inhibition of the water extract from the bean coat and from the whole bean. Conversely, no inhibition is displayed by the water extract of cotyledons. When SDH was used as a target enzyme, the Borlotto extract was the only one that inhibited the enzyme, with an IC_{50} of approximately 14.3 mg DBeq/mL. This feature, favoring polyalcohol accumulation, as it occurs, for example, in galactose-induced cataract (26, 27), would be deleterious for the cell. No SDH inhibition was observed with other beans at the maximal level tested of 28.6 DBeq mg/mL.

Although, to our knowledge, no toxicity data are reported for the Zolfino bean, it is well known that beans should not be eaten raw, due to the presence of antimetabolites and toxic compounds (28). Thus, the inhibitory action of different beans was measured on the supernatant of the suspending medium of the beans kept for 2 h at 100°C in a boiling water bath ('cooking medium'). These conditions simulate the process of beans being cooked, yet do not destroy the inhibitory potential, which actually seems to be enhanced. The cooking media of the Zolfino and Borlotto beans displayed an IC_{50} ranging from approximately 6.4 to 7.9 mg DBeq/mL. Although the inhibitory action of Cannellino and Corona beans was greater than when the incubation was performed at room temperature, it did not exceed 30–35% inhibition at the highest tested amount of approximately 10-DBeq mg/mL in the assay (Fig. 6c). The observed increase in the inhibitory ability of the beans after the thermal treatment may derive either from a more extensive release from the beans of the inhibitory species (the same or different species with respect to those extruded at room temperature) (see Supplementary Fig. 3) or from their modification under thermal treatment (see Supplementary Fig. 4). All options may also take place. In fact, the progressive increase in absorption of the cooking medium over time indicates that, as expected, cooking leads to a massive release of the internal bean components (with or without AR inhibitory action) (see Supplementary Fig. 3). On the contrary, the incubation at 100°C of the medium obtained at room temperature determined, for the Borlotto bean, both spectral changes (see Supplementary Fig. 4) and a significant increase of the inhibitory effect on AR (Fig. 6d). These effects were not observed with the Zolfino bean. Other factors must thus explain the comparable inhibitory action of the Zolfino and Borlotto beans when the whole beans were thermally treated (Fig. 6c). For example, some of the components extruded and activated, during the thermal treatment of the whole bean, may either contribute to the Zolfino inhibitory effect or mitigate the effect, as in the case of the Borlotto bean. This hypothesis, which we are currently investigating, may be supported by the results concerning the inhibitory potential of the water extracts of powdered beans (Fig. 7a). In this case, although Zolfino still appears to be the most active, all the bean extracts display a comparable AR inhibitory activity, and no marked increase of the inhibitory potential after the thermal stress was observed for any of them (Fig. 7b).

After thermal treatment, no inhibition of SDH activity was observed for any of the extracts, including the Borlotto bean (Fig. 6c). Consequently, after cooking the beans, the deleterious influence due to the inhibition of the sorbitol removal through the polyol pathway is, in any case, abolished.

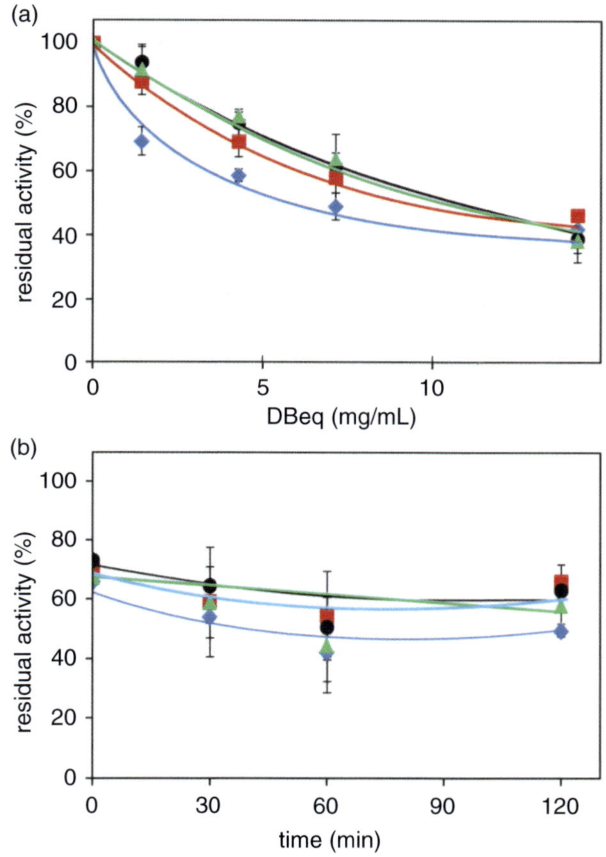

Fig. 7. Aldose reductase inhibition by water extract of bean flours. The effect of different extracts from the flour of Zolfino (◆), Borlotto (■), Cannellino (●), and Corona (▲) was tested on AR activity. The residual activity is reported as a percent of the activity in the absence of the effector, which accounts for 8 mU. Error bars (when not visible, these are within the symbol size) represent the standard deviation from three independent measurements. Bean seeds frozen in liquid nitrogen were powdered in a mortar, suspended (400 mg/mL) in water, and centrifuged (see Methods). Panel a: the indicated amounts of supernatants (expressed as DBeq mg/mL, see text) were used to test the AR inhibitory effectiveness. Panel b: the supernatants were subjected to incubation in a boiling water bath, and at the times indicated, aliquots were withdrawn and tested (4.3 DBeq mg/mL) for AR inhibition effectiveness.

A final comparison between the Zolfino and Borlotto beans, which were the most similar in terms of AR inhibition ability, was made after following specific recommendations for cooking the beans. Thus, Fig. 8 reports the AR inhibitory potential detectable in the cooking media of Borlotto beans previously soaked in water, as recommended in many recipes, and of Zolfino beans, cooked without soaking, as is also recommended. In this case, the Borlotto beans, having lost some inhibitory potential because of the preliminary soaking, are less efficient in acting on AR.

Conclusions

The known tenderness of the coat of the Zolfino bean, ease of cooking, excellent taste, mild flavor, and easy digestibility were good reasons for investigating this variety of bean. However, the particular pattern of the possible antioxidant metabolites shown in the Zolfino provided a further motivation for examining its properties as a functional food. In terms of the data characterizing the Zolfino with respect to other beans varieties, this study focused on the targets of AR and SDH, the two enzymes of the polyol pathway, in order to assess the potential of this bean to beneficially impact deleterious metabolic conditions. In terms of the extracts of thermally untreated beans, the AR inhibition data were useful in presenting the particular features of the different bean varieties, but the maintenance of the AR inhibitory potential of Zolfino after cooking is of special interest from a nutraceutical point of view. Zolfino's potential to reduce the flow of glucose, through the polyol pathway and without interfering with the SDH-dependent sorbitol removal, highlights that this bean can be exploited as a functional food. It suggests its ability to intervene in dysfunctions linked to the hyperactivity of AR, such as diabetic complications or/and inflammatory responses through AR-linked NF-kB cell signaling.

Further studies are required to correlate the observed AR inhibitory action of the well-defined components of raw beans, as well as those components that result from thermal treatment (that is, cooking). In this regard, work is in progress to examine the ability of different Zolfino components to differentially inhibit AR (13), which would increase its activity against diabetes complications and inflammation.

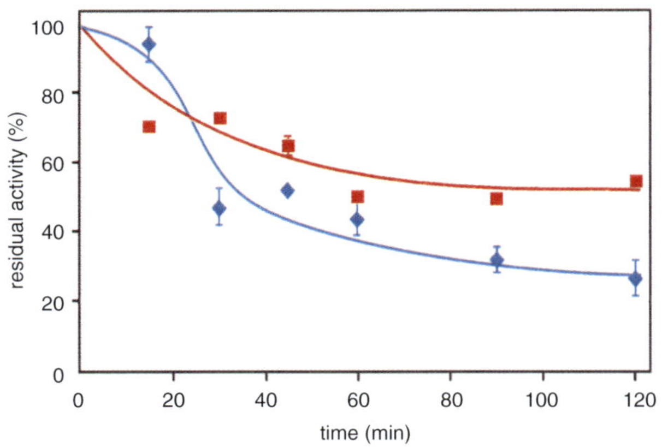

Fig. 8. Aldose reductase inhibition by the 'cooking media' of Zolfino and Borlotto. The suspending media of Zolfino directly incubated at 100°C (400 mg/mL) in water, and of Borlotto incubated as above after the removal of the water in which the bean (400 mg/mL) had been soaked overnight at room temperature. Residual AR activity was measured at different cooking times using 8.6-DBeq mg/mL and is reported as a percentage of the activity in the absence of the effector, which accounts for 8 mU. Error bars (when not visible, these are within the symbol size) represent the standard deviation from three independent measurements. (◆) and (■) refer to Zolfino and Borlotto, respectively.

Acknowledgements

This work was supported by Regione Toscana, Progetto IDARA.

The authors are grateful to Dr. Fiammetta Tanda for her valuable contribution to the graphical representation of the surface evaluation methods. Thanks are also due to Dr. Monica Pellegrini, Scuola Normale Superiore, Pisa, for her assistance in the imaging analysis.

Conflict of interest and funding

The authors declare that they have no conflict of interest.

References

1. Abala K. Beans: a history. Oxford: Berg; 2007, p. 188.
2. Piergiovanni AR, Lioi L. Italian common bean landraces: history, genetic diversity and seed quality. Diversity 2010; 2: 837–62.
3. Heimler D, Vignolini P, Dini MG, Romani A. Rapid test to assess the antioxidant activity of *Phaseolus vulgaris* L. dry beans. J Agric Food Chem 2005; 53: 3053–6.
4. Romani A, Vignolini P, Galardi C, Mulinacci N, Benedettelli S, Heimler D. Germplasm characterization of zolfino landraces (*Phaseolus vulgaris* L.) by flavonoid content. J Agric Food Chem 2004; 52: 3838–42.
5. Dinelli G, Bonetti A, Minelli M, Marotti I, Catizone P, Mazzanti A. Content of flavonols in Italian bean (*Phaseolus vulgaris* L.) ecotypes. Food Chem 2006; 99: 105–14.
6. Del Corso A, Cappiello M, Mura U. From a dull enzyme to something else: facts and perspectives regarding aldose reductase. Curr Med Chem 2008; 15: 1452–61.
7. El-Kabbani O, Darmanin C, Chung RP. Sorbitol dehydrogenase: structure, function and ligand design. Curr Med Chem 2004; 11: 465–76.
8. Alexiou P, Pegklidou K, Chatzopoulou M, Nicolaou I, Demopoulos VJ. Aldose reductase enzyme and its implication to major health problems of the 21(st) century. Curr Med Chem 2009; 16: 734–52.
9. Vander Jagt DL, Kolb NS, Vander Jagt TJ, Chino J, Martinez FJ, Hunsaker LA, et al. Substrate specificity of human aldose reductase: identification of 4-hydroxynonenal as an endogenous substrate. Biochim Biophys Acta 1995; 1249: 117–26.
10. Srivastava S, Chandra A, Bhatnagar A, Srivastava SK, Ansari NH. Lipid peroxidation product, 4-hydroxynonenal and its conjugate

with GSH are excellent substrates of bovine lens aldose reductase. Biochem Biophys Res Commun 1995; 217: 741–6.
11. Chatzopoulou M, Pegklidou K, Papastavrou N, Demopoulos VJ. Development of aldose reductase inhibitors for the treatment of inflammatory disorders. Expert Opin Drug Discov 2013; 8: 1365–80.
12. Maccari R, Ottanà R. Targeting aldose reductase for the treatment of diabetes complications and inflammatory diseases: new insights and future directions. J Med Chem 2015; 58: 2047–67.
13. Del Corso A, Balestri F, Di Bugno E, Moschini R, Cappiello M, Sartini S, et al. A new approach to control the enigmatic activity of aldose reductase. PLoS One 2013; 8: e74076. doi: http://dx.doi.org/10.1371/journal.pone.0074076
14. Balestri F, Cappiello M, Moschini R, Rotondo R, Buggiani I, Pelosi P, et al. L-Idose: an attractive substrate alternative to D-glucose for measuring aldose reductase activity. Biochem Biophys Res Commun 2015; 456: 891–5.
15. Del Corso A, Barsacchi D, Giannessi M, Tozzi MG, Camici M, Houben JL, et al. Bovine lens aldose reductase: tight binding of the pyridine coenzyme. Arch Biochem Biophys 1990; 283: 512–18.
16. Marini I, Bucchioni L, Borella P, Del Corso A, Mura U. Sorbitol dehydrogenase from bovine lens: purification and properties. Arch Biochem Biophys 1997; 340: 383–91.
17. Bradford MM. A rapid and sensitive method for the quantitation of microgram quantities of protein utilizing the principle of protein-dye binding. Anal Biochem 1976; 72: 248–54.
18. Laemmli UK. Cleavage of structural proteins during the assembly of the head of bacteriophage T4. Nature 1970; 227: 680–5.
19. Moïse JA, Han S, Gudynaitę-Savitch L, Johnson DA, Miki BLA. Seed coats: structure, development, composition and biotechnology. In Vitro Cell Dev Biol Plant 2005; 41: 620–44.
20. Debeaujon I, Léon-Kloosterziel KM, Koornneef M. Influence of the testa on seed dormancy, germination, and longevity in Arabidopsis. Plant Physiol 2000; 122: 403–14.
21. de Souza FHD, Marcos-Filho J. The seed coat as a modulator of seed-environment relationships in Fabaceae. Braz J Bot 2001; 24: 365–75.
22. Dall'Acqua S, Miolo G, Innocenti G, Caffieri S. The photodegradation of quercetin: relation to oxidation. Molecules 2012; 17: 8898–907.
23. Siddiq M, Ravi R, Harte JB, Dolan KD. Physical and functional characteristics of selected dry bean (*Phaseolus vulgaris* L.) flours. LWT Food Sci Technol 2010; 43: 232–7.
24. Samman N, Maldonado S, Alfaro ME, Farfan N, Gutierrez J. Composition of different bean varieties (*Phaseolus vulgaris*) of Northwestern Argentina (Region NOA): cultivation zone influence. J Agric Food Chem 1999; 47: 2685–9.
25. De La Fuente M, López-Pedrous M, Alonso J, Santalla M, De Ron AM, Álvarez G, et al. In-depth characterization of the phaseolin protein diversity of common bean (*Phaseolus vulgaris* L.) based on two-dimensional electrophoresis and mass spectrometry. Food Technol Biotechnol 2012; 50: 315–25.
26. Kador P, Inoue J, Secchi EF, Lizak MJ, Rodriguez L, Mori K. Effect of sorbitol dehydrogenase inhibition on sugar cataract formation in galactose-fed and diabetic rats. Exp Eye Res 1998; 67: 203–8.
27. Banditelli S, Boldrini E, Vilardo PG, Cecconi I, Cappiello M, Dal Monte M, et al. A new approach against sugar cataract through aldose reductase inhibitors. Exp Eye Res 1999; 69: 533–8.
28. Smartt J. Morphological, physiological and biochemical changes in Phaseolus beans under domestication. In: Gepts P, ed. Genetic resources of Phaseolus beans. Their maintenance, domestication, evolution and utilization. London: Kluwer Academic; 1988, pp. 143–62.

*Antonella Del-Corso
Biochemistry Unit
Department of Biology
University of Pisa
Via S. Zeno, 51
IT-56126
Pisa, Italy
Email: antonella.delcorso@unipi.it

19

Twelve-week-conjugated linoleic acid supplementation has no effects on the selected markers of atherosclerosis in obese and overweight women

Monika Dus-Zuchowska[1], Edyta Madry[2], Patrycja Krzyzanowska[1], Paweł Bogdanski[3] and Jaroslaw Walkowiak[1]*

[1]Department of Pediatric Gastroenterology and Metabolic Diseases, Poznan University of Medical Sciences, Poznan, Poland; [2]Department of Physiology, Poznan University of Medical Sciences, Poznan, Poland; [3]Department of Education and Obesity Treatment and Metabolic Disorders, Poznan University of Medical Sciences, Poznan, Poland

Abstract

Background: The antiatherogenic effect of conjugated linoleic acid (CLA) has been demonstrated in animal models. Although there are plenty of *in vitro* studies that suggest the profitable properties of CLA, the results in humans remain inconsistent.
Objective: In this study, we assessed the impact of CLA supplementation on the levels of atherosclerosis markers – high-sensitivity C-reactive protein (hs-CRP) and asymmetrical dimethylarginine (ADMA).
Design: Seventy-four adult female subjects with body mass index ≥ 25 kg/m^2 were enrolled in the double-blind, placebo-controlled nutritional intervention. The study participants were randomly assigned to receive 3 g/day CLA or placebo (sunflower oil) for 12 weeks. In all subjects, we measured hs-CRP and ADMA concentrations by using enzyme-linked immunosorbent assay.
Results: No significant differences were found in hs-CRP and ADMA levels before and after nutritional intervention between both groups. The changes in hs-CRP and ADMA concentration values (Δhs-CRP; ΔADMA median [interquartile range]) did not differ between subjects from the placebo (−0.1 [−0.8 to 0.3]; −0.02 [−0.12 to 0.14]) and CLA (0.2 [−0.7 to 0.9]; 0.04 [−0.14 to 0.13]) groups. The incidence of reduction of hs-CRP or ADMA concentration was not different in subjects of the CLA group compared to those of the placebo group (41.9% vs. 50%, relative risk [RR] = 0.8387, 95% confidence interval [CI] = 0.4887–1.4493, $p = 0.5232$ and 61.3% vs. 56.2%, RR = 1.0896, 95% CI = 0.7200–1.6589, $p = 0.6847$, respectively).
Conclusion: Twelve weeks of CLA supplementation had no effect on selected markers of atherosclerosis in obese and overweight women.

Keywords: *conjugated linoleic acid; atherosclerosis; high-sensitivity C-reactive protein; asymmetrical dimethylarginine*

Increased interest in functional foods has led to an improved understanding of their putative health benefits. In the omnipresent medication-based treatment of human problems and the inevitable side effects, natural products such as conjugated linoleic acid (CLA) could be a favorable, safe supplement therapy (1). CLA is a group of isomers of octadecadienoic acids, naturally produced in the gastrointestinal system of ruminants through microbial biotransformation of forage-derived fatty acids. The endogenous production of CLA in humans is possible from dietary-derived vaccenic acid, but CLA concentrations in human blood and tissues are low (2). The major sources of CLA for humans are dairy products and ruminant meats such as lamb and beef. There are also commercially available forms of CLA obtained through alkaline isomerization of linoleic acid–rich oils (3). The potential health benefits of CLA supplementation studied on animal models since 1987 include body fat reduction, improved insulin resistance, improved lipid profile, modulation of the immune system, stimulation of bone mineralization, anticarcinogenic effects, and prevention of atherogenesis (2, 4, 5). Bruen et al. (6) suggested the antiatherogenic effect of CLA is due to inhibition of the inflammatory response to the damage of the endothelium and modulation of circulating cholesterol. In animal models, the regression of the atherosclerotic lesions was associated with downregulation of proinflammatory genes and induction of apoptotic processes (7).

The advantages of CLA supplementation, shown in animal models, seem very attractive to the human population, especially with regard to its potential antiatherogenic effect. Since the last century, atherosclerosis (AT), with its wide spectrum of clinical manifestations, particularly ischemic heart disease and stroke, ranks among the top causes of death in the Western population. Obesity is one of the strongest risk factors of AT (8). According to World Health Organization data, in 2014 nearly two billion adults worldwide were overweight (39% of men and 40% of women), and, of these adults, more than half a billion were obese (11% of men and 15% of women) (9). These data obligates scientists to broaden the knowledge about possible new antiatherogenic and antiobesity agents such as CLA.

In this study, we assessed the impact of 12 weeks of supplementation of CLA on the levels of selected AT markers – high-sensitivity C-reactive protein (hs-CRP) and asymmetrical dimethylarginine (ADMA) in overweight and obese women.

Methods

Participant characteristics

Seventy-four female subjects aged over 18 years were enrolled in the study. Participants were recruited from the Obesity and Overweight Treatment Clinic of Poznan University of Medical Sciences, Poznan, Poland. Inclusion criteria were defined as follows: female sex, age over 18 years, and body mass index (BMI) $\geq$25 kg/m^2. Exclusion criteria included a history of chronic systemic disease (with the exception of hypertension [HT]); celiac disease; type 2 diabetes; pancreatic or liver disease, or both; current or recent (within the preceding month) treatment with CLA or agents interfering with fat digestion or absorption, or both (e.g. chitosan, orlistat, green tea); and pregnancy (10).

The flowchart illustrating the progression of participants through the study is presented in Fig. 1 (10, 11). Of the 187 registered women, 81 met the inclusion criteria of the study. Seven of those participants were excluded because of screening failures (shortage of time – 3; diarrhea, stomach pain – 1; difficulty in cooperation – 1; personal problems – 1; suspicion of ovarian cancer – 1). The randomization process included 74 participants. Thirty-seven of them formed the experimental CLA group and the rest were assigned to the placebo group. The dropout rate in the CLA group was comparable to the placebo group (13.51% vs. 16.22%). The dropouts included people who 1) missed the final study visit (3 women from the CLA group and 4 from the placebo group), 2) reported side effects (e.g. nausea) of the tested product (1 woman from the CLA group and 2 from the placebo group), and 3) became pregnant (1 woman from the CLA group).

A physical examination that included an evaluation of body weight, height, and BMI of each participant was conducted upon entry to the study. Baseline characteristics of the study group are summarized in Table 1.

Study design

This study was a randomized, double-blind, placebo-controlled nutrition trial. The study participants were randomly assigned to receive CLA or placebo (Olimp Laboratories, Debica, Poland). CLA and placebo products were identical (i.e. transparent capsules with a yellowish tint, packed in similar blisters). The CLA capsules contained 0.5 g of 80% CLA (50:50 *cis*-9, *trans*-11 and *trans*-10, *cis*-12 isomers), and placebo capsules contained 0.5 g of sunflower oil. The fatty acid compositions of both capsules were presented in our previous article (11).

During the randomization process, a computer-generated number was assigned to each study participant. The randomization codes were hidden from investigators and participants until the end of all data analyses.

All participants enrolled in the study were instructed to administer two capsules of the provided substance three times a day (3 g of CLA or placebo) with a meal for 12 weeks. The compliance was checked by 1) a monthly phone call to every participant by a member of the research group and 2) participants marking pill administration in a special calendar. The completion criterion was consumption of 75% of the supplement provided. The participants were asked to maintain their current lifestyle, including current physical activity and eating habits, during the trial period.

Biochemical analysis

A venous blood sample was collected, according to standardized methods, following an overnight fast and was immediately centrifuged. The plasma was poured into a tube and stored at -70°C until analyzed. In all study participants, hs-CRP and ADMA levels were measured by enzyme-linked immunosorbent assay (human ADMA, SunRed Biological Technology, Shanghai, China; hs-CRP, DRG International Inc., Springfield Township, New Jersey, USA).

Statistics

Results are presented as means $\pm$ standard errors of the mean and medians with interquartile ranges. Statistical analysis was carried out with STATISTICA 12 software (StatSoft Inc., Tulsa, OK, USA). The statistical significance of differences in hs-CRP and ADMA levels between the CLA and placebo groups was determined with Mann-Whitney *U* tests. The Wilcoxon-rank test was used for within-group analyses (baseline vs. 12 weeks). The significance level was set at $p < 0.05$. Assuming a potential drop-out rate of 20%, a significance level of 5%, and the detection power of 80%, the sample size was calculated as 37 for each group (10, 11).

This study was conducted according to Declaration of Helsinki guidelines and all procedures involving human

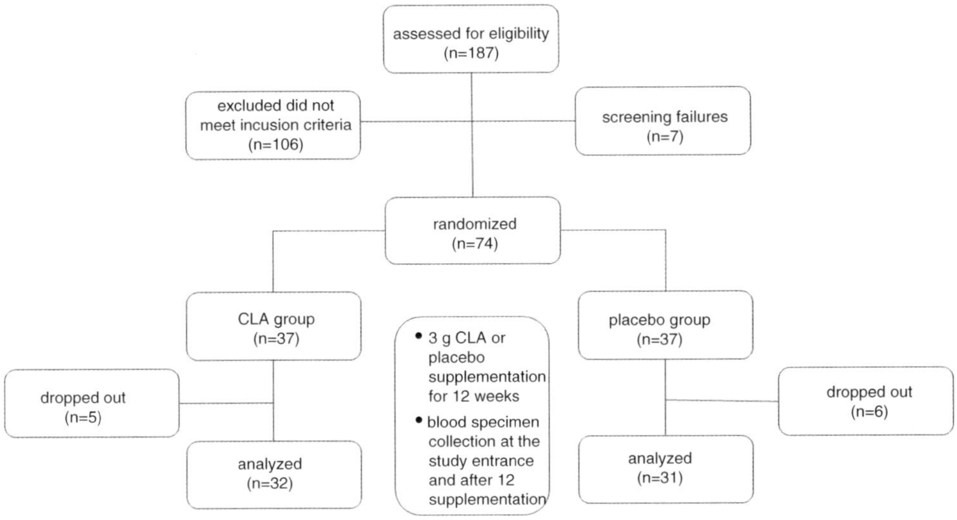

Fig. 1. Flowchart illustrating the progression of participants through the study.

subjects were approved by the local Bioethics Committee of the Institutional Review Board at the Poznan University of Medical Sciences, Poland (approval 358/14). Written, informed consent was obtained from all participants. The trial was registered in German Clinical Trials Register (DRKS-ID: DRKS00010469; www.germanctr.de/)

Results

hs-CRP

Before and after nutrition intervention, there were no significant differences in hs-CRP levels between both groups (Table 2). The changes in hs-CRP concentration (Δhs-CRP) did not differ between subjects from the placebo and CLA groups (Table 3). The incidence of reduction of hs-CRP concentration was not different in subjects in the CLA group compared with those in the placebo group (41.9% vs. 50%, relative risk [RR] = 0.8387, 95% confidence interval [CI] = 0.4887–1.4493, $p = 0.5232$).

ADMA

ADMA concentrations before and after supplementation in the CLA and placebo groups did not differ (Table 4). The changes in ADMA levels (ΔADMA) were not different in the groups studied (Table 5). The incidence of ADMA reduction was not different between the CLA group and the placebo group (61.3% vs. 56.2%, RR = 1.0896, 95% CI = 0.7200–1.6589, $p = 0.6847$).

Discussion

Our study assessed the potential antiatherogenic effect of CLA supplementation in obese and overweight women. We studied the concentrations of selected markers of AT, hs-CRP and ADMA, that mainly reflect inflammatory status and endothelial function. They are also the most important markers of plaque formation, which is strongly connected with cardiovascular risk (12, 13). Our results do not show any impact of CLA supplementation on the aforementioned circulatory markers of AT.

The strengths of our study include its randomized, double-blind, placebo-controlled character, which reduced the possibility of bias and a relatively large percentage of participants who completed the study (85.14%). Furthermore, the study was limited to female participants to eliminate potential sex-related differences (14). The median age of study participants was below the traditionally established age of increased risk of endothelial dysfunction and cardiovascular disease (CVD) (55 years for females). Diabetes was also an exclusion criterion because of its high impact on the risk of atherogenesis (15). To avoid the

Table 1. Baseline characteristics of the study group

	CLA group ($n = 37$)		Placebo group ($n = 37$)		
	Median	First–third quartile	Median	First–third quartile	p
Age (years)	54	43–59	54	45–61	0.9914
BMI (kg/m^2)	34.00	30.07–37.58	35.36	31.75–38.62	0.5049
CRP (mg/L)	2.7	1.4–3.6	2.9	1.5–4.0	0.5688
ADMA (nmol/mL)	1.55	0.58–2.62	1.42	0.65–2.37	0.9914

CLA, conjugated linoleic acid; BMI, body mass index; CRP, C-reactive protein; ADMA; asymmetrical dimethylarginine.

Table 2. Values of hs-CRP (mg/L) for CLA and placebo groups before and after the 12-week nutritional intervention

	CLA ($n = 31$)				Placebo ($n = 32$)				
	Median	First–third quartile	Mean	SEM	Median	First–third quartile	Mean	SEM	p
Before	2.7	1.3–3.7	3.1	0.5	3.1	1.3–4.0	3.5	0.5	0.5688
After	2.1	1.5–4.5	3.2	0.5	2.6	0.8–4.2	3.3	0.6	0.6375
p		0.6733				0.4537			

hs-CRP, high-sensitivity C-reactive protein; CLA, conjugated linoleic acid; SEM, standard error of the mean.

impact of exercise on AT markers, the study participants were instructed to maintain their standard level of physical activity throughout the study. HT is an important risk factor of AT (15). Because of the common coexistence of HT and obesity the selection of a large group of obese subjects without HT was impossible. A limitation of the study is the small number of participants, according to a restriction of the sample size calculation described in our previous article (11).

Previous *in vitro* studies discovered several antiathero-genic properties of CLA (16) and demonstrated the cellular and molecular mechanisms of CLA anti-inflammatory activity (17). However, the results of human studies remain inconsistent. Reynolds and Roche (17) suggested the discrepancy between human and animal experiments may result from genetic variability in humans and larger amounts of CLA provided to animals with artificially induced, closely controlled disease.

The present study is the first study designed to assess the effect of CLA supplementation on selected AT markers in the population of obese and overweight females. Although there were several studies that reported a potential effect of CLA supplementation on CRP levels, they were performed with different CLA dosages, at different intervention times, or with different inclusion criteria. Furthermore, none of the previous studies assessed the effect of CLA supplementation on ADMA levels.

Sluijs et al. (18) reported no significant impact of CLA on CRP in overweight and obese adults. Although the aforementioned project was the most similar to our study,

Table 3. Values of Δhs-CRP in the CLA and placebo groups

	Δhs-CRP		
	CLA	Placebo	p
Median	0.2	−0.1	0.4160
First–third quartile	−0.7 to −0.9	−0.8 to −0.3	
Mean	0	−0.2	
SEM	0.3	0.4	

Δhs-CRP, change in high-sensitivity C-reactive protein; CLA, conjugated linoleic acid; SEM, standard error of the mean.

it was conducted using capsules with different c9t11CLA and t10, c12 CLA ratios (80% vs. 20%, respectively), that might have influenced the results, because these isomers have different effects. Moreover, the potential sex differences were not eliminated, because the study included both females and males (18). Raff et al. (19) investigated the effect of a CLA-rich fat diet on risk markers of AT, inflammation, type 2 diabetes, and lipid peroxidation in 38 healthy men. The results of this randomized, parallel intervention study are in agreement with our analyses; however, the Raff et al. study was conducted on a smaller group, used only young male subjects, and supplemented a higher CLA dosage. The study by Moloney et al. (20) focused on patients with type 2 diabetes. Plasma CRP concentrations were not altered by CLA or control supplementation; however, the data should be interpreted with caution because of the small sample size (16 participants in every group).

Steck et al. (21) reported that the consumption of 3 g/day of 50:50 mixture of c9t11 and t10c12 CLA for 12 weeks had no effect on the inflammatory markers of CVD that is consistent with our results. However, in the same study, when a higher CLA dosage was applied (6.4 g/day), CRP levels increased markedly (21). The results should be interpreted with caution because of the small number of participants in every studied group ($n = 18$). Similarly, Smedman et al. (22) and Tholstrup et al. (23) showed the CRP level significantly increased after consumption of c9t11, t10c12 CLA mixture in high doses (4.2 g and 5.5 g, respectively).

There were only two studies performed with humans that demonstrated the decrease of CRP levels after CLA supplementation. Eftekhari et al. (24) studied the impact of CLA on inflammation in atherosclerotic patients. The 8-week-randomized clinical trial showed significant decreases in CRP concentration in the CLA group compared to the baseline, but this was not in comparison to the placebo group. Eftekhari et al. (24) suggested that the results were due to the low doses of t10,c12 CLA used in the trial, which has been reported as the isomer with several adverse effects on classical and novel markers of coronary vascular disease (2, 23). However, this hypothesis is not supported by the results of our study, because we used an identical dose and mixture ratio as Eftekhari

Table 4. Values of ADMA (nmol/mL) for the CLA and placebo groups before and after 12-week nutritional intervention

	CLA (n = 31)				Placebo (n = 32)				
	Median	First–third quartile	Mean	SEM	Median	First–third quartile	Mean	SEM	p
Before	1.58	0.56–2.75	1.65	0.19	1.36	0.59–2.29	1.57	0.19	0.9914
After	1.33	0.59–2.79	1.66	0.20	1.13	0.57–2.40	1.55	0.19	0.6771
p		0.7688				0.5632			

ADMA, asymmetrical dimethylarginine; CLA, conjugated linoleic acid; SEM, standard error of the mean.

et al. (24). Furthermore, they studied a group of non-obese volunteers with a history of angina, myocardial infarction, or bypass surgery. In Baghi et al. (25), the 2-week administration of CLA reduced serum concentrations of markers of inflammation (i.e. CRP, tumor necrosis factor-α) in healthy men after exhaustive exercise. However, their study is not comparable to our research because of a shorter time of CLA supplementation, different intervention characteristics (e.g. the participants underwent exhaustive exercise), and other inclusion criteria (e.g. young healthy males).

To our knowledge, this is the first study to assess the impact of CLA supplementation on ADMA levels, and it documents a lack of its action. ADMA is an endogenous inhibitor of endothelial nitric-oxide synthase. The reduction of nitric oxide results in endothelium dysfunction and local inflammation in consequence of activation of adhesion molecules and chemokines (26). Elevated plasma ADMA concentration has been identified as an independent risk factor for progression of AT and cardiovascular death (27). ADMA concentration is positively associated with low-density lipoprotein cholesterol concentration (28). Because CLA supplementation results in changes in the blood lipid profile (2, 29), we hypothesized that CLA may influence ADMA levels beneficially. However, we did not confirm this hypothesis.

The results of our research, as well as other clinical trials, do not confirm the positive results in animal studies. Therefore, further research on the effects and the safety of CLA supplementation should be conducted in large clinical trials.

Table 5. Values of ΔADMA in the CLA and placebo groups

	Δ ADMA		
	CLA	Placebo	p
Median	0.04	−0.02	0.9618
First–third quartile	−0.14 to −0.13	−0.12 to −0.14	
Mean	0.01	−0.02	
SEM	0.06	0.06	

ΔADMA, change in asymmetrical dimethylarginine; CLA, conjugated linoleic acid; SEM, standard error of the mean.

Acknowledgements

The project has been awarded a research grant from the Nutricia Foundation (number: 504-05-01103115-000-15-07588) and a Poznan University of Medical Sciences grant. The design, analysis of results, and the writing of this article were not affected by the Nutricia Foundation.

Conflict of interest and funding

The authors have not received any funding or benefits from industry or elsewhere to conduct this study.

References

1. Kim JH, Kim Y, Kim YJ, Park Y. Conjugated linoleic acid: potential health benefits as a functional food ingredient. Annu Rev Food Sci Technol 2016; 7: 221–44.
2. Benjamin S, Prakasan P, Sreedharan S, Wright A-DG, Spener F. Pros and cons of CLA consumption: an insight from clinical evidences. Nutr Metab 2015; 12: 4.
3. Christie WW, Dobson G, Adlof RO. A practical guide to the isolation, analysis and identification of conjugated linoleic acid. Lipids 2007; 42(12): 1073–84.
4. Whigham LD, Cook ME, Atkinson RL. Conjugated linoleic acid: implications for human health. Pharmacol Res 2000; 42(6): 503–10.
5. Pariza MW, Park Y, Cook ME. The biologically active isomers of conjugated linoleic acid. Prog Lipid Res 2001; 40(4): 283–98.
6. Bruen R, Fitzsimons S, Belton O. Atheroprotective effects of conjugated linoleic acid. Br J Clin Pharmacol 2016. doi: http://dx.doi.org/10.1111/bcp.12948 [Epub ahead of print].
7. Toomey S, Harhen B, Roche HM, Fitzgerald D, Belton O. Profound resolution of early atherosclerosis with conjugated linoleic acid. Atherosclerosis 2006; 187(1): 40–9.
8. Fruchart J-C, Nierman MC, Stroes ESG, Kastelein JJP, Duriez P. New risk factors for atherosclerosis and patient risk assessment. Circulation 2004; 109(23 Suppl 1): III15–19.
9. Available from: http://www.who.int/gho/ncd/risk_factors/overweight_text/en/
10. Lochocka K, Glapa A, Nowak JK, Duś-Żuchowska M, Grabańska K, Bogdański P, et al. Clinical outcomes of conjugated linoleic acid supplementation in the overweight and the obese: a study protocol. J Med Sci 2014; 83(4): 338–41.
11. Mądry E, Chudzicka-Strugała I, Grabańska-Martyńska K, Malikowska K, Grebowiec P, Lisowska A, et al. Twelve weeks CLA supplementation decreases the hip circumference in overweight and obese women. A double-blind, randomized, placebo-controlled trial. Acta Sci Pol Technol Aliment 2016; 15(1): 107–13.
12. Bălăşoiu M, Bălăşoiu AT, Stepan AE, Dinescu SN, Avrămescu CS, Dumitrescu D, et al. Proatherogenic adipocytokines levels

in metabolic syndrome. Romanian J Morphol Embryol Rev Roum Morphol Embryol 2014; 55(1): 29–33.
13. Lau DCW, Dhillon B, Yan H, Szmitko PE, Verma S. Adipokines: molecular links between obesity and atheroslcerosis. Am J Physiol Heart Circ Physiol 2005; 288(5): H2031–2041.
14. Vitale C, Miceli M, Rosano GMC. Gender-specific characteristics of atherosclerosis in menopausal women: risk factors, clinical course and strategies for prevention. Climacteric J Int Menopause Soc 2007; 10(Suppl 2): 16–20.
15. Vogel RA. Coronary risk factors, endothelial function, and atherosclerosis: a review. Clin Cardiol 1997; 20(5): 426–32.
16. Kritchevsky D, Tepper SA, Wright S, Czarnecki SK, Wilson TA, Nicolosi RJ. Conjugated linoleic acid isomer effects in atherosclerosis: growth and regression of lesions. Lipids 2004; 39(7): 611–16.
17. Reynolds CM, Roche HM. Conjugated linoleic acid and inflammatory cell signalling. Prostaglandins Leukot Essent Fatty Acids 2010; 82(4–6): 199–204.
18. Sluijs I, Plantinga Y, de Roos B, Mennen LI, Bots ML. Dietary supplementation with cis-9, trans-11 conjugated linoleic acid and aortic stiffness in overweight and obese adults. Am J Clin Nutr 2010; 91(1): 175–83.
19. Raff M, Tholstrup T, Basu S, Nonboe P, Sørensen MT, Straarup EM. A diet rich in conjugated linoleic acid and butter increases lipid peroxidation but does not affect atherosclerotic, inflammatory, or diabetic risk markers in healthy young men. J Nutr 2008; 138(3): 509–14.
20. Moloney F, Yeow T-P, Mullen A, Nolan JJ, Roche HM. Conjugated linoleic acid supplementation, insulin sensitivity, and lipoprotein metabolism in patients with type 2 diabetes mellitus. Am J Clin Nutr 2004; 80(4): 887–95.
21. Steck SE, Chalecki AM, Miller P, Conway J, Austin GL, Hardin JW, et al. Conjugated linoleic acid supplementation for twelve weeks increases lean body mass in obese humans. J Nutr 2007; 137(5): 1188–93.
22. Smedman A, Basu S, Jovinge S, Fredrikson GN, Vessby B. Conjugated linoleic acid increased C-reactive protein in human subjects. Br J Nutr 2005; 94(5): 791–5.
23. Tholstrup T, Raff M, Straarup EM, Lund P, Basu S, Bruun JM. An oil mixture with trans-10, cis-12 conjugated linoleic acid increases markers of inflammation and in vivo lipid peroxidation compared with cis-9, trans-11 conjugated linoleic acid in postmenopausal women. J Nutr 2008; 138(8): 1445–51.
24. Eftekhari MH, Aliasghari F, Beigi MAB, Hasanzadeh J. The effect of conjugated linoleic acids and omega-3 fatty acids supplementation on lipid profile in atherosclerosis. Adv Biomed Res 2014; 3: 15.
25. Baghi AN, Mazani M, Nemati A, Amani M, Alamolhoda S, Mogadam RA. Anti-inflammatory effects of conjugated linoleic acid on young athletic males. JPMA J Pak Med Assoc 2016; 66(3): 280–4.
26. De Gennaro Colonna V, Bianchi M, Pascale V, Ferrario P, Morelli F, Pascale W, et al. Asymmetric dimethylarginine (ADMA): an endogenous inhibitor of nitric oxide synthase and a novel cardiovascular risk molecule. Med Sci Monit Int Med J Exp Clin Res 2009; 15(4): A91–101.
27. Antoniades C, Shirodaria C, Leeson P, Antonopoulos A, Warrick N, Van-Assche T, et al. Association of plasma asymmetrical dimethylarginine (ADMA) with elevated vascular superoxide production and endothelial nitric oxide synthase uncoupling: implications for endothelial function in human atherosclerosis. Eur Heart J 2009; 30(9): 1142–50.
28. Böger RH, Sydow K, Borlak J, Thum T, Lenzen H, Schubert B, et al. LDL cholesterol upregulates synthesis of asymmetrical dimethylarginine in human endothelial cells: involvement of S-adenosylmethionine-dependent methyltransferases. Circ Res 2000; 87(2): 99–105.
29. Lehnen TE, da Silva MR, Camacho A, Marcadenti A, Lehnen AM. A review on effects of conjugated linoleic fatty acid (CLA) upon body composition and energetic metabolism. J Int Soc Sports Nutr 2015; 12: 36.

*Jaroslaw Walkowiak
Department of Pediatric Gastroenterology and Metabolic Diseases
Poznan University of Medical Sciences
Szpitalna 27/33, PO-60-572 Poznan
Poland
Email: jarwalk@ump.edu.pl

Permissions

All chapters in this book were first published in FNR, by Taylor & Francis Online; hereby published with permission under the Creative Commons Attribution License or equivalent. Every chapter published in this book has been scrutinized by our experts. Their significance has been extensively debated. The topics covered herein carry significant findings which will fuel the growth of the discipline. They may even be implemented as practical applications or may be referred to as a beginning point for another development.

The contributors of this book come from diverse backgrounds, making this book a truly international effort. This book will bring forth new frontiers with its revolutionizing research information and detailed analysis of the nascent developments around the world.

We would like to thank all the contributing authors for lending their expertise to make the book truly unique. They have played a crucial role in the development of this book. Without their invaluable contributions this book wouldn't have been possible. They have made vital efforts to compile up to date information on the varied aspects of this subject to make this book a valuable addition to the collection of many professionals and students.

This book was conceptualized with the vision of imparting up-to-date information and advanced data in this field. To ensure the same, a matchless editorial board was set up. Every individual on the board went through rigorous rounds of assessment to prove their worth. After which they invested a large part of their time researching and compiling the most relevant data for our readers.

The editorial board has been involved in producing this book since its inception. They have spent rigorous hours researching and exploring the diverse topics which have resulted in the successful publishing of this book. They have passed on their knowledge of decades through this book. To expedite this challenging task, the publisher supported the team at every step. A small team of assistant editors was also appointed to further simplify the editing procedure and attain best results for the readers.

Apart from the editorial board, the designing team has also invested a significant amount of their time in understanding the subject and creating the most relevant covers. They scrutinized every image to scout for the most suitable representation of the subject and create an appropriate cover for the book.

The publishing team has been an ardent support to the editorial, designing and production team. Their endless efforts to recruit the best for this project, has resulted in the accomplishment of this book. They are a veteran in the field of academics and their pool of knowledge is as vast as their experience in printing. Their expertise and guidance has proved useful at every step. Their uncompromising quality standards have made this book an exceptional effort. Their encouragement from time to time has been an inspiration for everyone.

The publisher and the editorial board hope that this book will prove to be a valuable piece of knowledge for researchers, students, practitioners and scholars across the globe.

List of Contributors

Gassan Darwiche, Bodil Roth and Bodil Ohlsson
Department of Clinical Sciences, Division of Internal Medicine, Lund University, Lund, Sweden
Skåne University Hospital, Malmö, Sweden

Peter Hö glund
Department of Laboratory Medicine, Division of Clinical Chemistry & Pharmacology, Lund University, Lund, Sweden
Skåne University Hospital, Lund, Sweden

Ewa Larsson, Trygve Sjöberg, Bjö rn Wohlfart and Stig Steen
Skåne University Hospital, Lund, Sweden
Department of Cardiothoracic Surgery, Clinical Sciences Lund, Lund University, Lund, Sweden

Laura Acevedo-Pacheco and Sergio O. Serna-SaldÍvar
Centro de BiotecnologÍa-FEMSA, Escuela de IngenierÍa y Ciencias, Tecnológico de Monterrey, Monterrey, México

Maike Linden and Katrin Helmbold
Clinic for Child and Adolescent Psychiatry, Psychosomatics and Psychotherapy, RWTH Aachen University, Aachen, Germany
JARA Translational Brain Medicine, Jülich Aachen Research Alliance, Jülich, Germany

Janina Kempf and Shabnam Sippas
Clinic for Child and Adolescent Psychiatry, Psychosomatics and Psychotherapy, RWTH Aachen University, Aachen, Germany
JARA Translational Brain Medicine, Jülich Aachen Research Alliance, Jülich, Germany
Faculty of Arts and Social Sciences, Maastricht University, Maastricht, The Netherlands

Christian Filss
Section JARA Brain, Jülich-Aachen Research Alliance (JARA), Jülich, Germany

Karl-Josef Langen
Section JARA Brain, Jülich-Aachen Research Alliance (JARA), Jülich, Germany
Institute of Neuroscience and Medicine (INM-3, -4, -5), Research Centre Juüich, Jülich, Germany
Department of Nuclear Medicine, RWTH Aachen University Hospital, Aachen, Germany

Albrecht Eisert
Department of Pharmacy, RWTH Aachen University, Aachen, Germany

Florian Daniel Zepf
Clinic for Child and Adolescent Psychiatry, Psychosomatics and Psychotherapy, RWTH Aachen University, Aachen, Germany
JARA Translational Brain Medicine, Jülich Aachen Research Alliance, Jülich, Germany
Centre and Discipline of Child and Adolescent Psychiatry, Psychosomatics and Psychotherapy, School of Psychiatry and Clinical Neurosciences & School of Paediatrics and Child Health, Faculty of Medicine, Dentistry and Health Sciences, The University of Western Australia, Perth, Australia
Specialised Child and Adolescent Mental Health Services (CAMHS), Department of Health in Western Australia, Perth, Australia

Elin W. Blakstad Astrid N. Almaas
Department of Pediatric and Adolescent Medicine, Akershus University Hospital, Lørenskog, Norway
Institute of Clinical Medicine, Campus Ahus, University of Oslo, Oslo, Norway
Department of Nutrition, Institute of Basic Medical Sciences, Faculty of Medicine, University of Oslo, Oslo, Norway

Sissel J. Moltu
Department of Nutrition, Institute of Basic Medical Sciences, Faculty of Medicine, University of Oslo, Oslo, Norway
Department of Neonatal Intensive Care, Women and Children's Division, Oslo University Hospital, Ullevål, Oslo, Norway

Britt Nakstad
Department of Pediatric and Adolescent Medicine, Akershus University Hospital, Lørenskog, Norway
Institute of Clinical Medicine, Campus Ahus, University of Oslo, Oslo, Norway

Marit B. Veierød
Department of Nutrition, Institute of Basic Medical Sciences, Faculty of Medicine, University of Oslo, Oslo, Norway

Oslo Centre of Biostatistics and Epidemiology, Department of Biostatistics, Institute of Basic Medical Sciences, Faculty of Medicine, University of Oslo, Oslo, Norway

Kenneth Strømmen
Department of Nutrition, Institute of Basic Medical Sciences, Faculty of Medicine, University of Oslo, Oslo, Norway
Department of Neonatal Intensive Care, Division of Paediatric and Adolescent Medicine, Oslo University Hospital, Rikshospitalet, Oslo, Norway

Pétur B. Júlíusson
Department of Clinical Science, University of Bergen, Bergen, Norway

Arild E. Rønnestad
Department of Neonatal Intensive Care, Division of Paediatric and Adolescent Medicine, Oslo University Hospital, Rikshospitalet, Oslo, Norway

Kristin Brække
Department of Neonatal Intensive Care, Women and Children's Division, Oslo University Hospital, Ullevål, Oslo, Norway

Christian A. Drevon and Per O. Iversen
Department of Nutrition, Institute of Basic Medical Sciences, Faculty of Medicine, University of Oslo, Oslo, Norway

Nurul Izzah Ahmad, Wan Rozita Wan Mahiyuddin, Cheong Yoon Ling, Siti Fatimah Daud, Nasriyah Che Hussein, Nor Aini Abdullah and Rafiza Shaharudin
Institute for Medical Research, Kuala Lumpur, Malaysia

Tengku Rozaina Tengku Mohamad
School of Food Science and Technology, Universiti Malaysia Terengganu, Kuala Terengganu, Malaysia

Lokman Hakim Sulaiman
Ministry of Health Malaysia, Federal Government Administration Centre, Putrajaya, Malaysia

Mekdes K. Gebremariam, Sigrun Henjum, Laura Terragni and Liv Elin Torheim
Department of Nursing and Health Promotion, Faculty of Health Sciences, Oslo and Akershus University College of Applied Sciences, Oslo, Norway

Marlene D. Kristensen,
Department of Nutrition, Exercise and Sports, Faculty of Science, University of Copenhagen, Copenhagen, Denmark
Novo Nordisk A/S, Bagsværd, Denmark

Nathalie T. Bendsen,
Department of Nutrition, Exercise and Sports, Faculty of Science, University of Copenhagen, Copenhagen, Denmark
Ferring Farmaceuticals A/S, Copenhagen, Denmark

Sheena M. Christensen, Arne Astrup and Anne Raben
Department of Nutrition, Exercise and Sports, Faculty of Science, University of Copenhagen, Copenhagen, Denmark
Novo Nordisk A/S, Bagsværd, Denmark
Ferring Farmaceuticals A/S, Copenhagen, Denmark

Shengli Yang
The College of Pharmaceutical Science, Zhejiang University of Technology, Hangzhou, People's Republic of China

Hui Zhang
Physical and Chemical Test Center, Zhejiang Institute of Quality Inspection Science, Hangzhou, China

Eric Lontchi-Yimagou
Laboratory for Molecular Medicine and Metabolism, Biotechnology Center, University of Yaoundé I, Yaoundé, Cameroon

Agatha Tanya
Department of Public Health, Faculty of Medicine and Biomedical Sciences, University of Yaoundé I, Yaoundé, Cameroon

Carine Tchankou, Judith Ngondi and Julius Oben
Laboratory of Nutrition and Nutritional Biochemistry, Faculty of Sciences, University of Yaoundé I, Yaoundé, Cameroon

Asmaa M. Zahran
Clinical Pathology Department, South Egypt Cancer Institute, Assiut University, Assiut, Egypt

Khalid I. Elsayh, Khaled Saad, Esraa M.A. Eloseily and Naglaa S. Osman
Pediatric Department, Faculty of Medicine, Assiut University, Assiut, Egypt

Mohamd A. Alblihed
Medical Biochemistry Department, College of Medicine, Taif University, Taif, Kingdom of Saudi Arabia

Gamal Badr
Zoology Department, Laboratory of Immunology & Molecular Physiology, Faculty of Science, Assiut University, Assiut, Egypt

Mohamed H. Mahmoud
Deanship of Scientific Research, King Saud University, Riyadh,Kingdom of Saudi Arabia
Food Science and Nutrition Department, National Research Center, Dokki, Cairo, Egypt

Jun Jiao, Shu-Fen Han, Wei Zhang and Xing Tong
Department of Nutrition and Food Hygiene, School of Public Health, Soochow University, Suzhou, China

Nicolai A. Lund-Blix
Department of Pediatric Research, Oslo University Hospital, Rikshospitalet, Oslo, Norway
Department of Nutrition, Institute of Basic Medical Sciences, University of Oslo, Oslo, Norway
Division of Epidemiology, Norwegian Institute of Public Health, Oslo, Norway

Kjersti S. Rønningen,
Department of Pediatric Research, Oslo University Hospital, Rikshospitalet, Oslo, Norway

Håkon Bøås3 and German Tapia
Division of Epidemiology, Norwegian Institute of Public Health, Oslo, Norway

Lene F. Andersen
Department of Nutrition, Institute of Basic Medical Sciences, University of Oslo, Oslo, Norway

Wenfeng Li, Yalong Lu, Di Huang, Xiao Han and Xingbin Yang
Shaanxi Engineering Laboratory for Food Green Processing and Safety Control, College of Food Engineering and Nutritional Science, Shaanxi Normal University, Xían, China

Masao Kanauchi
Department of Health and Nutrition, Faculty of Health Science, Kio University, Koryo-cho, Japan

Kimiko Kanauchi
Department of Internal Medicine, Narahigashi Hospital, Tenri, Japan

Aino-Maija Eloranta, Henna Jalkanen, Sanna Kiiskinen and Virpi Lindi
Department of Physiology, Institute of Biomedicine, School of Medicine, University of Eastern Finland, Kuopio, Finland

Taisa Venäläinen
Department of Physiology, Institute of Biomedicine, School of Medicine, University of Eastern Finland, Kuopio, Finland
Department of Clinical Nutrition, Institute of Public Health and Clinical Nutrition, School of Medicine, University of Eastern Finland, Kuopio, Finland

Sonja Soininen
Department of Physiology, Institute of Biomedicine, School of Medicine, University of Eastern Finland, Kuopio, Finland
Social and Health Center, City of Varkaus, Finland
Institute of Dentistry, School of Medicine, University of Eastern Finland, Kuopio, Finland

Ursula Schwab
Department of Clinical Nutrition, Institute of Public Health and Clinical Nutrition, School of Medicine, University of Eastern Finland, Kuopio, Finland
Department of Internal Medicine, Institute of Clinical Medicine, Kuopio University Hospital, Kuopio, Finland

Timo A. Lakka
Department of Physiology, Institute of Biomedicine, School of Medicine, University of Eastern Finland, Kuopio, Finland
Kuopio Research Institute of Exercise Medicine, Kuopio, Finland
Department of Clinical Physiology and Nuclear Medicine, Kuopio University Hospital, Kuopio, Finland

Sheng Li, Li-juan Yang, Yu-jiao He and Xiao-fei Shen
Chengdu Institute of Biology, Chinese Academy of Sciences, Chengdu, China

Jun-mei Huang
Chengdu Institute of Biology, Chinese Academy of Sciences, Chengdu, China
School of Chinese Pharmacy, Chengdu University of Traditional Chinese Medicine, Chengdu, China

Han-wei Liu
Ningbo Entry-Exit Inspection and Quarantine Bureau Technical Center, Ningbo, China

Fei Wang
Chengdu Institute of Biology, Chinese Academy of Sciences, Chengdu, China
Sichuan Translational Medicine Research Hospital, Chinese Academy of Sciences, Chengdu, China

Ping Wang
School of Chinese Pharmacy, Chengdu University of Traditional Chinese Medicine, Chengdu, China

Maria Waling, Cecilia Olsson1 and Agneta Hörnell
Department of Food and Nutrition, Umeå University, Umeå, Sweden

Anna S. Olafsdottir
School of Education, University of Iceland, Reykjavik, Iceland

Hanna Lagström and Sanna Talvia
Turku Institute of Child and Youth Research, University of Turku, Turku, Finland;

Hege Wergedahl, Eldbjørg Fossgard and Asle Holthe
Faculty of Education, Bergen University College, Bergen, Norway

Bert Jonsson
Department of Psychology, Umeå University, Umeå, Sweden

Ingibjorg Gunnarsdottir
Unit for Nutrition Research, Landspitali - The National University Hospital of Iceland and Faculty of Food Science and Nutrition, School of Health Sciences, University of Iceland, Reykjavík, Iceland

Francesco Balestri , Rossella Rotondo, Roberta Moschini, Mario Cappiello Carlo Sorce, Andrea Andreucci, Del-Corso and Umberto Mura
Department of Biology, University of Pisa, Pisa, Italy
Interdepartmental Research Center Nutrafood 'Nutraceuticals and Food for Health', University of Pisa, Pisa, Italy

Mario Pellegrino
Department of Translational Research on New Technologies in Medicine and Surgery, University of Pisa, Pisa, Italy

Vito Barracco and Livia Misuri
Department of Biology, University of Pisa, Pisa, Italy

Monika Dus-Zuchowska, Patrycja Krzyzanowska and Jaroslaw Walkowiak
Department of Pediatric Gastroenterology and Metabolic Diseases, Poznan University of Medical Sciences, Poznan, Poland

Edyta Madry
Department of Physiology, Poznan University of Medical Sciences, Poznan, Poland

Paweł Bogdanski
Department of Education and Obesity Treatment and Metabolic Disorders, Poznan University of Medical Sciences, Poznan, Poland

Lin-Xi Yuan and Xue-Bin Yin
Jiangsu Bio-Engineering Research Centre of Selenium, Suzhou, China

Li-Qiang Qin
Department of Nutrition and Food Hygiene, School of Public Health, Soochow University, Suzhou, China
Jiangsu Key Laboratory of Preventive and Translational Medicine for Geriatric Disease, Soochow University, Suzhou, China

Jia-Ying Xu
School of Radiation Medicine and Protection, Soochow University, Suzhou, China
Collaborative Innovation Center of Radiation Medicine of Jiangsu Higher Education Institutions, Soochow University, Suzhou, China

Index

A

Ad Libitum, 18, 75-76, 78-82

Adiponectin, 40-41, 43-50, 110, 112-113, 116-117

Adolescents, 25-26, 33, 37, 49, 62, 65-74, 123, 150, 153-155, 177

Aldose Reductase, 179-180, 182, 187-189

Anthropometry, 1-3, 64

Anti-hypercholesterolemia, 100

Anticarcinogenic, 190

Antineoplastic Drugs, 157

Antioxidants, 2

Apigenin Potentiates, 156, 164

Apoptosis, 41, 99-101, 103, 105-108, 157, 164-166

Appetite Parameters, 78

Appetite Sensations, 75-78, 80-82

Arteriosclerosis, 15, 92, 127

Autoantibodies, 99-100, 104-106, 122

B

Biomarkers, 9-10, 82, 119-120, 125-126, 135, 139, 142, 154, 167

Blood Adiponectin, 40, 46

Body Mass Index, 1-2, 7-8, 14, 28, 41, 49, 53, 76, 138, 145, 173-175, 190-191

Brown Adipose Tissue, 109-110, 115, 118

C

Casein, 16-22, 24, 80, 82, 85, 87

Catechins, 127, 129-130, 132-135

Chemopreventives, 156

Chicken Breasts, 84-85, 88-90

Cognitive Function, 168-169, 172, 175-177

Consumption Patterns, 52, 58, 61, 63-65, 82

D

Diabetes, 1-3, 7, 9, 11-15, 27, 82, 92-98, 105, 107, 109, 117, 119-125, 137, 142-143, 154, 188-189, 191, 193, 195

Dietary Assessment, 77, 119-120, 138, 142, 177

Dietary Behaviors, 66-69, 71-73

Dietary Culture, 76

Dietary Fibre, 14, 144-145, 147-150, 153

Dietary Tryptophan, 25, 37

Dietary Tryptophan Depletion, 25

Dyslipidemia, 1, 110, 114

E

Ecological Models, 66, 73

Efflux Transporter, 127, 133

Emulsifying, 17

Endogenous Synthesis, 120

Epidemiologic Study, 141

Ether Extract, 17

Ethnic Minorities, 68

Ethnicity, 2, 51-52, 55, 59, 69, 171

F

Fermentation, 11, 22, 84-86, 91, 135

Fiber Content, 7, 75, 77, 80-81

Flavonoids, 2, 17, 127, 131-132, 134-136, 156-157, 164-166, 180

Fructose, 85, 87, 127, 180, 182

G

Gastrointestinal, 2, 26, 76, 82, 190

Gender Differences, 144-145, 153

H

Hyperglycemia, 1, 12, 96

Hyperinsulinemia, 1, 11

Hyperlipidemia, 92

I

Immunomodulatory Properties, 100, 105

Inflammatory Disorders, 84, 189

Influx Rate, 25

Inoculation Volume, 85-87

Interferon Receptor Degradation, 156

Interventional Study, 1

Isoflavones, 17, 19, 22, 136, 180

L

Legumes, 4, 9, 24, 75-80, 137-138, 140-141

Leptin, 40-41, 43-44, 47-49, 109-110, 112-113, 116-117

Linear Regression, 66, 69-71, 185

Lipid Metabolism, 109-110, 112, 114-115, 117-118

M
Macronutrients, 76, 80-81, 117
Maize Tortillas, 16-23
Maltose, 85, 87
Metabolic Control, 1-2, 10
Metabolic Diseases, 137, 190, 195
Metabolic Syndrome, 13, 40, 47-49, 118, 142, 195
Micronutrients, 16-17, 143-144
Mortierella Alpine, 84, 90-91
Multivariable Regression, 69-70
Mycelial Growth, 84, 86
Mycelium Formation., 89
Mycoprotein Meal, 80

N
Nordic Diet, 1-5, 9, 12-13, 15, 81, 171, 177

O
Obesity, 1, 3, 7, 9, 11-15, 27, 41, 47, 50, 53, 61, 63, 65-66, 72-74, 82, 92, 97, 109-110, 112-114, 116-118, 137-139, 141-142, 170, 174-176, 178, 190-191, 193, 195
Octadecylsilane, 17
Okinawan Diet, 1, 3, 11, 14
Oxidative Stress, 22, 92-94, 96-98, 116, 143, 167, 180

P
Palatability, 36-37, 75-76, 78-81, 83, 85
Palatability Ratings, 81
Peptidase Activities, 164
Perceived Accessibility, 66, 68-72
Phaseolus Vulgaris, 179-180, 185, 188-189
Placebo-controlled, 76, 190, 194
Plasma Triglyceride, 123
Polyol Pathway, 179-180, 186-188
Polyunsaturated Fat, 144
Polyunsaturated Fatty Acids, 5, 41, 51, 84, 86-87, 89-91, 120, 139-140, 147, 149
Proteasome, 156-158, 160-166
Psychiatric Disorders, 27

Q
Quality Of Life, 1-2, 4, 9, 12, 14

R
Reproducibility, 73, 78, 82, 111, 119
Rheumatoid Arthritis, 84, 90, 105

S
Saponins, 17
Satiating, 11, 75, 78, 80-82
Serotonin, 25-26, 37-39
Socio-demographic, 52, 54, 178
Sorbitol Dehydrogenase, 179-180, 189
Soybean Proteins, 16-17, 23
Stachyose, 127-135
Sucrose, 5, 18, 85, 87, 135, 139-140, 144-145, 147, 149-150, 154, 171
Supplemented Leucine, 109, 111
Systemic Lupus Erythematosus, 99, 103-105, 107-108

T
Tea Catechins, 127, 130, 135
Type 2 Diabetes, 1-2, 9, 13-15, 92, 97, 143, 193, 195

U
Ubiquitination, 156-157, 160, 162-163, 165-166

W
Wheat Flour Tortillas, 16-23
White Adipose Tissue, 109-110, 113-115, 117